MENTAL MACHINERY

Mental Machinery

The Origins and Consequences of Psychological Ideas

Part 1: 1600–1850

GRAHAM RICHARDS

The Johns Hopkins University Press
Baltimore

Printed in Great Britain

First published in the United States of America,
1992, with the generous assistance of
the Karl and Edith Pribram Endowment.

The Johns Hopkins University Press
701 West 40th Street
Baltimore, Maryland 21211–2190

Library of Congress Cataloging-in-Publication Data

Richards, Graham.
Mental machinery: the origins and consequences of psychological ideas: part one, 1600–1850 / Graham Richards.
p. cm.
Includes bibliographical references and index.
ISBN 0-8018-4544-0 (hc)
1. Psychology--History. 2. Psychology--Philosophy--History.
I. Title.
[DNLM: 1. History of Medicine, 17th Century. 2. History of Medicine, 18th Century. 3. Psychology--history. BF 81 R515m]
BF95.R53 1992
150'.9'032--dc20
DNLM/DLC
for Library of Congress 92-1552

Contents

Preface ix

Introduction: Some Problems of Psychology 1

PART ONE THE SEVENTEENTH CENTURY

Chapter 1 Vast Confusions and New Paradoxes

I Introduction 15
II Epistemization 26
III Mechanization 36
IV From Faith to Reason 45
V The Invention of Privacy 50
VI The Language Problem 54
VII Forgotten Anticipations of Psychology 66
VIII Spinoza and Leibniz 81
IX Seventeenth-Century Psychology: A Revised Version 89

PART TWO PSYCHOLOGICAL IDEAS IN THE EIGHTEENTH CENTURY

Introduction 97

Chapter 2 The Vehicle of Conjecture: Ideas of Language from Locke to Tooke 104
Chapter 3 Sensible Reasoning: Philosophical Moves towards Psychology 134
Chapter 4 Practical Pressures: Nerves, Madness, Sex and Education 194
Chapter 5 Rethinking Eighteenth-Century Psychology 231
Chapter 6 Reading the Body and Ruling the Mind: The First 'Scientific' Psychologies 249

PART THREE 1800–50: THREE ROUTES TO PSYCHOLOGY

Introduction 289

Chapter 7 The German Route:
Between Matter and Metaphysics 291
Chapter 8 The British Route: The Nervous Empire 325
Chapter 9 The French Route: Degenerating Dreams 375
Chapter 10 Conclusion: Making the Mind Up 1600–1850 390

Notes 407
Appendix 431
Bibliography 435
Proper Name Index 472
Subject Index 482

It is not speech which we should want to know: we should know the speaker.
It is not things seen which we should want to know: we should know the seer.
It is not sounds which we should want to know: we should know the hearer.
It is not the mind which we should want to know: we should know the thinker.

Kaushitaku Upanishad 3.8

The more abstract the truth you want to teach the more you must seduce the senses to it.

Nietzsche

Welcome my son, welcome to the machine.

Pink Floyd

FOR THREE DEAR FRIENDS

Alexandra Yardley, Rob Man and Gerry Gaden

Preface

This work has presented me with a challenge I have as yet but half met, in that the present volume concerns only the period from 1600 to 1850, the eve of Psychology's appearance as a discipline in Germany and Britain. A second volume covering the subsequent period is planned. In the course of writing the present one, the scale required of the project has seemed to expand continually – at times uncontrollably. It is both more and less than the book I originally envisaged; more because the enquiry raised numerous unexpected questions (and suggested some answers) which I do not believe have been properly acknowledged before, less because the comprehensive account of specific ideas which I intended frequently eluded me. An empirical philological survey of English psychological language was also planned as an extended appendix; this will now have to await Part II.

During the last decade or so the history of Psychology has been dramatically changed by writers such as Kurt Danziger, Thomas Leahey, David Leary, Nikolas Rose, Roger Smith and Bill Woodward. Albeit belatedly, an exploration of the perspectives of social constructionism and other contextual approaches has begun. The present work is a further extension of this. However much the interpretational frameworks and the perceived tasks of history of Psychology have changed, those of us working in this area still remain indebted to the scholarship of such earlier writers as G.S. Brett, Fay Berger Karpf, A.A. Roback and, of course, Edwin Boring, whose works remain as indispensable secondary sources and repositories of information on which even the post-modernest of us find ourselves continuing to draw for names and dates and signposts to forgotten, still unexplored, material. More directly we owe a great debt to Michel Foucault and his many successors in the History of Psychiatry field, not least for opening our eyes to our own previous failures to see the full psychological dimension of the History of Psychology.

While identifying myself with this new history of Psychology,

I have tried to deploy my own 'metapsychological' perspective to demonstrate the need for a yet more radical reappraisal and reinterpretation of our discipline's past. I have also resisted the temptation not to indulge in occasional gratuitous digressions and personal asides in the interests of maintaining a po-faced dignified academic stance – I have always found that these are what makes the works of others digestible, and hope their presence here serves my readers similarly. That's my excuse, anyway.

The number of people to whom this work is in one way or another indebted is considerable. First I would like to thank Roy Porter for triggering the whole project off and Simon Schaffer for turning my head around at various points as well as being ever-helpful and encouraging. Some day his Boswell will come. Others who have helped include Mary Boyle, John Christie, Rob Farr, Clive Gabriel, Michael Hunter, Ludmilla Jordanova (on physiognomy), Julian Martin (for bureaucratic Bacon), Mary Midgley, John Radford, George MacDonald Ross, Vivian Salmon (on Wilkins & Co.), Roger Smith, and Elizabeth Valentine. (Any omissions from this list are quite inadvertent.) The British Library has continued to serve me (and all its other users) well under mounting difficulties of its own, and I am also grateful to the Wellcome History of Medicine Library, Cambridge University Library, and not least the Polytechnic of East London Library at Maryland House. To all those who have kept me supplied with offprints of their journal papers I owe a particular thanks, since without their generosity I would have remained in the dark about more topics than I care to enumerate. In a less definable but none the less pervasive way I owe much to my fellow members of the British Psychological Society's History and Philosophy Section for providing such a congenial academic forum and home base. My colleagues and students at the Polytechnic of East London have continued to provide moral support. Sabrina Izzard's maintenance of my second-hand book supplies has been absolutely crucial (and Any Amount of Books in Charing Cross Road has been pretty useful too). Finally here I would like to thank Brian Southam at The Athlone Press for being so understanding in the face of an ever-retreating deadline. This book was written without the help of any grant-giving agencies and I did all my own word-processing. And thanks to Carol O'Dea for processing the printout and tearing off all those strips down the side with holes in.

And of course, without Maura's loving support and quite outrageous ego-boosting skills I am sure this work would never have been finished.

Responsibility for the contents of the book and any errors therein rests entirely on me.

Graham Richards
Tunbridge Wells, July 1992.

Introduction: Some Problems of Psychology

> It's only by thinking even more crazily than philosophers do that you can solve their problems.
>
> (Wittgenstein, *Culture and Value*, p.75e)

1 What is Psychology?

There currently exists a discipline called Psychology[1], the defining characteristics of which may be summarized as follows:

(a) a commitment to a programme of empirical research into 'the psychological' conducted according to what are taken to be the prevailing criteria of 'good scientific method';
(b) the utilization of this programme to evaluate and generate theories of 'the psychological' according to what are taken to be the prevailing criteria of 'scientific theory construction and testing';
(c) the use of the findings thereby gained to generate and develop applied technologies and expertise for the management of 'the psychological' e.g. management of deviance, child-rearing, ability evaluation, psychopathology, education, etc.

Defining the actual subject matter, 'psychology' or 'the psychological', of this discipline is notoriously difficult; nevertheless we may perhaps define it as 'behaviour and its covert determinants'. 'Covert determinants' include wishes, plans, motives, traits, cognitions, schemata, perceptions, memories, emotions, conditionings, feelings, instincts, etc., whether consciously- or unconsciously-located, and the physiological substrates of these. It is essential to this enterprise that this subject matter be accorded the same ontological status as the subject matters of other scientific disciplines – i.e. that 'the psychological' really exists as a natural object for this kind of enquiry, that there are indeed some such entities as those just listed (although their individual status in this respect is often highly controversial among discipline members). It is the assumed presence of such covert determinants which renders a behaviour 'psychologically' significant even when the research strategy (as in J.B. Watson's Behaviorism) apparently ignores them; a tremor caused by Parkinson's disease is thus not, *per se*, part of Psychology's subject matter because its covert determinants are deemed purely physiological and thus neither consciously nor unconsciously intentional or meaningful. The problem of which kinds of covert determinant are 'psychological' nevertheless remains, especially if we reject dualistic notions of the mind–body relationship. Nor does the above definition exclude, in principle, the phenomenological study of consciousness – indeed, the presence of a phenomenological dimension is perhaps crucial.

The sheer heterogeneity of Psychology regarding both topics researched and types of theory testifies to the intractability of the underlying conceptual difficulties in reaching a consensus regarding the ways in which its subject matter is to be 'scientifically' conceptualized. So acute has this problem become that an impending disappearance, or at least fission, of the discipline is now foreseen in many quarters. Nevertheless, the essentially reflexive character of Psychology, or of any successor discipline, cannot be evaded.

And here we encounter our first major difficulty. In order to elucidate this it is necessary to return to basics, in this case the nature of language. As I have discussed elsewhere (Richards, 1989a), the use of modern human language entails a trio of linguistic roles; speaker/listeners (the agents who are using the language), referents (that about which they are discoursing) and utterances (the actual words, or other signals, being used). The contents of a linguistically construed universe can all be assigned one or other of these roles; precisely which one varies according to the exigencies of the situation. In order to communicate about themselves, speakers have to use language reflexively. If the things about themselves (or other speakers) to which they wish to refer are not public (e.g. a dream or an intention) they can do so (given the meaninglessness of private language[2]) only by reflexively applying to themselves (or others) the language used for referring to the public world. In effect (although this is something of an oversimplification) they say, 'I am like *that*'. The upshot of this, I argued, is a process of what I termed 'physiomorphism' – namely, that speakers assimilate to themselves the properties of the public world. It is not my task in this book to reiterate the case in full (see Richards, *ibid.*, 1989b for fuller accounts). One implication of this must, though, be immediately insisted upon: any concept which refers to the public world possesses (if only potentially) a reflexive (some would say 'indexical') meaning as a way of referring to a speaker-property.

In short, our species has, since it evolved modern lexical, syntactic language (probably around 40,000 years ago), been engaged in reflexive discourse. Over time a body of language which I have called Psychological (or, perhaps better, Person) Language (PL) developed, which, while overlapping with the 'World Language' (WL) to a great extent, acquired a distinctive lexicon of its own. This PL cumulatively enshrines in the received linguistic repertoire the physiomorphic history of the linguistic community. Although the etymologies of some of the terms in the distinctive PL lexicon may be lost in the smog of time, the WL origins of others may be readily identified and, crucially, no new term can be identified as entering PL except by this route. PL is clearly in constant flux, although its expansion rate seems to outstrip obsolescence[3], as novel experience and changing sociocultural and technological circumstance alter the terms in which reflexive discourse is conducted.

Clearly, then, our first difficulty is the assumption that 'the psychological' can be accorded the same status as an ostensible natural object of enquiry, as is the case in the physical sciences[4]. 'The psychological' exists primarily as the terms in which reflexive discourse is conducted. If Psychology alters the terms of this discourse it has thus, in so doing, changed the nature of its subject matter. Even more problematically, the introduction of the term 'psychological' as an umbrella term for that 'realm' of phenomena partly listed above itself alters the situation, ascribing to it a coherence which reflexive discourse did not previously recognize.

This augurs ill for any attempt at writing a history of Psychology. As Roger Smith (1988) has wisely observed, Psychology has existed as a discipline (in the terms we identified at the outset) only since the late nineteenth century, while the texts traditionally invoked in histories of Psychology to fill out the discipline's 'long past' as opposed to its 'short history' do not constitute a continuous intellectual tradition, nor were they putatively concerned with addressing the same questions as Psychology (although odd anticipations may be located). A sentence like the following, from Kantor's *The Scientific Evolution of Psychology* (1963), is thus radically misleading:

> As we shall see, as late as the seventeenth century the representatives of modern psychology, Descartes, Hobbes, Locke, and Leibniz, basked in the moonlight of Aristotelian psychology as transformed by St. Thomas. (p.155)

It is misleading not because of what it says about the influence of St. Thomas Aquinas on the famed philosophical quartet, but in terming them 'representatives of modern psychology'. They can hardly represent something which did not exist, and if the term 'psychology' is read in the subject-matter sense the proposition is a straight contradiction in terms; they can have been representatives only of seventeenth-century psychology. Even a highly sophisticated writer like Yolton can refer to the 'psychological theories' of seventeenth- and eighteenth-century philosophers (particularly in relation to their accounts of perception). In the present work I will, *faute de mieux*, use the term 'psychological idea' to refer to the terms in which pre-Psychological reflexive discourse has been conducted, but this does not, anachronistically, imply the contemporary presence of a category 'psychological'.

True, some historians of Psychology, notably Leahey (1987), have attempted to address the contextual issue, but they are confronted with a genre problem. Since they are writing primarily for North American undergraduates, the task of offering a contextualized interpretation of the discipline becomes conflated with that of providing basic historical knowledge regarding, for example, the seventeenth-century 'scientific revolution' or nineteenth-century European culture. Within the limited space available, genuine contextual analysis becomes little more than a matter of innuendo. While general histories of Psychology tend to be written by those identifying themselves primarily as Psychologists, the relevant specialist monographs and journal papers on pre-twentieth-century topics often tend to be written by historians of science, philosophy, literature, or 'ideas' operating within somewhat different intellectual agendas and at levels of focused historical scholarship which the psychologist may find difficult to handle. Of the fourteen contributors to Fox's collection *Psychology and Literature in the Eighteenth Century* (1987), for example, ten are in departments of English, two are philosophers, one a pathologist and one a librarian. Ash and Woodward's *Psychology in Twentieth-Century Thought and Society* (1987), by contrast, has a ratio of nine psychologists to four historians.

The messages coming from these two kinds of source, general history textbook and specialist monograph, are, unsurprisingly, somewhat inconsistent. The former continue to tell stories of ultimately progressive linearity and continuity, legitimating the current state of the discipline. The latter increasingly give the lie to this perspective. The *Journal of the History of the Behavioral Sciences*, the only journal exclusively devoted to the topic, admittedly falls into a somewhat intermediate category, but its editorial allegiance appears until recently to have been to a fairly conservative and traditional concept of history of science. I have argued elsewhere (Richards, 1987a) that the establishment of a 'History of Psychology' subdiscipline within Psychology in the USA constituted a self-legitimating manoeuvre in its own right – if a branch of History of Science called History of Psychology can be created, then the scientific character of Psychology is further endorsed. R.I. Watson's founding of the *Journal of the History of the Behavioral Sciences* occurred in this context.

To return to the founding of Psychology, Nikolas Rose (1987) has shown how the discipline owes its existence to sociocultural conditions prevailing in late-nineteenth-century Europe and North America, in which a need for the 'management of individuality' surfaced acutely on a number of practical fronts, primarily education and child-rearing, subnormality and crime – in a phrase, 'social welfare'. Contemporaneous studies of perception, learning and motivation may also be understood in the contexts of advancing industrial technology and social and political trauma (especially surrounding the First World War). Current historians of science are in general becoming chary of 'tunnel-vision' disciplinary histories; historians of Psychology must be even more so. If we are to find a way out of this impasse, two possibilities offer themselves:

(a) We can reconstrue the task as being that of writing a

history of reflexive discourse. This would solve the problems of spurious continuity, disciplinary self-legitimation, and unselfconscious presentism which have vitiated orthodox history of Psychology (R. Smith, 1988; Rose, 1985; Richards, 1987a). It would also meet the requirement that we construe past 'Psychological' texts as data rather than Psychology (Richards, *ibid.*) – i.e. as evidence regarding the nature of our subject matter ('psychology') in pre-Psychological times. (This latter 'extension of sampling', however, may be viewed as attempting backhandedly to recoup the notion of a 'natural object of enquiry'.)

(b) We can readdress the canonical texts (of Descartes, Hobbes, Locke, Hartley, Hume, the Mills, etc.) in order to disclose the conditions under which they were produced, the issues they were intended (and contemporarily understood) to be addressing, and their general *non*-Psychologicality in the modern sense. This would serve as a corrective counter-history in relation to orthodox histories of Psychology. To establish the non-Psychologicality of earlier reflexive discourse further we would also spread our net somewhat wider to consider lesser-known texts which might appear to be protoPsychological but are usually omitted from the historian of Psychology's purview.

These are not, of course, clearly distinct strategies; the second would achieve at least some of the goals of the first, and is a necessary condition for accomplishing them. In the present book I have, especially in tackling the very difficult seventeenth century, opted for a compromise course, although the bias has been towards the latter for two reasons. First, because putting the familiar canonical texts in their place appears to be the more urgent desideratum as well as providing a bridge between orthodox concerns and a more generalized analysis of reflexive discourse as such. Secondly – and more practically – because recent scholarship in the histories of science, ideas and philosophy provides a fairly developed body of secondary literature, often of a highly sophisticated character, upon which to draw in addressing such an agenda. By contrast, materials for studying the history of British (if not French) *mentalités* or collective representations in reflexive discourse are sparse (John Morgan, 1986 is an important exception). A critique of the canon appears to be the logical first step towards a broader consideration of reflexive discourse.

2 Goals of Psychology

A second angle from which psychology becomes problematical needs to be noted here – namely, what it is for. We have already mentioned Rose's argument that it is about producing technologies for managing individuality. From the perspective of the Frankfurt School, however, the situation is rather more complex. K.O. Apel (1977) identified three 'critical interests of knowledge'. First, we may be seeking 'manipulative understanding' – we are concerned with asking of our subject matter 'how it works', how to predict its future behaviour and, if possible, acquiring control over it. This is the orthodox 'prediction and control' goal of the physical sciences. The appropriate methods involve objectifying experimentation, identification of mechanical cause–effect relationships, etc. Secondly, we may seek 'communicative understanding'. We want to enhance our management of our social relations and understand one another. This goal generates the humanities: history, literary criticism, the study of art, cultural studies, etc; in Psychology it typically yields such areas as 'counselling', 'art therapy' and 'assertiveness training'. Finally, we may be after what Apel, in fine Teutonic fashion, terms 'critically emancipatory self-reflection': we want to enhance our own self-understanding by identifying and liberating ourselves from forces which currently enchain us. Here Apel instances both psychoanalysis and Marxism.

The bind in which Psychology finds itself is that at one level the cultural demands on it are to meet goals of types two and three, while authority to do so can be achieved only by successfully presenting itself as 'scientific' – i.e. as a goal-one-orientated endeavour. Unfortunately, the objectification of the subject so central to goal-one interests is fundamentally incompatible with satisfying goal-three interests, to which the self-transformation of the subject is equally central. Successful pursuit of goal-two interests may on occasion involve subsidiary goal-one-type activities (e.g. acquiring manipulative understanding of self-expressive techniques), but again this is not the point of the pursuit.

Certainly within post-World War II Psychology there have been moves to escape this bind (e.g. by Humanistic Psychology) by attempting to downgrade the 'scientific' commitment and align with the humanities or philosophy. This has proved difficult to carry through, not least because the arena of activity in which this approach usually operates tends to be psychopathology, and unless the Psychologist is willing to break away completely and become a fringe-cult guru, he or she must retain credibility as a quasi-medical practitioner – an area subject to heavy intellectual policing. I do not intend to explore this further at this point, except to say that it places a question mark even over the adequacy of such broad characterizations of the nature of Psychology as those with which I opened. As a taxonomy of goals, the Apel list may nevertheless prove heuristically useful as one framework for differentiating the ostensible purposes of modern Psychologists from those of the earlier writers routinely depicted as their intellectual ancestors. While explicitly cited on only a few occasions, Apel's analysis has had a considerable influence on my own thinking and is covertly present throughout.

3 The Range of the Present Work

The period 1600 to 1850 encompasses change at all levels on a Europe-wide scale. Given the linguistic nature of the approach being adopted, the present work has a somewhat Anglocentric character. This is especially so in the coverage of the seventeenth century. There is an additional justification for this, however, in that it is widely held that it was in Britain during that century that the 'modern' mentality had its origins. Descartes, Leibniz and Spinoza necessarily concern us, but the broader dynamics of the British situation remain central in determining the subsequent character of European proto-Psychological thought. In France it is Locke who provides the *philosophes* with their starting point, and in Germany it is Locke and Newton who serve as Leibniz's intellectual foils. In the eighteenth century it is in Britain that the Industrial Revolution and the development of parliamentary democracy (of a sort) set the direction which Western culture in general will later take – again, therefore, the most significant changes in psychological ideas also tend to occur there. I have, however, attempted to take cognizance throughout of the major continental figures, and essayed a more detailed comparison between the British, German and French situations.

As far as North America is concerned, there is little to be said regarding the pre-1850 period. Prior to the New England Transcendentalist movement of Emerson and Thoreau the only native-born figures who might be considered are Jonathan Edwards and Benjamin Rush. Apart from them, North America served more as dumping ground for European ideas of all kinds – some of which eventually took root, some of which, like some good wines, simply did not travel well. One reads with sympathy the introduction to poor Frederick Rauch's *Psychology; or a view of the Human Soul; including Anthropology, adapted for the use of Colleges* (1844) – fleeing from Heidelberg for political reasons in 1831, in his mid twenties, with a message of Christian piety infused with *Naturphilosophie*, he became President of Marshall College Pennsylvania but died in his mid thirties, leaving his book like a geological erratic bearing little relationship to the intellectual terrain around it and, notwithstanding some contemporary success, devoid of consequence. (Many American universities did, of course, provide courses on 'Mental and Moral Science', strongly influenced by Scottish Enlightenment thought.) I am not insensitive to the deeper native roots of later US Psychology, but on balance I felt it better to reserve the North American story *in toto* for the second half of this project.

The amount of space devoted to different figures and topics here is not a direct reflection of my rating of their 'importance' in some objective sense. In several cases I have devoted relatively more space to a person or topic (such as Reid or phrenology) than is usual. This occurs for two reasons: (a) the need to redress past neglect; or (b) because they present an opportunity for seeing the process whereby psychological ideas are generated, even if from other perspectives the long-term impact was minimal or the individual's reputation has not survived the verdict of history. The notion that there is some correct 'weighting' ideally to be adhered to is in any case problematical. Apart from involving a begging of the question, the whole direction of post-modern thought is to challenge the viability of such canons and recognize them as serving rhetorical functions in relation to the historical situation of a discipline at a particular time. Where writers have been 'honoured' with a place in the canon, this is of course a historical fact in its own right, but it does not mean that their works will necessarily bear upon the questions we are now addressing more significantly than those of others less honoured. I am not trying here to *amend* Psychology's canon so much as use historical research in a way different to those uses which generated the canon in the first place. This involves critiquing the significance of canonical figures in relation to the questions I am addressing. As it turns out, my 'weightings' are not quite so quirky as all this may portend. The general point is simply that to change the agenda is to change the canon, and that there are no agenda-free canons.

4 Metapsychology and Self-Disclosure

A further paradox must be noted. The book is itself premissed on a Psychological theory regarding the generation of 'the psychological'. Although this is better construed as 'metapsychology' than 'Psychology', it nevertheless implies that I have retained a toe in the 'empirical Psychology' camp. On the one hand, I am hoping that it will provide some sort of Archimedean point from which to construe the emergence of modern p/Psychology; on the other, I would not, in the final analysis, wish to insist on its status as being other than an invitation to view affairs in a certain way. But then, to a Wittgensteinian, the mistake of scientific positivism was to assume that scientific propositions could ever be anything else. To expand further on this here would pre-empt matters dealt with in the final chapter.

Finally, in the spirit of the enterprise, I will – albeit obliquely – try to contextualize myself. As Roger Smith (1988) points out, there are two senses to the term 'presentism'. Negatively, it refers to histories written in order to legitimate the present state of the discipline, or to demonstrate that the author's own theoretical constituency within it represents the authentic voice of the discipline's central 'progressive' tradition. But we can none of us escape the present; we are writing in the present, for the present, with our own political – in the broadest sense – agendas. Positively, we do best to articulate these and render them visible, rather than adopt a pose of transcendental detachment. My 'political agenda' is to contribute towards the emergence of a genuinely multidisciplinary approach to the task of enhancing our understanding of ourselves, an approach in which particular disciplines are viewed as perspectives to have in one's repertoire rather than sources of personal identity for their members. (More generally, the book itself has finally emerged as a piece of 'critically emancipatory self-reflection' on the scientific *mentalité* itself – but that belongs to the last, not the first, chapter.) As I tried to indicate in *On Psychological Language,* the 'physiomorphic' perspective has a potentially powerful integrating role in this, drawing together such apparently diverse fields as human evolution, the nature of religion, anthropology and – the focus of our concern here – the histories of both Psychology and its subject matter. Expressed in these terms, it might seem a relatively simple, if overambitious, goal. The underlying message to be discerned, though, is that this approach itself will play a part in initiating a new, more consciously reflexive (though not navel-gazing) move in the very story it purports to tell.

I ended my book *Human Evolution* by saying that we have to get ourselves under control. This is perhaps platitudinous, but rightly places me in the green doom-watching camp, for which I make no apology. The points of greatest leverage for effecting control are not always obvious, nor are the vectors via which they work immediately evident. Devoting one's energies to unravelling the nature of reflexive discourse will, I hope, prove to be just such a case. There can, after all, be few things more fundamental to our overall behaviour than our beliefs about what we are – however difficult it sometimes is to differentiate the roles of chicken and egg regarding the relationship between the two[5].

PART ONE
The Seventeenth Century

1
Vast Confusions and New Paradoxes

> I hear new news every day, and those ordinary rumours of war, plagues, fires, inundations, thefts, murders, massacres, meteors, comets, spectrums, prodigies, apparitions, of towns taken cities besieged in France, Germany, Turkey, Persia, Poland &c. daily musters and preparations, and such like, which these tempestuous times afford, battles fought, so many men slain, monomachies, shipwrecks, piracies, and sea-fights, peace, leagues, stratagems and fresh alarms. A vast confusion of vows, wishes, actions, edicts, petitions, lawsuits, pleas, laws, proclamations, complaints, grievances are daily brought to our ears. New books every day, pamphlets, currantoes, stories, whole catalogues of volumes of all sorts, new paradoxes, opinions, schisms, heresies, controversies in philosophy, religion etc. Now come tidings of weddings, maskings, mummeries, entertainments, jubilees, embassies, tilts and tournaments, trophies, triumphs, revels, sports, plays: then again, as in a new shifted scene, treasons, cheating tricks, robberies, enormous villainies in all kinds, funerals, burials, deaths of princes . . .
>
> (Robert Burton, *The Anatomy of Melancholy*, Democritus to the Reader, p.15[1])

I INTRODUCTION

1 The Absence of Psychology in the Seventeenth Century

With some interesting but quite minor exceptions (considered in Section VII), the seventeenth century is devoid of texts comparable in aims or method to modern Psychology, an absence generally ignored by historians of Psychology eager to identify its roots in the Scientific Revolution. Like a Mormon's ancestors, Bacon, Robert Burton, Descartes, Hobbes and Locke (even Malebranche, Spinoza and Leibniz, though rarely Pascal) are retrospectively converted into Psychologists. What did exist, of course, as it always has, was reflexive discourse – discourse about the nature of human beings – which, as ever, took varied forms. Most important were theological writings about the nature of the human soul, dominated by a moral concern with Christian salvation. Closely related to this genre are a number of (usually Aristotelian) treatises on the 'passions' of a classificatory and moral nature[2]. Other forms of reflexive discourse included (apart from drama and poetry) characterologies [3] and physiognomical works[4], medical texts on psychopathology (e.g. melancholy)[5], and a variety of books on education[6], proto-anthropology[7], child-rearing[8] and language[9]. These last constitute but a minute fraction of the total number of publications before 1700[10]. Philosophy, while separate from theology, had long been subordinated to the latter, but now starts to regain its autonomy (especially in Bacon and Hobbes, although the earlier-sixteenth-century Neo-Platonists had begun the move; Descartes, as we will see, is a more complicated case). The 'essay' as represented by Bacon and Montaigne is an intermediate category, half secular moral philosophy and half literary exercise.

To get our bearings, it will help to consider Bacon at the outset. The two major accounts he gives us of his views on psychological matters are in Aphorisms 39–56 of the *Novum Organum* and Books IV–V of *The Advancement of Learning*[11]. The former explores the four 'Idols of the Mind' – the various sources of errors in understanding. These comprise the Idols of the Tribe (innate failings common to all, such as believing that 'the sense of man is the measure of things'), of the Cave (individual idiosyncratic foibles and biases due to education, temperament, etc.), of the Market-place ('the ill and unfit choice of words' due to acceptance of their common use 'according to the apprehension of the vulgar') and the Theatre (dogmatic acceptance of received philosophies: '. . . in my judgment all the received systems are but so many stage plays, representing worlds of their own creation after an unreal and scenic fashion'). Note here the focus on epistemological failings, as one would expect in what is, canonically, the first text in modern philosophy of science. It is from the *Advancement of Learning*, though, that Bacon earned his place in histories of Psychology, for it is commonly maintained that he therein identified the need for such a discipline within the overall scheme of the sciences. It is of interest, then, to turn to the text and see how he envisaged his 'general science concerning the Nature and State of Man' (p.373, *Works* IV). What unfolds is quite unlike anything since undertaken by Psychologists. We start with a division between the 'nature of man undivided' (the Person of Man) and the 'League', i.e. the connections between the mind or soul and the body. The first 'takes into consideration two subjects principally; the Miseries of the human race, and the Prerogatives or Excellencies of the same' (p.374, *ibid.*). He envisages a collection of 'ultimities': '... the miracles of human nature, and its highest powers and virtues in mind and body, should be collected into a volume, which should serve for a register of the Triumphs of Man' (p.375, *ibid.*). On this basis the *Guinness Book of Records* would constitute a primary Psychological text.

The League 'or Common Bond between Soul and Body' is subdivided into (a) how the workings of one disclose the other; and (b) how they 'work the one upon the other'. In expanding on (a), however, Bacon identifies physiognomy and interpretation of dreams as the major themes. Turning to (b), he insists that the soul retains its final 'sovereignty' (pp.377–8, *ibid.*), invoking a comparison with 'monarchs who, though powerful, are sometimes controlled by their servants, and yet without abatement of their majesty royal'. Enquiries are also urgently needed 'concerning the proper seats and domiciles which the several faculties of the mind occupy in the body and its organs'. Questions regarding the mind–body relationship itself he evades: 'in the end all such must be handed over to religion to be determined and defined' (p.398, *ibid.*). Investigation of the well-known 'faculties' of Understanding, Reason, Will, Appetite and Affections is assigned to the separate disciplines of Logic (the first two) and Ethics, although 'it is true indeed that the imagination performs the office of an agent or messenger or proctor in both provinces, both the judicial and the ministerial' (p.405, *ibid.*). His discussion of memory is concerned mainly with its improvement. He also delves into 'Divination' (astrology) and 'Fascination' (pp.399–400, *ibid.*).

Bacon's 'Psychology' is only intermittently congruent with the discipline's present concerns; his priorities are different, his approach is essentially a normative or moral philosophical one, his view of existing categories and concepts uncritical. His image of the mind, as some of the quoted passages indicate, is what one might call 'bureaucratic' – the sovereign soul (in a 'League' with the body) is surrounded by advisers and servants who are engaged in performing various 'offices', and are 'invested' with various degrees of 'authority', though he also compares remembering to '. . . the hunting of a deer within an enclosure' (p. 436, *ibid.*). Nobody in the ensuing century (apart, maybe, from the forgotten John Bulwer [see below, pp. 70–73]), actually made any attempt to create a 'Philosophy of Humanity' according to Bacon's agenda. It is thus misleading to depict Bacon's 'Psychological' passages as constituting the foundation stones for the modern discipline. A third text in which he sketches a 'Psychological' agenda more programmatically is *Parasceve*, which is appended to the *Novum Organum*. Here, it is true, a 'History of Vision and things Visible', a 'History of Venus, as a species of Touch' and a 'History of the Intellectual Faculties' are among the enquiries called for. P.B. Wood (1990) notes this, and the other passages, as being especially influential in Scotland in the following century (notably on John Gregory; see below, p. 229). The direct Baconian impact on psychological thought, such as it was, is thus delayed by over a century until it is taken up in the Scottish Enlightenment. This is ironic since, as we shall see, the Scottish Enlightenment contribution (bar Hume's) has, in its turn, been overneglected by historians of Psychology.

The inclination of contemporary authors of general history of Psychology texts to assimilate seventeenth-century reflexive discourse into the discipline stems directly from their question-begging assumption that modern Psychology is a *bona fide* 'science'. If that is the case, then its genealogy must necessarily be traceable to the beginnings of 'science' in the Scientific Revolution (hence Bacon, Galileo, Descartes, etc., earn inclusion simply by virtue of being leading figures in that revolution). Furthermore, as a 'natural science' it must also have a natural object of enquiry as its subject matter – thus, however faulty earlier studies of this subject matter, the subject matter did actually exist and was already the focus of – albeit crude – study. Neither of these conclusions is self-evidently valid. To clarify the situation, we need to reconsider the nature of 'reflexive discourse'.

2 'Reflexive Discourse' and a Digression on English

Elsewhere I have argued that 'human nature' is essentially 'physiomorphic' in character[12]. Philosophical and linguistic considerations led me to propose that, for modern *Homo sapiens sapiens* at least, 'psychological' properties are generated by a reflexive discourse which has to depend on the reflexive application of the terms used in what I called 'World Language'. This raises fundamental difficulties for any notion of the 'psychological' as a natural object of enquiry. Whatever we understand by the 'psychological' exists only at the level of the reflexive discourse which creates, encodes and determines the qualities and phenomena which we ascribe to ourselves and use to construe our experiences of ourselves and others. It follows that changes in the terms of such discourse (typically initiated by encounters with the novel in the public world) constitute changes in the 'psychological' itself. *Even the move of formulating the category 'psychological' constitutes such a change.* This is not to deny that some 'natural' properties – lurking, as it were, behind the language – may underlie the phenomena we now call, for example, emotions, instincts, etc. It is, though, to assert that as objects of enquiry such phenomena are knowable only as linguistically encoded – which means as physiomorphically constructed from public 'world' (which includes the social world) phenomena. The alternative is a physiological reductionism which eschews the 'psychological' altogether.

One essential prerequisite for a discipline of 'Psychology' is the creation of the category 'the psychological' or 'psychology' as a viable subject matter. The significance of seventeenth-century reflexive discourse for Psychology rests largely on the role it played in the eventual emergence of this superordinate category. Even so, the modern category 'psychology' did not exist in the seventeenth century (though the word as an isolated, and generally unadopted, neologism did), nor even in the eighteenth, at any rate with its modern connotations[13]. What existed were 'Pneumatology' (the science of the soul) and numerous works on the Passions, Understanding, Wit, Conscience, Character, the 'Microcosm', and Minde.

A digression on the state of English at the beginning of our period is apposite here. (As noted in the Introduction, I will use the anachronistic adjective 'psychological' in referring to terms used in reflexive discourse, this being an unfortunately cumbersome technical expression. In doing so I suppose I am proposing yet a further meaning for the term 'psychological', i.e. 'the subject matter of reflexive discourse'.) Past knowledge as yet still unrefuted and new discoveries by now undeniable, the turn of the sixteenth and seventeenth centuries found learned Europeans, and especially learned Englishmen, in a peculiar state of intellectual – and, indeed, spiritual – weightlessness. Sharing in this condition, the greatest English writers were able to perform manoeuvres of the imagination of unsurpassed dexterity; freshly translated ancient wisdoms and freshly reported contemporary novelties serving equally to fuel the creative task. In little over half a century the linguistic resources of the English language had been revolutionized, and in no area more profoundly than in the realm of psychological expression and exploration. In 1545 the physician T. Phayre, still feeling the dearth of English medical texts, defends himself for writing in English and seeks 'to provoke them that are of better lerning to utter theyr knowledge in lyke attemptes'.[14]. By 1600 this battle has long been won, and writers of all kinds are luxuriating in the new-found versatility of their language. Only English underwent a revolution on quite this scale and of quite this kind, and elsewhere in Europe Latin remained the primary medium for philosophy, medicine and Natural Philosophy (even if vernacular translations ensued). Neither in England nor in France did the switch occur overnight, but in both the use of the vernacular became increasingly acceptable for philosophical work over the first decades of the century, Bacon, Hobbes and Descartes writing both in Latin and in their native tongues.

The reasons why English was capable of revolutionizing itself are complex, but four factors were central: first, a final abandonment of inflection in the early sixteenth century which consolidated the grammatical flexibility English had acquired in the Middle Ages; second, its already heterogeneous nature, combining as it did both Anglo-Saxon and Norman French vocabularies; and third, the post-Humanist spread of literacy in the classical languages among the newly educated secular middle classes. In combination these latter two factors resulted in a massive expansion of the vocabulary as writers such as Roger Ascham, Thomas More, Thomas Elyot, and Richard Mulcaster injected the language with terms of Latin and Greek derivation, while others, notably Edmund Spenser, rediscovered the resources of Middle English and dialect vocabularies. The Fourth factor, of course, was printing which, as well as its more obviously dramatic effects, inevitably entailed a progressive standardization of spelling. Not that this was achieved overnight, and well into the seventeenth century one finds variations within the same sentence; Earle (1628) on 'A downe-right scholler', for instance, writes: '. . . his fault is onely this, that his minde is somewhat much taken up with his mind' (Character 21). (One almost senses a deliberate play on two senses of the word 'mind/e' here, but this is surely illusory.) Taken together, these factors created a fertile climate for neologisms and stylistic experiment.

This linguistic story amounted to a breakdown in the psychological barriers between the Latin-speaking intellectuals (hitherto, but no longer, almost all churchmen) and the rest of the population. The sophisticated repertoire of psychological concepts encoded in Latin and Greek philosophy and theology was transplanted wholesale into the English vernacular (though slow seepage from Latin had been going on long before). Baugh (1959) cites the following as among the terms introduced by Thomas More: *absurdity, anticipate, comprehensible, exact, exaggerate, explain, fact(!), frivolous, paradox* and *pretext*. Elyot is credited with, among many others: *accommodate, analogy, exhaust, to experience, frugality, inimitable, irritate* and *modesty*. The rising educated middle class now have at their disposal a range of psychological concepts as large and complex as that of the Schoolman, Philosopher or Theologian who had hitherto operated in cloistered isolation. More than that, the vocabularies could now interact and fuse in a way which had been impossible when the learned had always to discourse in one of two quite distinct modes: Latin or the vernacular. Freely floating, late Renaissance English writers could take the language in any direction they wished. Significantly, by the end of the sixteenth century literacy rates in the south east of England may have been as high as 80 per cent, London probably being Europe's most literate city[15].

While it would be unwise to consider this linguistic situation as unconnected with the background sociopolitical factors, it would be equally unwise to see it as a mere epiphenomenon. There were clearly some quite distinct and unique features characterizing the condition of English in the early sixteenth century and relating only tenuously to local sociopolitical circumstances: its grammar, its etymologically diverse vocabulary, and the conjunction of these with Europe-wide developments such as printing and Humanism. More, Elyot and Mulcaster, as leaders in vernacularizing the classical lexicon, were striving to advance the broad Humanist programme, a Europe-wide imperative. They would also have been familiar with the complex medieval and Renaissance 'Psychologies' of Averroës, Avicenna and Aquinas (E.R. Harvey, 1975). Significantly, it was in More's circle and the new educational curricula of schools such as Eton and Merchant Taylors (under Mulcaster) that the roots of Elizabethan drama were struck (Boas, 1950).

To review the entire English psychological vocabulary here would be too extensive an undertaking. It incorporated terms from many sources in addition to the basic physical and sensory property words, such as crafts (e.g. weaving and husbandry), Hippocratic and Galenic medicine, social roles, law and economics, Classical philosophy and, of course, Christian theology. And this richness provided the resources exploited with such awesome success by Shakespeare, Donne and their literary contemporaries. Two especially interesting sources of novel imagery for describing psychological processes were alchemy and Paracelsian iatrochemistry, both at their height in Britain from around 1580 to 1620. As Nicholl (1980) shows, the literary impact of this complex and exotic *topos* on poets, dramatists and satirists from Shakespeare down to Nashe was enormous. It provided a rich language for characterizing psychological, as much as physical, change and transformation. (This is to leave aside the deeper Jungian argument that fundamentally alchemy was itself a vehicle of personal spiritual transformation.) Pervasive though the impact of alchemical language was, it did not initially affect philosophical thinking about psychological topics such as the 'passions'. Not until the Restoration did schemata drawn ultimately from this source impact on Natural Philosophical accounts of psychological phenomena, and then, as we will see, via their deployment in physiological theorizing.

3 The Orthodox Story and Its Limitations

Standard History of Psychology texts from Boring and Murphy down to Murray, Schultz, Robinson and Leahey (albeit more cautiously in the last case) have presented a relatively simple story of the discipline's seventeenth century roots centring on Descartes, Hobbes and Locke[16]. Descartes's role is seen as twofold: his commitment to mechanistic explanations of material phenomena and his complementary distinction of the mind as a separate immaterial unextended substance knowable by reason. Since he offered speculative physiological accounts of the 'passions', perception and memory, he is cast as the founding father of physiological Psychology and originator of the reflex concept[17]. Over and above this, as a major star of the Scientific Revolution he must naturally figure in a broader sense as initiator of that scientific project of which Psychology is assumed to be a part. Hobbes then takes the mechanistic model a stage further, rejecting Cartesian dualism, so becoming a proto-behaviourist or at least a proto-empirical Psychologist. The story culminates in Locke as offering the first systematic mechanistic Psychology, a Psychology in which quasi-atomic 'ideas' originating in sensory experience combine to create all psychological phenomena. Although he uses the term only in passing (and in a very restricted sense) he is accorded the status of founder of Associationism, allegedly to dominate British Psychological thought until the late nineteenth century. The major European philosophers Malebranche, Gassendi, Spinoza and Leibniz are mentioned primarily as representing rival approaches which petered out. Additional figures such as Robert Burton, Willis and the Spaniard Huarte are also occasionally cited in passing as respectively pioneering or anticipating clinical, physiological and applied Psychology. An impression is created that from Descartes onwards there was an identifiable tradition of investigating the psychological in a 'scientific' way. The key word is 'mechanization' – there was a 'mechanization of the world view', brought about by the Scientific Revolution, in which Psychological thought participated. This image is seriously flawed.

Although the respects in which it is flawed will concern us throughout this chapter, three must immediately be noted.

(a) It is grossly oversimplified in that it selects from the seminal texts those contents retrospectively construable as

Psychological while ignoring the authors' goals and the contemporary debates in which they were engaged. It also mistakes the adoption of a 'mechanistic' style of analytic discourse for the adoption of a proto-scientific *method* as such. The consequence of this is to present the story as more simply 'progressive' and continuous than in fact it was. More on this in due course.

(b) Although some writers have made gestures towards contextualizing and nods at social constructionism, they have, as noted in the Introduction, been hampered by the requirements of the 'History of Psychology' textbook genre. Contextualization has become conflated with – and overwhelmed by – the pedagogic task of conveying some rudimentary historical background knowledge to North American freshmen and sophomores, vitiating any genuine contextual analysis. The real psychological distance between the seventeenth and twentieth centuries is masked by a need to render past events comprehensible to a contemporary – and non-European – readership.

(c) In seeking to depict seventeenth century writers as early pioneers in studying 'psychology' as a natural object of enquiry, a number of embarrassing features of the reflexive discourse of the period are overlooked: as G.M. Ross (1988) has recently made clear, there was no modern concept of 'consciousness' in play; the term 'idea' was extremely slippery to put it mildly; the 'mind–body problem' was not so labelled and the issue was treated as a purely conceptual, philosophical riddle with theological implications, not an empirical one; and, most patently of all, everyone was talking about the soul. Terms such as 'passion', 'apprehension' and 'resentment' were frequently, if not always, used in contexts where we want to read 'emotion', 'perception' and 'feeling' respectively (e.g. in the 1650 translation of Descartes's *Passions of the Soul*; see below p. 40). But how far such modernization of the vocabulary distorts the meaning of the original is at least worth asking. Can we really treat a text on 'passions' as a text on 'emotion'? The answer to this, at least, is an unambiguous 'no', for originally the 'passions' denote passivity on the subject's part (e.g. fear), while 'emotions' move or spur them to action (e.g. anger). This distinction is progressively lost sight of over the course of the eighteenth century, and both 'passion' and 'emotion' may be used for both, until passion finally yields the field sometime around 1800, retaining only a more restricted usage to refer to deeply held and strongly expressed emotions. With the loss of 'passion' in the original sense modern Psychology has lost the passive/active distinction. And what, in modern terms, was Descartes's '*l'Ame*'? Soul? Mind? Consciousness?

If we are to recover the historical significance for modern Psychology of seventeenth century 'Psychological' texts, the orthodox story must needs be set aside. As it stands it merely assumes what it sets out to prove – that a continuous tradition of Psychological discourse can be traced back to the seventeenth century, and that the apparent 'anticipations' of later Psychology to be found there are indeed real, intentional, and directly ancestral to modern Psychological treatments of the same themes.

4 An Alternative Approach

The alternative approach adopted here is to identify the major features of the extremely complex process whereby 'psychological' discourse was transformed during the seventeenth century. In doing this I will be focusing primarily on Britain, although the psychological transformation in question was in many respects Europe-wide. This shifts attention from Psychology in the discipline sense, to 'psychology' in the modern subject-matter sense – which for the moment we now have no choice but to retroject. I have identified five such features or facets of this transformation, but these are in many respects artificially differentiated and are not intended as in any way definitive, nor am I claiming that they were deployed as 'categories' by seventeenth century writers themselves. They are:

(a) 'Epistemization'. The shift in focus of philosophical concern from the moral and ontological to the epistemological.
(b) Mechanization. Accepting that there was a 'mechanization' of reflexive discourse, we need to examine exactly what this meant.
(c) Rationalization. The resolution of the faith versus reason tension in favour of the latter (closely related to [a]).

(d) The Invention of Privacy. This has been discussed discussed by David Morse (1989), and its implications for the origins of Psychology are considered. It also offers us an opportunity to look at Robert Burton.

(e) The Language Question. A stylistic move from the 'synthetic' and 'discursive' to the 'analytic' in the seventeenth century is widely recognized (Burton and Locke may be taken as representative of these poles). This is related to a crucial debate on the nature of language, extending from Hobbes via Wilkins to Locke, which has a vital bearing on the whole issue of the conceptualization of the psychological.

Following these we will consider some generally forgotten instances of what may more legitimately be considered as proto-Psychology, and address the question of why they did *not* in fact inaugurate the discipline. In the final section I will try to pull the various threads together and propose a revised reading of the role of the seventeenth century in the history of Psychology.

II EPISTEMIZATION

By the end of the seventeenth century the central philosophical issue, both in Britain and on the Continent, had become the nature of knowledge – its sources, acquisition, kinds and status. One might argue that therein lies its major contribution to future Psychology – in providing the basis for making 'information processing' the essence of the psychological. So deeply has this penetrated modern Psychology (and not only its overtly 'cognitive' versions) that we need to remind ourselves that it was not always thus. There are other options, of which the theological has been the most historically salient. 'For puritans', as Morgan (1986) tells us, 'the central fact of human existence was . . . the relationship, in all its intricacies, of the individual and God, not the free being in control of his own destiny' (p.77). And not only for Puritans – the 'central fact' for almost all writers in 1600 was the fate of the soul, and reflexive discourse had the moral as its abiding focus, whether at the folk level of the Seven Deadly Sins or the heights of Aquinian philosophy. In Protestant theology the need for detailed analysis of the soul's predicament was rendered more intensely acute, and the Puritan's 'central fact' became bestowal of Grace in a mystical conversion experience of direct contact with God. (See also Section

IV below.) How did the moral, and ontological, became displaced by the epistemological as the dominant psychological theme? Neither Locke nor anyone else, of course, was using the category 'epistemology', which originated in 1854 (J.G. Buikerood, 1985). What we term 'epistemology' long remains undifferentiated from, or subsumed under, 'logic' in philosophical discourse.

1 Ontology to Epistemology

In morally orientated, fundamentally theological, philosophical analyses, ontological issues inevitably loomed large. First there was the eternal issue of the existence of God, and the nature of His existence. Second came the equally eternal conundrum of the nature of the immortal soul itself. Couple this with acceptance of Aristotle's doctrine of the tripartite soul which had become grafted onto Christian metaphysical orthodoxy in the Middle Ages, and ontological issues become inescapable. This is the intellectual context in which Descartes's philosophical work is initially embedded. As the earliest major figure in the orthodox canon, Descartes has received universal acclaim as a proto-Psychologist. The *Meditations* is cited as crucial evidence of this, and thus provides a sort of test case for the received account.

Note first that the full title of the 1680 English edition is *Six Metaphysical Meditations; wherein it is proved that there is a God.* I cannot resist quoting the following passage from Molyneux's Preface as indicating how he, at any rate, viewed the work:

> I cannot resemble his Performance herein better than to the Six Days Work of the Supream Architect....In the first Meditation we are Presented with a Rude and Indigested Choas [sic] of Errours and Doubts, till the Divine spirit of the Noble *Des-Cartes* (pardon the boldness of the Expression) *moves upon the confused face of these waters*, and thereout produces some *clear* and *distinct* Light; by which *Sun-shine* he proceeds to bring forth and cherish other *Branches of Truth*; Till at last by a six Days Labour he Establishes this Fair Fabrick (as I may call it) of the *Intellectual World* on foundations that shall never be shaken. Then sitting down with rest and satisfaction he looks upon this his Off-Spring and pronounces it GOOD. (pp. [10/11])

The contemporary significance of the *Meditations*, then, was clearly theological; it represented the first attempt at a fully rational theology. And such it was intended to be, from the prefatory address 'To The Most Wise and Illustrious the Dean and Doctors of the Sacred Faculty of Theology in Paris' (wherein he argues the necessity, if infidels are to be converted, of proving 'by means of natural reason' both the soul's immortality and the existence of God), via the 'Synopsis of the Six Following Meditations' in which the contents of four of them (2, 3, 5, 6) are summarized as concerning the proof of God's existence. And so through to the content of the Meditations themselves, where this issue constitutes the explicit ground and context for even the most extended passages of 'pure philosophizing' (as I may call it) regarding the limits of doubt and the nature of the body–mind relationship, by virtue of which the work gained its philosophical eminence. The burden of Meditation Six (considered by Robinson [1981], along with Meditation Two, as the most 'psychological') is to prove the existence of material things and reconcile Divine honesty with human perceptual fallibility, the argument hinging at a crucial point on the fact that 'God is not a deceiver, and that consequently He has not permitted any falsity to exist in my opinion which He has not likewise given me the faculty of correcting' (1967 edn, p. 191) (proved in Meditation Four).

The technical philosophical issue at stake in Descartes's effort to differentiate the infallibly known properties of the mind and its innate ideas from those which are dubitable is, in fact, a quite traditional one. To quote G.M. Ross (1988): 'If the *Meditations* are read without any modern presuppositions, then it should be obvious that Descartes' primary concern was with the old Platonic distinction between universal truths of which we have knowledge, and physical particulars about which we have mere belief' (p. 219). Clearly, then, Descartes is by now unable to address the central theological and ontological questions without getting embroiled in epistemological issues.

The appearance of the *Meditations* in 1641 coincided with the outbreak of Civil War in Britain. Hobbes, in Parisian exile, responded immediately with a series of *Objections* (his first philosophical publication). In these he aimed to undermine Descartes's ontological differentiation between the soul and the body and argued (as he continued to do at length in *Human Nature* and *Leviathan*) that even those phenomena Descartes ascribed to the soul alone (Reason, Will, Imagining) admitted of material 'mechanistic' explanations. This position entails adopting a purely empirical epistemology – there is nothing 'innate', our reflexive knowledge consists of linguistically encoded sensory input, existing as residual material motion in the brain. The problem of 'will' was resolved by the use of the Latin term '*conatus*' (translated into English as 'endeavour') for physical movement and 'will' alike (see Section VI below). He can maintain this because unlike Descartes, for whom matter was passive, requiring *external* agency to move it (i.e., ultimately, God), Hobbes held motion to be a property of matter. (One of the complications of the notion of 'mechanism' to be discussed below.)

Yet Hobbes's materialism did not mean that he had abandoned moral philosophy. On the contrary, the function of Hobbes's 'Psychological' writing was to underpin his political philosophy - as a conduit via which he could derive a 'social cosmology' from the new physical cosmology of Galileo (see Verdon, 1982). (Again, see Section VI below.) The joint presence in the intellectual arena of the opposed positions of Descartes (a Jesuit-trained Catholic after all) and Hobbes (widely seen as atheistical) could not but provoke English Protestant orthodoxy into trying to formulate a response. It is from their struggles to do so, during the middle decades of the century, that epistemology finally emerges as central. Descartes and Hobbes had between them made this an unavoidable component of future theological and moral philosophical debate. Each presented a metaphysical system with distinct epistemological implications and containing unambiguous epistemological propositions. Descartes had concluded, from his ontological demonstration of God's existence, that the individual divine soul was endowed with a potentially infallible Reasoning faculty operating in terms of 'clear and distinct' innate ideas. This alone could guarantee knowledge of the reality underlying the fickle testimony of the senses. Hobbes concluded from his ontological refutation of the need to postulate an 'immaterial' soul that knowledge arose from linguistic reasoning about sensory experience. We must, even so, stress that these epistemological positions had arisen in the context of moral philosophy: for Descartes, the immediate goal was to demonstrate how Reason could secure Faith; for Hobbes, it was to provide a rigorous theoretical basis for a system of social order, a realm ungoverned by any divinely ordained natural laws. For Hobbes, morality had to be socially constructed and his task, in a context of fanatical social strife and fratricidal anarchy, was to show how.

2 Theology to Philosophy

The philosophical problem certain divines (pre-eminently, but not exclusively, the Cambridge Neo-Platonists Henry More and Ralph Cudworth) now had to face was threefold: (a) refuting Hobbes's apparently atheistical materialism; (b) redressing the deficiency of Cartesianism with respect to God's attenuated role in the affairs of His mechanized material world; and (c) doing this in a way consistent with nascent Natural Philosophy. This philosophical problem was being posed in a climate of intense doctrinal confusion, in turn embedded in issues of political power. By the Restoration the spectrum ranged from remnants of extreme radical sects (such as the Fifth Monarchists) to re-enthroned High Church Anglican Archbishops. Any acceptable solution was therefore constrained; it had to avoid the excesses of both radical fanatical 'enthusiasm' and autocratic doctrinal dogmatism.

The Achilles heel of their situation was, as we will be considering further, a felt need to engage in *reasoned* argument purged of appeals to authority and rhetorical casuistry. If Hobbes, Descartes and their followers (not many in Hobbes's case, but sceptical and heretical philosophical voices abounded) were to be refuted their arguments must be engaged directly. The theologians now found themselves fighting on unfamiliar ground. Hobbes's identification was with the Natural Philosophers, the Baconians, not with theology. Descartes's core identification was less clear – certainly it was with theology, as we have seen, but his task (in the works we are concerned with) was to reconcile orthodox theological doctrines to Natural Philosophy – with which he also centrally identified. This, ironically, meant that his theology was highly unorthodox. Each, in his different way, held Reason as the final arbiter.

Having to argue on several fronts (with Natural Philosophers, conservative co-religionists, radical co-religionists, 'Atheists' – for which read Hobbes – and Cartesians) the Cambridge Neo-Platonists sought refuge in a new theology of their own: 'a bold rejection of the entire Western theological tradition from St.Augustine through the medieval schoolmen to the classic Protestantism of Luther, Calvin, and their variegated followers in the seventeenth century'[18]. But neither they nor any other theologians could evade two questions in particular which now loomed large on the theological agenda: (a) what is the nature of our knowledge of God? (Or 'What is the origin of our idea of God?') and (b) What is the relationship between God and the material world? But once embarked on trying to answer such questions rationally, the Cambridge Neo-Platonists and all other theologians engaged in the debate were faced with others of a more general nature which underlay them: (a) What is the nature of any knowledge at all? (Or 'What is the origin of ideas in general?') and (b) How can we identify the principles by which the material world is governed? 'Pneumatology', the 'science of the soul', thus met Natural Philosophy.

Theologians increasingly found themselves debating these questions with Natural Philosophers such as Robert Boyle and Robert Hooke. This was not, in all cases, confrontational. Both parties acknowledged the urgency of the task of providing a rational basis for religion in the face of what they saw as a rising tide of scepticism, but Natural Philosophers (e.g. Boyle[19]) were disinclined to endorse the – to them – amateurish cosmologies speculatively invented by theologians. A truly rational religion would have to be based on a scientifically credible cosmology, consistent with experimental evidence[20]. Further exploration of the basic epistemological questions required a more analytic approach by someone in tune with Natural Philosophy. Natural Philosophers, too, had need of an epistemological model; they needed to be able to differentiate conceptually between knowledge and belief, between data and hypotheses, and above all between the kinds of question which were answerable and those which were not. Divines like Stillingfleet and Tillotson were, by the 1680s, doggedly sticking to the view that the idea of God could not be derived from sensory experience and was thus innately implanted along with the self-evidently true premisses of logic, but they rejected Descartes's crude mechanism.

It is at this point, and in this context, that Locke's *Essay on Human Understanding* finally appeared after long gestation. Locke was a political radical, an exiled plotter against James II, supporter of the Monmouth Rebellion and William of Orange and conduit of funds for subversive purposes. The aim of the *Essay* was equally radical, though it is hard to discern at this distance and has required detailed exegesis to uncover. In many respects it is a cunning and dissembling book as well as a philosophical masterpiece. Like Hobbes's *Human Nature*, it was a prelude to an explicitly political work, the *Two Treatises on Government*. Locke's targets were the 'latitudinarian' divines who, while opposed to James II's Catholicism and tyrannical style of government, felt themselves doctrinally obliged to acquiesce, since Kings occupied their thrones by virtue of Divine Providence. And these are precisely the same people who are defending innate ideas, seeing Natural Philosophy as potentially or actually atheistic in tendency, and are generally bogged down in mealy-mouthed moderation.

Now Locke, by focusing *exclusively* on epistemology, was able radically to subvert the terms of the entire debate. The innateness of the idea of God is dismissed in a page, on the simple grounds that there are plenty of cases of people with no such notion. 'And . . . if we should with attention mind the lives and discourses of people not so far off, we should have too much reason to fear that many . . . have no very strong and clear impressions of a Deity upon their minds; and' (he adds archly) 'that the complaints of atheism made from the pulpit are not without reason' (I. 4. 8). A single paragraph later suffices to explain how we get the Idea of God via 'the simple ideas we receive from reflection' (II. 23. 33) (though he does extend the discussion for a further three). Understood – and meant to be understood – in the context of contemporary theological debate, the *Essay* is provocative precisely because its author so glaringly omits to make theology the central issue, his discussion of God coming almost peripherally. What is so often depicted as the rational outcome of nearly fifty years of progressive and lofty philosophical consideration of the nature of the human mind – naturally emerging as it were from some intellectual chrysalis – was nothing of the kind. It was a consciously provocative, even aggressive, publication of revolutionary intent. And theology did not quietly go its way thereafter, the contemporary critical response to the *Essay* was a barrage of theological attack on Locke's perceived 'Deism', even his 'Atheism'. Nor was such criticism a misunderstanding (as one might argue that Wilberforce's response to Darwin was) – Locke's critics knew perfectly well what he was up to, and how well he had succeeded. Locke's *Essay* does not, then, constitute a simple abandonment of theologically orientated philosophy and the *de novo* birth of secular mechanistic epistemology so much as an active flinging down of the gauntlet – a move (albeit subversive) *within* the existing philosophical framework rather than a rejection of it.

3 Sensational Ideas

Locke's central epistemological concept was 'Idea'. 'Idea' is a word with a complex history. Long used in the ordinary-language sense to refer vaguely to any specific mental content, as a technical philosophical term it variously meant an image, a Platonic archetype, or an impression in the brain. The problem which came to the fore after Descartes was precisely how 'ideas' were to be conceptualized as occurring – whether they existed in the 'immaterial' mind (or soul), as 'corporeal' modifications of the brain, or perhaps were of both kinds. The epistemological issue of how ideas came to be formed was, of course, part and parcel of the same debate, raising the issue of the relationship between sensory information and ideas. A sensationalist epistemology could easily lead, as Descartes well knew, to scepticism, a belief that the qualities and properties of material phenomena as known via the senses were only 'ideas' constructed by the mind, with no provable correspondence to real properties of matter. For Descartes the solution here was to adopt the distinction between primary properties (such as form) and secondary properties (such as colour, sound, smell) – the former being 'real' and the latter (on Yolton's recent reading of the issue) being ideas which signified the real properties in a way analogous to the relationship holding between words and their referents[21].

The mid-century debates over the corporeality or otherwise of ideas, the existence of innate ideas and the idea–sensation relationship, are extremely tangled and again infused with theological connotations. The twists and turns of these debates are only now being unravelled by historians of philosophy (not of Psychology)[22]. Locke's highly generalized use of 'Idea' to cover everything from simple sensations and perceptions to the most complex abstract notions was a move aimed at undercutting the existing confusion, enabling him to reanalyse the nature of human understanding with a minimum of preconceived assumptions. On whether matter can think Locke's position is not entirely clear-cut. In Book II. 23. 23 *et seq.* he seems to dodge the issue by arguing, basically, that the question is as wrapped in obscurity as that of how objects can have the property of extension: 'These ideas, the one of the body, the other of our minds, every day's experience clearly furnishes us with: but if here we again enquire how this is done, we are equally in the dark' (II. 23. 28). In Book IV. 10. 10 *et seq.*, however, he argues that matter as such can no more think than move without external intervention. God supplies both motion and the power of thought. Nevertheless, this does not place him in the dualist camp since he does not accept 'Mind' as a separate substance – it is at least conceivable, he controversially suggests, that the power of thought has, rather, been infused *into* matter by God, just as motion has been. Since the overt aim of the *Essay* is identifying the limits of human understanding, to delimit the boundaries of the knowable, he can in effect call a halt to the debate on the grounds that this is precisely one of the issues falling on the 'unknowable' side of the fence. As to the *ontological* status of Ideas, this is simply a pointless question.

While Locke's famous *tabula rasa* image is easily read as signifying his wholesale commitment to a sensationalist empirical epistemology – all knowledge comes via the senses, all ideas are built up from 'ideas of sensation' – he nevertheless has to posit certain 'ideas of reflection' of an intuitive nature if the process of building up complex ideas is to get off the ground at all, and uses phrases like 'the common light of reason'. His position with regard to Reason is ultimately not too far from Descartes's – it is 'natural *revelation* whereby the eternal Father of light and Fountain of all knowledge, communicates to mankind that portion of truth which he has laid within reach of their natural faculties' (IV. 19. 4). Only in the next century is the attempt made, especially by Condillac and other French *philosophes* to carry the sensationalist analysis through to the 'ideas of reflection' also (see below, pp. 108–110). What is obvious, however, is that in Locke's *Essay* the central psychological issue has become 'understanding', epistemology, not salvation or the ontological status of the soul. We have also entered a relatively austere and abstract realm of technical discourse about 'ideas', 'modes', 'relations', 'substances' and 'sensations' (although elucidatory metaphors are sometimes drawn from contemporary Natural Philosophy). The authority of ancient learning has evaporated; gone are the hanging shoulder notes citing other authors – the four Books are entitled plainly 'Of Innate Notions', 'Of Ideas', 'Of Words' and 'Of Knowledge and Opinion'. Even the 'Passions' are nowhere in sight (though they were soon to return).

The 'Epistemization' of philosophical discourse over the course of the seventeenth century, while associated with the rise of Natural Philosophy, appears to have had a good measure of internal momentum of its own. In attempting to find theological formulations of the interrelationship between God, the soul and the material world capable of meeting changed standards of rational rigour and a totally transformed cosmological picture, philosophers and theologians found themselves embroiled in tortuous debates concerning the nature of ideas, the nature of knowledge, the nature of substance, and the soul's transactions with the senses. Apparently abstruse conceptual points became loaded with theological import, exacerbated by the doctrinal paranoia of the years from 1640 to the 1688 'Glorious Revolution'. Natural Philosophers themselves became drawn into the debate: as these proto-scientists struggled with the nature of matter, motion, mechanism and method, so theological and Natural Philosophical thought became increasingly co-ordinated. To have credibility, especially in Britain, any theological solution had to be consistent with those on offer in Natural Philosophy. Conversely, pious Natural Philosophers such as Boyle felt driven to find solutions supportive of doctrinal theological aims. As Margaret Jacob has shown, the Newtonian cosmology was seen by many Latitudinarian churchmen as meeting this need and formed the basis on which a new orthodoxy, a 'Rational Religion', was built[23]. But the epistemological debate as such had reached a level of technical complexity rendering theology extremely vulnerable to the attentions of an analytically adept, secularly minded radical such as Locke, politically motivated to restrict Religion's evidently calamitous role in civil affairs. Though intellectually allied, in part, with some of those engaged in formulating the new consensus, Locke's own position is clearly to the left of it. Following the 1688 Revolution, restored to England, newly acquainted with Newton (a secret Unitarian), and fairly sympathetic to the political aims of 'Rational Religion', Locke adopted a placatory tone in the face of the ecclesiastical attacks his *Essay* had elicited from such men as Bishop Stillingfleet, distancing himself from John Toland's 'deistic' *Christianity not Mysterious* (1696), and publishing his own *Reasonableness of Christianity* in 1695.

Locke's *Essay* is not Natural Philosophy, even though he clearly identifies with the Natural Philosophical project. It stands as a meta-text, providing a secular analysis of the process of gaining knowledge as such. But in devising a new account of the mind for philosophical purposes, was Locke doing anything directly ancestral to Psychology? Or, more broadly, is epistemological discourse necessarily also Psychological discourse? The answer must be 'no'. Locke's account is arrived at purely analytically, and although the end-product is a complex, rationally constructed, system it is not a 'scientific theory'. This much would probably be admitted by orthodox historians of Psychology, who would argue that Locke, although not 'scientific', shared modern Psychologists' concerns – the difference being only methodological. But as I have tried to indicate, this is not the case: Locke's aims, the rationale for his *Essay* and the factors which brought epistemology to the forefront of philosophical concern, have little in common with anything currently concerning Psychology. One may, though, concede that what a writer achieves may differ from what was intended. As founder of Associationism – which did at the end of its long career metamorphose into a genuinely Psychological theory – Locke cannot be denied his ancestral significance for the discipline. But that does not justify viewing the *Essay* itself as Psychology. His *Some Thoughts Concerning Education* (1693) bears a much closer resemblance to it, but is usually discussed only in histories of education.

III MECHANIZATION

1 The Orthodox Version

Until recently there was virtual unanimity among historians of science that the seventeenth century saw a 'mechanization of the world-view'[24]. There is similar unanimity among historians of Psychology that psychological thought participated in this trend[25]. It would be churlish to offer an outright denial of either proposition. Even so, recent historiography reveals some serious shortcomings in both. The problem, in a nutshell, is 'what did they mean by mechanism?' Conventionally this has been taken to mean Descartes's basic 'inertial impact' version, odd exceptions being viewed as regressive anomalies. In a dramatically reductionist move, Descartes proposed that the phenomena of the material world could all ultimately be accounted for by solid particles knocking into one another like snooker balls. Outcomes of such impacts are determined by the force of the impact and the shapes of the particles. The kinds of machine Descartes knew were things like clocks, hydraulic fountains, windmills, cranes and similar artefacts involving cog-wheels, pulleys, levers, and water-pressure. (This move had a covert significance, which I cannot explore here, in reversing the significance traditionally ascribed to machines; far from being seen as yielding insights into Nature, human made machines were essentially embodiments of cunning artifice, even deceit.) It is important to bear this in mind, since today the term actually means little except that a process is governed by physical laws. It retains a reductionist ring, but has little cash value as a genuine description. Only with Newton's acceptance of 'action at a distance' is it conceded that this concept underwent serious modification. The impression given is that Natural Philosophers proceeded to explore the potential of this simple mechanistic paradigm until Newton came up against gravity. The concept of mechanism is thus unproblematic. For Psychologists the significance of this lies in the elaborate 'physiological Psychologies' of Descartes and Hobbes, in which are identified the seeds of Behaviourism and the reflex concept. But how coherent was the concept of 'mechanism'?

2 The Varieties of Machinery

The essential merit of Descartes's concept of 'mechanism' has traditionally been seen to lie in the fact that with its advent 'occult' explanatory principles such as 'sympathy', 'congruity', 'powers' and the like were abandoned, these frequently amounting to no more than a technical sounding redescription of the phenomenon to be explained (Molière famously parodying this by explaining that morphine induced sleep because it had 'dormitive powers'). Henceforth, we learn, such principles rapidly disappeared from Natural Philosophy. Unfortunately for this version of events, historians of science have come to recognize that Descartes's concept of 'mechanism' was only one of several with which Natural Philosophers were juggling.

First, there was the controversy (with, as we saw, theological overtones) about whether matter was passive or active. Was motion necessarily supplied from outside (Descartes), or was it somehow inherent in matter (e.g. Hobbes and, later, Leibniz, as well as Hooke, in places at least)? Secondly, as Henry (1989) demonstrates in Hooke's case, the 'occult powers' identified by the Hermetic and Paracelsian magi of the sixteenth century were not abandoned, especially in relation to chemical phenomena, but reworked and refined. Experimentalists could adopt a much broader notion of 'mechanism', wherein readily demonstrable macro-phenomena (particularly sympathetic resonance, or magnetism) could be used as models for explaining invisible micro-phenomena. If this can occur in the visible world, the implicit argument goes, there is nothing unreasonable in supposing that something like it occurs in realms beyond sensible access. The fact that such macro-phenomena were themselves inexplicable in terms of Cartesian mechanics did not prevent them being seen as representing types of mechanism in their own right. As Schaffer (1987) demonstrates, by the 1670s the foci of Natural Philosophical enquiry in England (linked with experimental pneumatics) had become formulating the role of an 'aetherial' vitalistic spirit in animating the universe, and incorporating (while constraining within the terms of experimental Natural Philosophical practice) a theologically viable notion of spirit. In this debate the boundary between physical and spiritual virtually disappeared, as did that between 'particles' and 'fluids'. Whatever else they were doing, Newton, Boyle, Hooke, Mayow and their fellows were *not* simply elaborating on Cartesian, Gassendist or Hobbesist corpuscular mechanism. A *non-materialist* concept of 'mechanism' was the very aim of their endeavours. 'If a mechanical philosophy was to be possible, the minimum condition was the establishment of a proper place for spirit.'[26]

According to Henry (1989), the gulf between 'Natural Magic' and 'Natural Philosophy' is far from wide, and the hard-headed reaction against 'magic' is largely a myth; it is rather that the definition of 'magic' became retrospectively narrowed to cover only those things which Natural Philosophers did not adopt from the Natural Magic tradition – which were actually its peripheral rather than central features. Wilkins could entitle a book *Mathematical Magic* without qualms, while works such as Wecker's popular *18 Books of the Secrets of Art and Nature* (1660) mingled old-fashioned magic and new 'science' quite merrily[27]. The still controversial – and hugely documented – topic of the relationship between Science and the 'occult' traditions during the Scientific Revolution must however be left aside here[28].

A central implication of Cartesian mechanism was its commitment to a corpuscular or atomistic view of matter. This was reinforced by the testimony of the microscope, which revealed ever descending levels of corpuscularity[29]. Cartesian mechanism could be saved in one way by invoking covert atomic-level mechanisms to explain those macro-phenomena which appeared to involve action at a distance. But this path led only to speculative hypothesizing of a kind which experimentalists were loath to engage in and saw as a vain indulgence. (Descartes's own physical cosmology involving vortices of invisible particles, a notable failure, being a case in point.) And by the Restoration, the leading English Natural Philosophers had, as just mentioned, abandoned the corpuscular cosmology in its initial simple form. The lesson from this for us is that to talk of a 'mechanization of the world-view' conveys a misleading impression of uniformity, begging the question, very much at issue at the time, of what 'mechanism' actually meant. Fortunately, perhaps, for the subsequent development of the physical sciences, there was certainly no simple Cartesian consensus.

3 Mechanism and Psychology

What, though, of 'physiological Psychology'? We must differentiate between the Cartesian and Hobbesian versions. The most relevant Cartesian text is *The Passions of the Soul*, reluctantly published in 1649 and translated into English the following year. His more detailed *Treatise on Man (Traité de l'homme)* did not appear in an English translation during the seventeenth century, and by the time of its posthumous publication (1664) the Cartesian paradigm of mechanism was already obsolescent in English natural philosophy. Undoubtedly a classic physiological text – 'the first modern book entirely devoted to the subject' according to Singer (1928) – much of it was in the process of being rendered out of date by experimentalists (such as Borelli, Swammerdam and Stahl) and practising anatomists such as Willis, though his account of reflexes remained influential. It added little to his previous writings as far as psychological matters are concerned. I therefore feel justified in focusing on the earlier and more widely accessible work. Given the crucial place of this text in disciplinary histories we need to consider it at some length.

In a prefatory letter Descartes tells us: 'my design was not to lay open the Passions like an Oratour, nor yet a Morall Philosopher, but only as a Physician' (1650 B3). Yet it turns out to be an extremely heterogeneous work in which several aims are interwoven: (a) philosophical differentiation of mental phenomena properly belonging exclusively to the immaterial non-extended soul from those properly ascribable to the body: (b) elaborating a physiological account of the latter of these and their interaction with the former in the pineal gland or 'kernel' (as the 1650 translation had it); and (c) more traditional moral philosophizing in the latter part of Book Two and throughout Book Three on the functions and control of the individual 'passions'. At the outset we are confronted with the problem of what he means the term 'passions' to signify, for in places it seems far from being a simple synonym for what we now term 'emotions'; we read in Article XVII that '. . . we may usually term one's passions all those kinds of perception or forms of knowledge which are found in us . . .' (1967, p. 340); when they are enumerated later, however, 'passions' do become almost identical to modern 'emotions' ('emotions', when used, by contrast, seems only to denote 'movements'). Given, as noted above, that passions and emotions are actually quite distinct concepts anyway, the former denoting passivity and the latter motivation to action, the relationship between Descartes's concerns and those of contemporary students of 'emotion and motivation' is even more problematical.

It is worth remarking here that if we compare the standard 1911 Haldane and Ross (1967) translation to the 1650 one, with which contemporary English thinkers would have been acquainted, we are aware of a subtle shifting of tenor arising from the use of a less 'Psychological' vocabulary; Haldane and Ross's 'perceptions' are 'apprehensions', 'desires' are 'wills', 'feelings' are 'resentments', 'clear cognition' is 'evident knowledges' (Art. XXVIII), while 'regret' and 'shame' are 'grief' and 'dishonour' (Art. XLV). Somewhat puzzlingly, the 1650 version refers only to 'spirits' where Haldane and Ross have 'animal spirits', and their 'passion of apprehension' was, in 1650, plain 'fear' (Art. XXXVI). The crucial primary passion they called 'wonder' was 'admiration' in 1650. Not surprisingly, the cumulative effect of these, coupled with numerous other less salient vocabulary and syntactic differences, is to distance the 1650 text further from modern Psychological discourse than a reading of the later translation would suggest, even though such distancing is hard to quantify.

Understandably, psychologists of a Behaviourist bent perceive in the physiological passages of *Passions of the Soul* (and the account of the reflexes given in the *Traité de l'homme*) some ancestral anticipation of their own position. On closer examination, though, the similarities tend to fade. Descartes's entire orientation throughout the *Passions of the Soul*'s physiological passages is aprioristically to contrive or deduce the physiological mechanisms whereby everything, from blushing and swooning to memory (given a particularly incoherent treatment in Art. XLII), is brought about – or how the soul – dangling, as it were, in the pineal gland (even if also, in some fashion, all-pervasive) – may somehow be envisaged as being both affectable by and capable of affecting the behaviour of the all-powerful animal spirits.

Two points are to be noted about this: (a) there is no suggestion that the account is in any way deficient – Descartes has deduced it all purely logically from current physiological knowledge, with which he seems entirely happy. He does not admit areas of ignorance or obscurity, he never thinks that 'further research is needed'. His role-model, as we know from the first Meditation, was Aristotle – given enough peace and quiet, he believed, he could personally provide a complete account of the natural world to replace Aristotle's. So it is here – he is not offering a theory or tentative suggestions, he is telling the reader how things are, and have to be. Nor is there any suggestion that this knowledge may provide the basis for a psychophysiological technology. (b) The physiological explanation of psychological states (especially 'passions') is in itself nothing new, it was no more than the Hippocratic/Galenian orthodoxy to explain mood and character in terms of humours and animal spirits.

The originality of the *Passions* lies in Descartes's attempt to clarify the borderline between psychological phenomena dependent on the body and those properly and exclusively ascribable to the soul. His insistence on the soul's unity leads him to reject orthodox scholastic accounts in two respects. First, he rejects the idea of strife between the soul's higher (rational) and lower (sensuous) parts. This apparent strife is due to contrary movements of the pineal gland by the soul and the material animal spirits. Secondly, on the same grounds, he rejects the classification of the 'passions' into the 'concupiscent' (positive, e.g. desire) and 'irascible' (negative, e.g. aversion). Traditionally the classification of 'passions' had involved their derivation from these 'two appetites' of the soul. For Descartes the soul possesses only faculties, not parts, and while these faculties include desire and anger, there is no need to consider these two as more primary than its faculties for 'wondering, loving, hoping, fearing'. (It is unclear to me why this move should be seen as a 'progressive' or pioneering advance by modern masters of positive and negative reinforcement!) In a manner consistent with the soul's unity, he prefers to derive all passions ultimately from 'wonder' ('admiration' 1650): '. . . a sudden surprise of the soul which causes it to apply itself to consider with attention the objects which seem to it rare and extraordinary' (Art. LXX), a passion in which – uniquely, he believes – the body plays no part. Wonder, love, hatred, desire, joy and sadness comprise the 'six primitive passions'. Original though this is, at this distance it looks less like a revolutionary break from the traditional accounts than their technical rectification.

From the *Passions,* then we emerge believing that all apparently intrapsychic conflict is in fact misconstrued conflict between soul and body. Understanding this provides us, furthermore, with 'a general remedy against the Passions' (Art. CCXI) of a faintly Buddhist character: 'we should . . . recollect that all that presents itself before the imagination tends to delude the soul and causes the reasons which serve to urge it to accomplish the object of its passion to appear much stronger than they are, and those which serve to dissuade it to be much weaker. . . . [w]e ought to abstain from pronouncing any judgment on the spot, and to divert ourselves by other thoughts until time and rest have entirely calmed the emotion which is in the blood' (1967, p. 426). Wise counsel, perhaps (reflecting, no doubt, the common seventeenth-century respect for the Stoics, which Descartes shared), but hardly pioneering psychotherapy – let alone behaviour modification.

In seventeenth-century terms *The Passions of the Soul* is not entirely distinct in character from other works in what was a well-established genre, mostly bearing somewhat similar titles[30]. While cutting the cake in somewhat different fashion and couched in terms of Descartes's distinctive metaphysical system, it is not evident why its novelties mark it out as peculiarly proto-Psychological. His aim was the very opposite, incorporating 'mind' (up to a point) into 'mechanical science'. As for the 'great impetus' he is alleged to have provided for proto-physiological Psychology, the principal figure via whom such impetus would have been transmitted in Britain, Willis (see Section VII), was not a Cartesian at all, while his continental successors such as Stahl and, later, Haller were to depart significantly from him on central doctrines about the soul–body relationship. Descartes does not belong at all obviously in the seventeenth-century tradition of physiological *research* (as opposed to theorizing), which often (e.g. in Stahl and Willis) remained far from clearly demarcated from the Paracelsian and Hermetic traditions, and had a different concept of mechanism. Descartes was not an 'iatrochemist' of any description. What we are left with is a distant exercise in speculative psychophysiological reductionism undertaken for ends which are ultimately theological and moral.

Hobbes's physiological account differs from Descartes's most patently in extending it to those phenomena Descartes had reserved for the soul. What is remarkable, given the huge significance ascribed to Hobbes's role in the 'mechanization of the mind', is how minimal is the textual basis for this. Except for about eight pages in the *Elements of Philosophy* there is virtually no hard physiology in the entire ten volumes of his writings. What we do find, in *Leviathan*, *Human Nature* and *Elements of Philosophy*, are a number of passages (somewhat repetitive) in which the mechanistic case is argued in more or less *a priori* terms, or deduced in a schematic fashion. As well as the more familiar openning account in *Leviathan* in which Imagination, Memory, etc., are accounted for in terms of inertial inward continuation of motion (with no physiological detail), the following from *Human Nature* is typical:

> . . . conceptions and apparitions are nothing really, but motion in some internal substance of the head; which motion not stopping there but proceeding to the heart, of necessity must then either help or hinder the motion which is called Vital; when it helpeth it is called delight, contentment, or pleasure, which is nothing really but motion about the heart, as conception is nothing but motion in the head: . . . when such motion weakeneth or hindereth the vital motion, then it is called pain.
> (Molesworth edition of English works [EW] IV, p. 31)

As is this, from *Elements of Philosophy*, Part IV, Chapter xxv:

> . . . when that endeavour inwards is the last action in the act of sense, then from the reaction, how little soever the duration it be, a phantasm or idea hath its being; which, by reason that the endeavour is now outwards, doth always appear as something situate without the organ. (EW I, p. 391)

The thrust of Hobbes's 'mechanistic Psychology' is only that such an account is logically sustainable and plausible, with no genuinely extended physiological explanations of how the mechanism is embodied in flesh and sinew (his account of perception being the sole exception). As stressed above, his top priority was political; basic psychological matters are of interest because 'the principles of politics consist in the knowledge of the motions of the mind, and the knowledge of these motions from the knowledge of sense and imagination' (*ibid.*, p. 74). But nowhere does Hobbes demonstrate such 'knowledge'; all he demonstrates is what it would look like if he did have it. In Section V we will look at Hobbes's 'Psychology' from a different perspective, for the present it seems to me that his acclaimed role as pioneer mental mechanist, herald of Behaviourism and harbinger of the reflex, is grossly overplayed. In spite of such reductionist phrases as 'conceptions and apparitions are nothing really, but motion' he nowhere envisages a truly reductionist translation of our psychological language into one restricted to references to such motions, comparable to the modern Behaviourists's vocabulary of conditioning, reinforcement, and 'fractional anticipatory goal-responses'.

Finally, we return to Locke. Is the *Essay* mechanistic? Though he was trained as a physician, Locke spends little time on physiology, but the work does have a mechanistic 'feel' to it, deriving primarily from the atomistic character of his analysis. Conscious phenomena are analysable into simple quasi-corpuscular ideas of sensation, which are then 'combined' in various ways to form complex ideas of sensation, juxtaposed to yield ideas of relation, and otherwise manipulated to create general and abstract ideas, and ideas of reflection. If this is 'mechanistic' in addition to being atomistic (which it certainly is), it is so in an oddly rudimentary way – more like building a wall. But the essence of machines, however mechanism is conceived, is surely motion, and of this there is very little in the *Essay*, at least in explaining the fortunes of 'ideas'. (Locke does, of course, discuss the *idea* of motion.) The more closely one examines the *Essay*, the more elusive its mechanistic character becomes; Locke rarely deploys mechanistic concepts or images in an explanatory role, and his vocabulary is primarily analytic (modes, relations, qualities, forms, etc.). Since the *Essay* obviously does not descend from the *physiological* speculations of

Hobbes and Descartes, it is difficult to see how its traditional role as the culmination of a grand process of 'mechanizing the psychological' can be rigorously sustained. Perhaps mechanism and atomism have been conflated by previous students of the topic, and rational analysis has been equated to science. The fact that Locke is writing in an intellectual climate dominated by Natural Philosophy and identifies with its aims does not of itself make him a Natural Philosopher of the mind. As we will see in Section VI, the 'mechanization of the mind' took a somewhat different route.

IV FROM FAITH TO REASON[31]

We saw in Section II that theological and religious considerations pervaded the philosophical debates leading to the 'epistemization' of psychological discourse. To understand why this was so, we need to look a little more closely at the factors impelling Protestant religious thought along a trajectory from faith to reason. This section may appear to be a digression since it does not deal with psychological texts, but I believe it is essential for a grasp of the broader psychological context in which the texts we have been discussing were produced. (And since the issue it deals with is a case of psychological change, it falls within Psychology's orbit of professional interest.)

Lutheran and, even more, Calvinist theology placed personal conversion and experience of Divine Grace at the heart of Christianity. According to predestinarian Calvinist doctrine, God had already chosen those who were to be saved, hence the central question for a believer was assurance of one's place among these Elect. This could be guaranteed only by personal knowledge of Christ in a conversion experience. Good works alone did not suffice (although they were perhaps a necessary condition). For 'Covenanters' this was the moment when a covenant was made with God: a personal quasi-legal agreement, as it were, to obey God's laws and commands in return for salvation. Achievement of Grace might involve many years of preparation by devout Bible study and prayer before the spiritual pilgrim's faith was rewarded. Grace was available to all equally, regardless of social status and learning. At the heart of Protestant – and especially puritan – faith there thus lay an essentially irrational core in the form of a profound and ineffable psychological event – conversion. This event transformed the believer's perceptions of both self and world; the self becoming a vehicle for implementing God's will and the world infused with Divine meaning. Fervency and 'enthusiasm' could easily ensue.

By the end of the sixteenth century the established Church's Puritan wing was faced with the extremist and irrationalist fervour of radical sects outside it who had taken the doctrine of personal knowledge of election to its logical conclusion and rejected all forms of institutional religious authority. At the same time they were striving for internal reform of the Anglican Church to improve the spiritual quality of the clergy, and for involvement with Church policy and formulation of doctrine.

One can readily appreciate therefore the tension developing between irrational faith and reason. Negatively, reason alone – however learned and clever – could not achieve salvation. Without commitment to the central spiritual quest in which life's meaning ultimately resided, without acceptance of the fundamentally arbitrary and irrational experience of personal election, a person was damned. Learning could even seduce people into amassing a worldly knowledge valueless unless illumined by the Divine light vouchsafed to the true believer. Reason had its place in managing worldly affairs, but it was irrelevant to the fate of the soul. On the positive side, 'regenerated Reason', reason transmuted by Divine illumination, was of spiritual value, enabling inspired exegesis of the biblical Word and its effective propagation, as well as helping the devout man (and they do all seem to have been men) of learning to out-argue doctrinal opponents such as Jesuits. Reason was thus firmly subordinated to faith, its arena of action strictly delimited.

Eminent Puritans, having to survive in the more ruthless higher echelons of ecclesiastical and political power-broking, needed all the 'Reason' they could muster. John Morgan (1986) has provided a highly documented account of the ambivalence of 'Puritan Attitudes towards Reason, Learning, and Education' (as his subtitle has it)[32]. Simultaneously striving for a better-educated and university-trained clergy, yet capable of ferociously anti-intellectual outbursts, mainstream puritan divines prior to 1640 had to tack furiously between emphasizing faith or reason – confronted by fanatical Brownists or rapturous Ranters, they spoke for reason; confronted by Laudian doctrinal autocracy, they spoke for faith.

But when the chips were down, as at the outbreak of the Civil War, faith necessarily took priority. (So we can see why Descartes's *Meditations* evoked such opposition, for here was a man who did indeed claim that reason could, unaided, confirm faith and knowledge of God.)

With the Civil War, 'irrationalist' forces could flourish unchecked. Gripped by the twin convictions that the Last Days of scriptural prophecy were unfolding and that they were the Saints therein referred to, the radical sects fused religious fanaticism with an utopian social vision. The varieties and fates of these Ranters, Levellers, Diggers, Muggletonians, Fifth Monarchy Men and Quakers have been lovingly chronicled and analysed in numerous works by Christopher Hill, rendering unnecessary any further account of them here[33]. But a belief that the final phase of the Christian historical plot was unravelling, that Antichrist was abroad and Armageddon impending, was not the monopoly of the radicals. From Milton downwards, few appear to have remained totally immune (except, probably, Hobbes). The quashing of the radicals, the factional dissent of the last days of the Commonwealth and the final indignity of the Restoration in 1660 dealt a fatal blow to the spiritual self-confidence of the erstwhile Saints. Blind personal faith had had its chance and been found wanting. How, then, could a Christian orthodoxy re-establish itself? For those royalist High Church bishops who had suffered most during the interregnum, the answer was a return to dogmatic formulation of doctrine from the top. This, not surprisingly, was unacceptable to those, now disenchanted and disillusioned, who had shared and understood the radical spiritual aspirations of the 1640s and retained an inner loyalty to them. But they understood too that the intellectual climate had changed on a Europe-wide scale. The answer that now appeared inescapable was a truly Rational Religion, congruent with the new 'scientific' cosmology, discouraging 'enthusiasm' and providing a rationale for social order. For the remaining saints the quest for Glory was transformed into a personal 'Pilgrim's Progress' – there was to be no participation in the collective inversion of the order of the world, only solitary negotiation of its pitfalls and temptations.

One area of psychological importance which felt the impact of this shift was the construal of madness. Michael MacDonald (1981) has argued that the post-Restoration rise to dominance of medical models of madness was primarily due to the hostility of the new religious and political establishment towards all forms of religious enthusiasm. Earlier eclectic approaches (such as those of MacDonald's subject, Richard Napier) had incorporated and integrated spiritual- and physical-level explanations. Reports by victims of madness that Satan had appeared to them, that they were assailed by demons, or that their good angel had been vanquished were not rejected out of hand and served at least to render their experiences meaningful (both to themselves and to those around them) in a broader religious cosmological context. By the end of the century such reports were coming to be seen as insane delusions in themselves. Madness was now physical in nature and probably rooted in immorality. Far from leading directly to any therapeutic improvements, the abandonment of often efficacious – albeit irrational or quasi-magical – earlier treatments left the mad at the mercy of almost universally inefficacious physical treatments. Prayerful fasting, astrological amulets and witchcraft-deterrency rituals disappeared from official view, to be replaced by whippings, scarification and incarceration.

A Rational Religion was, as mentioned above, eventually formulated in the 1690s by Latitudinarian divines influenced by Newton and Boyle, and promoted thereafter in the influential 'Boyle Lectures'. It extended the notion of divinely ordained Natural Laws to the civil realm; there was a natural social order to which Christians must conform. If this order was overthrown, not only the human but the natural realm too was endangered, for both formed part of the Great Architect's harmonious design. (Margaret Jacob [1976] has the fullest account of this, although the role she ascribes to Newton himself is disputed.)

The ensuing Age of Reason did not, therefore, arise exclusively from the successes of the Natural Philosophers or from John Locke, there was a much deeper psychological shift in orientation (of which Natural Philosophy and Locke's *Essay* were themselves overt expressions) towards the rational and away from the passionate and irrational. Perhaps the religious tension between faith and reason was in turn but one form in which an even deeper and more general psychological tension, rooted in a combination of socioeconomic and cosmological upheaval, expressed itself (see, for example, Barbu's rather sweeping psychohistorical account[34]). The religious level is nevertheless the form in which it is most easily accessible.

How far can the above analysis be extended beyond Britain? After all, the epistemization of philosophical discourse was surely a Europe-wide phenomenon? By contrast with Britain the tendency of French philosophy during the mid seventeenth century was (a) towards an intensification of concern with the nature of faith, and defence of Catholic orthodoxy (e.g. Pascal and Malebranche) and (b) towards a more Aristotelian interest in pure logic as a formal discipline in the work of the Port Royal logicians. Overt religious controversy within France, heart of the Counter-Reformation, remained primarily an inter-Catholic affair, with dissenting Protestant voices audible only from the Low Countries to the north. The hegemony of the Catholic Church culminated in the revocation of the Edict of Nantes in 1685, and the subsequent exodus of Protestant Huguenots to Holland and Britain. Francophone religious and philosophical radicals such as the encyclopaedist Bayle operated for the most part as exiles, Holland becoming the main publishing centre for Protestant writings.

Even so, materialist Natural Philosophy flourished under the aegis of the newly established Acadèmie de Sciences (founded 1666) and, unlike in Britain, with a fairly doctrinaire commitment to Cartesian mechanism. It is not, though, until after Pierre Coste's 1700 translation of Locke (published in Amsterdam) that the change in philosophical orientation wrought by English writers is re-exported to the Continent (where Hobbes and Locke had both lived while writing their most important works). This is not to say that French philosophy after Descartes had no role in the epistemization of philosophical discourse – far from it, both Malebranche and Gassendi were instrumental in developing the terms of philosophical discussion (Norton, 1981). It is, rather, that the complex English climate provided the cultural context in which the final moves could be made.

The two other major philosophical figures of this period, Leibniz and Spinoza, will be discussed separately below. Both are very much thinkers *sui generis*, and their full intellectual influence was long delayed. In Leibniz particularly the new concern with epistemology is very apparent, but his philosophical and scientific work in general was stimulated primarily via his international contacts with English and French intellectuals (such as Samuel Clarke and the Jansenist Port Royal theologian Antoine Arnauld) rather than by anything going on in the court of Hanover. But few philosophical systems could be more different from Locke's than those of Spinoza and Leibniz, and it was the Lockean one which, in the event, was to call the tune for the next half-century.

In brief, however multinational the input into the debates, the actual emancipation of philosophy from theological concerns and the most systematic replacement of faith in faith by faith in reason occurred in Britain, or at any rate in the works of English writers writing in English.

But in all this turmoil there was another, subtler development occurring in which we may perhaps detect the historical beginnings of the creation of Psychology's autonomous, self-conscious, self-contained individual subject. To this we turn next.

V. THE INVENTION OF PRIVACY[35]

The polarity between public and private has become so natural to us that it takes us aback a little to remember that it had specific cultural and historical origins. We take it for granted that each of us requires (even if they do not always enjoy) a private personal space. But privacy is not only, or even primarily, physical; it arises, as Morse (1989) says, as 'a new mode of consciousness' (p. 256) during the Renaissance. At first it is those, like Thomas More, whose eminent public lives required constant pragmatic dissembling, compromise and tongue-biting who experience the need for a compensatory space insulated from public inspection and secure from unwelcome intrusion in which they can be honest, both to those around them and to themselves. An alternative, private realm is constructed where the individual can exercise intellectual and creative freedom, can observe and criticize the public world, can introspect and explore their own thoughts and feelings. Morse, noting the French essayist Montaigne as a classic early example, describes his library (located in a tower) as 'a theatre of self-exploration where he can mull over what he has read in his books and capture his thoughts even at the very moment when they come to him, often in a quasi-divine frenzy of inspiration' (pp. 258–9).

From now on we can detect the presence in European – and especially British – culture of a series of 'counter-texts' originating in the private libraries, rectories and gardens of scholars, divines, physicians, housebound women, and independent gentlemen whose public lives are of no great moment in contemporary public affairs. These texts are not moves in public controversies, nor are they always intended for pedagogic edification or career advancement. Some were published only posthumously. Morse focuses on three writers, John Donne, Robert Burton and Thomas Browne, as representative of this essentially heterogeneous genre. Of these Burton is of most interest here, since his *Anatomy of Melancholy* is frequently cited as a proto-Psychological text. This is both more and less than the truth. Burton, an unmarried, impoverished Cambridge scholar whose clerical career had been thwarted (he finally got a living in the 1630s) was already in his forties when the first edition appeared in 1621. This first edition concentrated in the main on the ostensible subject of its title, Melancholy, surveying it with unprecedented thoroughness, but already spilling over into misanthropic criticisms of human society. By the final, sixth, edition it had broken these bounds completely, comprising (in the Shilleto edition) over thirteen hundred pages of unrelenting diatribe, lament, humour, consolation, advice, sarcasm, irony and expostulation regarding the human condition, performed with an unrelenting display of encyclopaedic learning. The scaffolding for this is what at first glance appears to be a highly detailed analysis, based on the method of the French logician Ramus, in which the contents are classified according to successively minor subdivisions of major themes. Thus Symptoms are classified as General or Simple, General Symptoms as of Body or Minde, the latter as Common or Particular etc. As Renaker (1971) shows, however, the work totally subverts the clarity and order which this method aimed to achieve; instead, it enables Burton to digress and ramble as he pleases.

Burton's relationship to his reader is totally ambivalent – on the one hand he claims: 'I look for no favour at thy hands, I am independant, I fear not.' Then he immediately recants; 'No, I recant . . . I care, I fear, I confess my fault, acknowledge a great offence . . .' (p. 140); 'I earnestly request every private man, as *Scaliger* did *Cardan*, not to take offence' (p. 141). He writes behind the persona of Democritus Junior, identifying with the Greek philosopher Democritus, famed for his amused contempt for the follies of human life, but in the event his temper in the work ranges across a wide spectrum of moods and attitudes. Melancholy becomes a peg on which to hang ruminations about everything from love philtres and clothes to demonic possession and the quality of the air, from the futility of warfare to phlebotomy and basil. At one point he unleashes a page-long list of 102 misogynist epithets on the foul features of women (Vol. 3, pp. 178–9) which it is hard to forgive. Eventually of course it made Burton a celebrity, 'Yet' – to quote Morse again – 'the strangest osmosis of all is that *The Anatomy of Melancholy*, a book that takes all the world and all human history for its province, is somehow transformed into a celebration of private man – of Democritus Junior in his study' (p. 306). Or, as an anonymous *Times Literary Supplement* writer somewhat overkindly put it: 'There in the centre of the labyrinth he is to be found, wise, tender, romantic, sensitive and charitable, hopelessly at odds with a world of which he was afraid' (28 April 1921, p. 266)[36]. And the epigraph to this chapter surely in some ways marks the beginning of whatever we mean by 'modern consciousness'. If *The Anatomy of Melancholy* is Psychology, so is *Finnegans Wake*.

Browne's *Religio Medici*, by contrast, comes across on first reading as a smug, self-satisfied, patronizing and even intellectually cowardly work, while his vast *Pseudodoxia Epidemica* ('Vulgar Errors') presents us with a compendium of miscellaneous learning and speculation comparable to Burton's. His works too, though, are a celebration of the autonomous private mind wryly detached from the turmoils of the age, quietly content with a fairly undogmatic private faith and sceptical of popular opinions[37].

Another genre testifying to the growth of the private is the diary, first adopted by Puritans to record their day-to-day religious travails (though not all were written without at least one eye on publication). The diary provides a portable private refuge in which the individual can reassert authenticity, monitor their feelings, confess their true responses and public dishonesties. John Evelyn is one famous case, but it was Samuel Pepys, of course, who took the final step of actually writing in a private code. Other English 'private persons' of the period would include the poet Thomas Traherne, much of whose work remained in manuscript until the present century, and perhaps the strange Margaret Cavendish, Duchess of Newcastle, whose massive and largely forgotten folios present an extraordinary miscellany of poems, stories, philosophy and scientific speculation in dire need of scholarly attention[38].

This rise of privacy, linked to Protestant belief in a personal relationship with God, constitutes an important, if neglected, facet of seventeenth-century psychological change. It is not exclusively Protestant, even so – in France, for example, the trend continues from Montaigne to the very different religious introspectiveness of Blaise Pascal's *Pensées*. It constitutes the culturally visible beginning of the idea that the individuated ego or personality is the carrier of the authentic self. And this move counterpoints the growing importance of the public person, the public figure whose position rests on their individual efforts and character rather than inherited status or facility at traditional role-playing. There is also a sense in which the notion that the *real* person was the private person reverses a traditional view that one is most 'real' when performing in public – testifying from the pulpit or in court, or from the parliamentary benches, or even in the alehouse. It would be absurd to picture Cromwell seeking, like a modern US Presidential candidate, to enhance his appeal by introducing Mrs Cromwell, little Richard, and the family beagle to the platform and issuing information about his favourite puddings. Such behaviour would have met with uncomprehending derision. Today the *sine qua non* of public credibility is belief in private authenticity; in the seventeenth century it was, rather, the opposite – achievement of public authenticity still rendered the private largely irrelevant.

Behind these changes lie demographic and social factors, particularly those relating to the character of the family, and Morse's observations on the rise of privacy must be understood in the light of Lawrence Stone's monumental analysis of such factors which carries the story through to the end of the following century (Stone, 1977). Finally, the rise of privacy being addressed here must be differentiated from a debate going back to classical times between the respective merits of the active life [*vis activa*] and the contemplative life [*vis contemplativa*], although the reactivation of this debate in some quarters was perhaps not unconnected with it; the exchange between Sir George Mackenzie (1665) and John Evelyn (1667) on the issue does not, however, suggest that the terms of the argument had changed significantly (Vickers, 1985).

The significance of privacy for Psychology is that its invention was a necessary step on the road to creating the 'psychological subject' as an object of enquiry. Only when the existence of a private psychological realm as the locus of personal authenticity and 'being' has become culturally accepted can the events, processes and phenomena of this realm be conceived of as natural objects of scientific scrutiny. The seventeenth century contains the beginnings of this, although it did not come to fruition until the end of the following century at the earliest – a century we may note which saw English gentlemen eternally prey to Burtonian Melancholy, the Black Dog, exorcized by then of its metaphysical profundity.

Again, then, the role of a classic 'Psychological' text, in this case Burton's *Anatomy of Melancholy*, emerges from current historical scholarship as lying in the 'subject matter' rather than 'discipline' sense. It was not a book *about* Psychology, it was the expression of a particular psychological condition. Of course it has a historical place in the 'discipline' sense too in so far as we can cull from it much information about contemporary views on the causes and treatment of 'Melancholy' (virtually everything as it turns out!), but this is to ignore the nature of the text as a whole – as an often bitter affirmation of the power and primacy of the private[39].

VI. THE LANGUAGE PROBLEM

1 A Strange Absence of Innovation

In this section I am concerned with an issue which I briefly considered in *On Psychological Language*. If Psychological Language (PL) is physiomorphic in character, we would predict – and the prediction is generally borne out – that innovations in the language used for referring to the external world will be fairly quickly incorporated into it. In the seventeenth century we appear to find, on the contrary, that the PL used by, say, Locke at the end is a considerably depleted one in comparison with that used by, for example, Burton (not to mention Shakespeare and Donne) in its earlier decades. Furthermore there is little evidence of any large scale incorporation into PL of the language used by Natural Philosophers in labelling and discussing their discoveries. In part this failure may simply be an aspect of a shift from synthetic to analytic styles of discourse, widely recognized as occurring around mid century (the various versions of Glanville's *Vanity of Dogmatizing* have been seen as tracking this change). Although this is true, on closer scrutiny the more immediate explanation appears to lie in the attitude towards language of Hobbes, John Wilkins and the early

Fellows of the Royal Society – an attitude which, in Britain, largely brought about the shift from synthetic to analytic usage (although the same shift occurred throughout Europe and was a much more deeply rooted phenomenon than we can examine here – see Reiss [1982] for a wrestle with what appears to be more or less the same issue). My argument is that their understanding of the nature of language and the recommendations for linguistic reform which stemmed from it were incompatible with PL innovation of the usual kind. I further argue that the physiomorphic process outflanked this damming, primarily via changes in the terms in which physiological phenomena were construed, but also at a rather different 'meta' level by using the social role of Natural Philosopher as such, as a model for the nature of mind, a model facilitating the 'epistemization' process discussed earlier.

2 The Quest for Linguistic Perfection (i): Hobbes

Hobbes, once again, proves to be a crucial figure. As mentioned, for Hobbes the supreme human faculty of reason derived from – was even identical with – language. His account of language is provided in Chapters IV–VI of Leviathan[40]. Language is first of all an act of naming, if it is to be used successfully, there must thus be agreement on the definitions of words: '. . . in the right definition of names lies the first use of speech; which is the acquisition of science: and in wrong, or no definitions, lies the first abuse; from which proceed all false and senseless tenets' (ch. IV). He cites geometry: 'And therefore in geometry, which is the only science that it hath pleased God hitherto to bestow on mankind, men begin at settling the significations of their words; which settling of significations they call "definitions," and place them at the beginning of their reckoning' (ch. IV). It is at this level that many errors enter: 'By this it appears how necessary it is for any man that aspires to true knowledge, to examine the definitions of former authors . . . For the errors of definitions multiply themselves according as the reckoning proceeds, and lead men into absurdities . . .' (*ibid.*). All reasoning is a form of 'reckoning' in the mathematical sense: 'For "reason," in this sense, [i.e. as a 'faculty of the mind'] is nothing but "reckoning," that is adding or subtracting, of the consequences of general names agreed upon for the "marking" and "signifying" of our thoughts; I say "marking" them when we reckon by ourselves, and "signifying," when we demonstrate or approve our reckonings to other men.' (ch. V).

There are four categories of 'general name' by means of which things may 'enter into account': (a) pertaining to body or matter; (b) 'accidents' or qualities of matter; (c) 'properties of our own bodies' ('as when anything is seen by us, we reckon not the thing itself, but the sight, the colour, the idea of it in the fancy . . . and such are names of fancies' – by this, I understand, he is trying to include sensation terms in a materialist framework, but this kind of obscurity is very much the point at issue); (d) names given to "names" themselves (e.g. ' "narration," "syllogism," "sermon," "oration" '). Two kinds of error can arise at this point: new terms the meaning of which is not explained by definition, and contradictory and inconsistent 'significations' such as (digging at Descartes) '"incorporeal body"' which is as meaningless as '"round quadrangle"'. A further list of eight errors follows in Chapter V, of which two (the second and seventh) need to concern us here: '. . . giving of names of "bodies" to "accidents;" or of "accidents" to "bodies;" as they do that say, "faith is infused," or "inspired;" when nothing can be "poured" or "breathed" into anything, but body'; and secondly: '. . . the use of metaphors, tropes, and other rhetorical figures, instead of words proper'.

Errors in reasoning are thus essentially linguistic in origin, stemming from failure to adhere rigorously to the canons of unambiguous definition and the confusion of 'names' which belong to different categories ('category mistakes' in modern philosophical parlance). Among these are the muddling of 'bodies' and 'accidents', and figurative language in general. The message in all this is that if reason and science are to succeed in acquiring 'true knowledge' they must, so to speak, clean up their linguistic acts – they must avoid, among other things, all flowery figurative language and maintain a clear distinction between names of 'bodies' themselves and names of their 'accidents' (i.e. qualities or properties): 'To conclude, the light of human minds is perspicuous words, but by exact definitions first snuffed, and purged from ambiguity; "reason" is the "pace;" increase of "science," the "way;" and benefit of mankind, the "end." ' (ch. V).

By adopting this stance Hobbes can, I must stress, evade a central difficulty of the kind of philosophical analysis of 'human nature' in which he, Descartes and other philosophers were engaged –

i.e. the ontological status of the referents of reflexive discourse. Since all is ultimately a question of matter in motion, the terms of such discourse are references to 'properties of our bodies'. He is thus able, in Chapter VI, to make a trouble-free transition from discussing 'vital' and 'voluntary' motions, via 'appetites' to a survey of the 'passions' and the 'Speeches by which they are expressed'. Yet, while affirming that it *is* physical, he never genuinely *reduces* the psychological to the physical, nor does the problem of 'consciousness' even raise its head (the modern sense of the term not being in his repertoire, as we saw above). 'For Hobbes, reason is nothing other than computation with words, and human consciousness is nothing other than the accompaniment or substitution of imagery by language' (Ross, 1988, p. 228).

The implication of the Hobbesian programme of linguistic reform for PL generation is clear – since PL generation can occur only by means of what to Hobbes and his contemporaries would look like 'metaphors' and 'tropes', it is implicitly ruled out. Paradoxically, though, Hobbes's refusal to acknowledge a distinction between physical and psychological was precisely what enabled him to translate the emerging Natural Philosophical cosmology of Galileo and Descartes into psychological and social terms. Michel Verdon (1982), for example, sees in the famous 'state of nature' (starting point for Hobbes's political philosophy, in which life is 'nasty, brutish and short') a direct emulation of Galileo's thought-experiment of motion in a vacuum: 'Hobbes similarly imagined the motion (behavior) of individuals in a *social* vacuum (the "state of nature" . . .) to discover the first laws of *human* nature' (p. 657). The apparently neutral term '*conatus*' or 'endeavour' (defined in geometrical rather than simple physical terms as 'motion made through length of a point, and in an instant or point of time') enables him to assimilate 'will' to physical motion, as noted previously[41]. From the present theoretical perspective, Verdon's systematic mapping of the parallels between Hobbes's moral and political philosophy and the Galilean/Cartesian physical cosmology looks very much as one would expect physiomorphic assimilation of novel world concepts into psychological terms to look. In fact it would be hard to find a clearer example. Having done it, however, Hobbes bolts the door behind him, rejecting the very features of language which enabled him to do it as poisoned wellsprings of error, henceforth to be assiduously avoided.

This view of language as a bewitching source of confusion for the seeker after knowledge was not exclusive to Hobbes. Descartes, Mersenne, Hartlib and the educationist Comenius were all mooting the possibility of an improved and universal 'philosophical language' designed to encode the truth clearly and unambiguously. And they, like Hobbes, saw the incorrigible ambiguity of normal language as the source of the problem. Surely a language could be devised in which the words possessed only one clearly defined meaning, a language in which words and their referents could be matched up in a one-to-one fashion? This would ensure clear thinking on the one side and a direct conversion of thoughts into unambiguous words on the other. Mutual misunderstanding would become impossible. The Royal Society was also aware of the need for 'a close, naked, natural way of speaking' without 'amplifications, digressions, and swellings of style', as Thomas Sprat put it. Among those closely connected with the Royal Society – indeed he was a founding member – was John Wilkins, to whose realization of this dream of linguistic perfection we now turn.

3 The Quest for Linguistic Perfection (ii): Wilkins

Wilkins first tackled the issue in his *Mercury* (1641), a text dominated by his fascination with cryptography, and over the next two decades he continued to explore the topic in collaboration with George Dalgarno, an Oxford schoolmaster who had independantly begun a similar project. Others in the Oxford circle, such as Seth Ward, William Petty, Cyprian Kinner and John Wallis (and even Archbishop Ussher), also became enthusiastic. In 1654 Ward published *Vindiciae academiarum*, in which the scope of the project was expanded:

> Ward's concern is no longer simply with a set of common symbols for simultaneous translation of conventional verbal usages in existing languages, but with the creation of a whole new language, each of whose words would refer to a single, scientifically observed phenomenon or philosophically constructed concept, without the penumbra of vagueness and imprecision introduced into conventional languages by varying usages and faulty observation. (Shapiro, 1969, p. 209)

In 1657 Cave Beck also tackled the task in his *Universal Character by which all Nations may Understand One Anothers Conceptions* (curiously, Thomas Urquhart, the hyper-loquacious translator of Rabelais, also mooted a universal language). Wilkins and Dalgarno continued to work at a more comprehensive, version, Dalgarno publishing *Ars Signorum* in 1661. This still fell short of Wilkins's ambitions, his own scheme finally appearing in 1668 (the first manuscript having been lost in the Fire of London of 1666) as *An Essay Towards a Real Character and a Philosophical Language*, issued with the Royal Society imprimatur. This is among the most curious products of England's 'scientific revolution'.

The first feature of Wilkins's invention to be noted is the primacy of the *written* script, or 'character'. Although he proceeded to assign phonetic values to his symbols, it is the symbol system itself which is fundamental; language has been transformed from a matter of speech to a matter of written signs. Now, given that these signs are intended as univalent, corresponding directly to their referents, this amounts to a belief that the world can be converted into a universal text. The author in a sense disappears behind a purely 'objective' symbolic representation of the matters to which he or she is referring. As Tony Davies (1987) observes, Wilkins wanted 'to abolish language altogether', replacing it with a character that, in his own words, would 'not signifie *words* but *things* and *notions*', thereby 'inverting the traditional relationship between speech and writing' (pp. 86–87). Behind this scheme lies the vital assumption that 'all men's minds operated in the same way and had a similar "apprehension of things"' (Shapiro, 1969, p. 214). This assumption in turn, as far as language is concerned, rested on unswerving acceptance of the doctrine of an original, universally understood, God-given, Adamic language, destroyed when God inflicted a confusion of tongues upon us as punishment for the Tower of Babel. Indeed, as Aarsleff (1976) observes, there is a covert link with the mystical doctrine of a Divine Adamic language proposed by figures like Jacob Boehme, who in all other respects are polar opposites to the devotees of reason.

The second central feature of the system is that in order to construct such a 'character' Wilkins had to classify all the phenomena of the universe, along with all abstract concepts, which he undertook adopting the Aristotelian distinction between genera and subspecies. This was not without a direct scientific pay-off, particularly in biology and zoology, in initiating the systematic classification of life-forms which, via John Ray (with whom Wilkins worked), was perfected by Linnaeus. Nothing was excluded. The universe had been comprehensively and rigorously catalogued, classified and encoded. This was no solitary exercise; Wilkins had the assistance of at least Pepys (an interesting link in view of Pepys's own invention of a new 'character' for his diary), Ray, Willoughby and the Duke of Buckingham. The scientific community was almost universal in its endorsement of the project's aims – even Newton and Locke took it seriously. Wilkins and his friend John Wallis actually used the character in correspondence. Following Wilkins's death in 1672 numerous figures continued to work on its development. The *Essay Towards a Real Character and a Philosophical Language* was not, therefore, an eccentric product of one man's obsession but a crucial articulation of the Natural Philosophers' view of language which elicited minimal dissent from his intellectual colleagues and associates. Aarsleff sees in it 'the chief source of Royal Society doctrines about language and style' (1976, p. 362). Including *en route* an engraving of Noah's Ark and an explanation of how all the animals fitted into it, plus translations into the *Real Character* of the Lord's Prayer and Creed, it was also infused with piety, as befitted a future Bishop of Chester. Wilkins's motivation was as much religious as scientific, for he, like many contemporaries, saw in the 'universal character' a route towards ending the deadly religious and doctrinal disputes which were racking European culture, and creating a Rational Religion.

4 Implications for Psychological Language

In Wittgensteinian retrospect, it is easy to see how the entire project was based on a totally flawed understanding of the nature of language. (And even though subsequent Western thought has been peppered with universal language projects to the present day, universal *character* projects are rare.) The error was a failure to recognize that language is *essentially* multivalent, that its usage always occurs in specific situations (even the writing of books) in which a particular user–listener/reader relationship is involved. The 'meanings' of terms are always, in principle, being *explored* and are thus subject to choice, renegotiation and change. The assumption that operations of the mind are universally identical is a vast begged question. What the error boils down to, in fact, is a failure to appreciate that the world is meaningfully constructed *by* our language, and that no such construction is self-evidently 'truer' than any other – even though it may be superior for certain purposes[42].

As far as PL is concerned, the Wilkins project, if universally adopted by scientists, would entirely paralyse the 'scientific Psychology' project. There could be no 'metaphorical' transfer of terms from the physical to the psychological domain, no reflexive application of world properties and phenomena, no alterations in the way in which one experienced oneself or others, or construed one's inner life. Only meat could be tender, and only trains could go off the rails. Even less could I recognize that I had repressed libidinal drives or that someone's short-term memory store was damaged; repressed, drive, short-term, store would be represented by signs admitting of one meaning only. The contrast with the earlier Hermetic vision of the magus assimilating into himself the properties of the universe, a vision in which physical and psychological constantly signify each other, could not be more marked.

In fact it is hard to see how even the physical sciences could flourish under such a tyrannical linguistic regime, since theorizing continuously involves the analogical and metaphorical transfer of terms from one area of discourse to another. Wilkins does, albeit faintly, appreciate the utility of metaphor and devotes Part III, Chapters VI and VII to discussing it. His solution to the problem is simplicity itself:

> The note of *Metaphorical* affixed to any Character, will signifie the enlarging the sense of that word, from that restrained acception which it had in the Tables, to a more universal comprehensive signification: By this common Metaphors may be legitimated retaining their elegancy, and being freed from their ambiguity. (p. 323)

Yet in spite of a thorough survey and categorization of what we would consider psychological concepts (in Part II, chs VIII–X) under such heads as 'Actions of the Understanding and Judgment', 'Corporeal Actions belonging to Sensitive Bodies', 'Of Habit' and 'Of Manners', there is no hint that he is aware of a problem regarding the generation and definition of reflexive terms. He fails to develop any real theory of meaning beyond a crude 'picture theory':

> That *conceit* which men have in their minds concerning a Horse or Tree, is the Notion or *mental Image* of that Beast or Natural thing, of such a nature, shape and use. (p. 20, original emphasis)

How one might have a 'Notion' or 'mental Image' of phenomena in the realm of thought and imaging itself, without embarking on an infinite regress, he does not explain. In fact the earliest clear appreciation of this I have found is in Bishop Browne (1728) (see below p. 138).

The belief that linguistic errors were the main barrier to knowledge, and that a rationally constructed language or character would eliminate them, was uncritically accepted by seventeenth-century virtuosi from Bacon on. The world consisted of things, and words could surely be made to refer to them unambiguously by classifying them into uniquely named classes. Possible relations between them could be similarly dealt with, *and the received repertoire of 'psychological' concepts could also be likewise systematized.* The 'ruins of Babel' could be 'repaired'. 'Psychological things' were no more problematical than physical ones, since they were universally apprehended in the same way. If psychological language was muddled it was for the same reason that all language was muddled – sloppy definitions, irresponsible use of metaphors, contradictory combinations of terms and the like – hence the solution was the same. Leaving aside the question of how metaphor and analogy could occur in the Wilkins scheme even regarding public phenomena, if (as I am claiming) *all* reflexive discourse is conducted ultimately in just these terms, such a programme of reform in relation to PL is scotched from the start.

Oddly enough, although Locke shared Hobbes's hostility to rhetoric and metaphor (see Bennington, 1987) and respected the Wilkins project, there is a sense in which his position could be interpreted as physiomorphic (see especially *Essay*, Book III, ch. 1, below pp. 106–108), for in his system our ideas about the nature of our minds are (at first sight) as equally rooted in ideas of sensation as any others. The spartan quality of Locke's technical analytical language clearly reflects that linguistic wariness of his intellectual peers in Natural Philosophy of which Wilkins's *Real Character* was the supreme expression. But a radically Empiricist epistemology such as Locke's necessarily implies that psychological ideas must derive from ideas of sensation – which amounts to a physiomorphic concept of mind. The stumbling block is that Locke's epistemology regarding the psychological was *not* as radically Empiricist as is often assumed, for there is indeed a 'common light of reason', a 'faculty of reasoning', 'intuitive knowledge' universally shared. Once this is granted the traditional corpus of philosophical PL 'ideas' becomes less problematical (albeit in need of clarification or more rigorous reformulation) since they can be construed as originating in the application of this 'common light' to our (also common) self-experience. Thus 'understanding' and 'will' are indeed *faculties* of the mind, but we err in (as we might now say) reifying them into agents – rather, they are 'powers' (Essay II. 21. 6). Genuine PL *innovation* thus remains stultified notwithstanding Locke's empiricism. This is explored further in Chapter 2 below.

Wilkins's dream of a perfect philosophical character was not confined to British Empiricists; Leibniz pondered a similar scheme, albeit on a radically different basis (see below, p. 84). In the event, despite the labours of a number of his associates and followers during the late seventeenth century (Aubrey, Hooke, Francis Lodowyck, Andrew Paschall, Thomas Pigott, Ray, Wren and others), efforts to develop Wilkins's scheme petered out as realization of its practical futility dawned[43].

5 The Bypass

One might therefore find it even more remarkable that Psychology's historians see its birth in the Scientific Revolution; not only had Descartes defined the realm of scientific enquiry so as to exclude the soul from its purview, but the Natural Philosophical concept of language saw the very process by which psychological ideas are generated as an egregious error. This was a Canute-like posture. Direct PL-generation within Natural Philosophy was inhibited, but an alternative channel existed. If 'Psychology' was ruled out, physiology was very much in the picture. The link between medico-physiological enquiry and the mechanistic (in whatever terms) enquiries of the Royal Society is complex; the medical establishment often eyed the Royal Society with suspicion as a potential rival, and their research traditions had somewhat different origins. While Harvey's discovery of the circulation of the blood had dramatic psychological effects in changing the meaning of the heart (Romanyshyn, 1982; Richards, 1989a), physiological research had seen no overturning of traditional wisdom comparable to that achieved in physics and astronomy since Copernicus. As with chemistry (with which it had close connections via the apothecary), the transformation of older Galenian (in the case of medicine), Paracelsian and Hermetic approaches into 'modern' experimental and empirical science was protracted and confused. The phenomena did not (for all Descartes's physiological speculations) really lend themselves to easy explanation in simple 'physical impact' mechanistic terms. As the century proceeded, physiologists and 'iatrochemists' continued to elaborate on the vocabulary of 'animal spirits' and 'humours' while drawing eclectically on analogies from other proto-sciences – especially from chemistry, but also from physics and elsewhere.

For Psychology the most important text is Samuel Pordage's English (from Latin) translation of Willis's *The Anatomy of the Brain* (1681), which will be discussed in the next section. By the end of the century the combination of novel physiological accounts, Boyle's chemistry and Locke's atomistic account of the mind was radically affecting the terms in which psychological phenomena were being explained and experienced (see Chapter 2). What is happening here is that the wealth of proto-scientific conceptual innovations emanating from physics and chemistry is being incorporated first into an account of the body. Bodily phenomena are reconceptualized as being determined not by a few simple humours or vaguely immaterial external forces impinging on the humoral economy, but as a vast chemical laboratory-cum-hydraulic-engine in which distillations, fermentations, rarefactions and sublimations of numerous fluids and spirits of varying subtlety are forever coursing down tubes, seeping through pores, evaporating and condensing, and causing muscles to swell and shrink to manipulate the diverse cords and levers governing movement. The body is thus constantly threatened by blockages of pores, inappropriate thickenings or thinnings of the fluids, overloaded vessels and violently turbulent chemical reactions in the guts due to overheating. And these misfortunes can be variously triggered by the air inhaled, the food and drink ingested, unhealthy habits or unwonted exertions. In short, it was a recipe for rampant hypochondria.

But once we start identifying these phenomena within us, interpreting our bodily sensations, feelings and health in terms of this new physiological vocabulary, the boundary between physical and psychological is breached. To put it at its simplest: if you believe that the heart serves to heat the blood, then to describe someone as 'hot-blooded' (or 'warm-hearted') is hardly a mere metaphor. Some 'psychological' meaning of the term is inevitably and rapidly established. This source had long contributed to PL; humoral physiology had already enabled people to be melancholic, sanguine, bilious and choleric; as well as being in a particular 'humour', they could also be 'high- (or low-) spirited'. By 1700, however, the 'mechanized' universe, having become introjected into a mechanized body, was ready for the final metamorphosis into a mechanized mind.

This, of course, is what historians of Psychology have always noted, but they have misread the story. The 'mechanization of the mind' was not an intellectual achievement, nor part of the evolution of a discipline called Psychology. Ironically, it arose because, even if it figured as an aspiration, such a discipline was unimplementable in Natural Philosophical terms. The inevitable incorporation of WL innovations into psychological discourse is a collective linguistic process, able to sweep round the barrier erected by Wilkins and Hobbes by restricting its flow for a while in the already well-worn 'body language' channel. And if any kind of language is patently bivalent between physical and psychological, it is that used for the body. 'Mechanization of the mind' occurred in spite of, not because of, the Natural Philosophers. Such an interpretation helps to clarify difficulties historians have had in untangling the significance of seventeenth-century 'physiological psychology'. Fox (1987), for example, still feels bound to consider Descartes (in the *Treatise of Man* in particular, where his 'machine' model of the body is most fully articulated) as giving 'mechanical explanations for what we would call psychological events' (p. 6), and cites an unpublished Ph.D. dissertation by B.C. Ross (1970), 'Psychological Thought Within the Context of the Scientific Revolution: 1665–1700', in which the author 'suggested that the first real psychologists were not philosophers but physiologists'. In the light of our present argument it is clear that the one thing Descartes was *not* explaining was the *psychologicality* of such events, i.e. their *conscious* construal, while any would-be 'real psychologists' later in the century had no option but to study physiology instead. Here the theoretical allegiances of historians of Psychology play a crucial role; for a radical Behaviourist their perceived reductionism is precisely what makes Descartes and Hobbes great pioneers, while for those in other camps they seem only distantly to anticipate Behaviourism's errors.

There is, though, a final 'meta' dimension to all this which I wish to introduce here, although it will be more fully developed in the final chapter: one source of PL has always been public social roles (hence 'magisterial', 'lordly', and 'maternal'). In referring to the relationship between soul and body, in trying to symbolize the 'self', people have frequently adopted one such role as an epitome of the universal condition, thus the self may be seen as a King, Farmer, Pilgrim, Captain of a ship, Father or Knight (but rarely a 'queen' or 'mother' in male-authored texts). What I want to suggest here is that the Lockean epistemization of the mind represents something of a similar move with regard to the role of Natural Philosophy itself. For the Natural Philosopher the central psychological fact is not ruling, producing or spiritual navigation, but gaining knowledge. The 'epistemization' (if not the mechanization) of mind may thus be read as a move which universalizes the Natural Philosopher's mode of consciousness into representing the human mode of consciousness in general. People have long intuitively sensed something like this, and have been arguing the matter with science ever since. But how could an account of consciousness produced in the Natural Philosophical climate have been anything else?

VII.FORGOTTEN ANTICIPATIONS OF PSYCHOLOGY

The strong line adopted so far is not a claim that proto-Psychological texts were absent. My aim has been to show how those texts usually so classified ought not to be included in this category, since their goals and methods were fundamentally different from those of Psychology. Here I wish to disinter some of the few exceptions. These have been largely forgotten by general historians of Psychology, although I hasten to add that some, at any rate, are well known in other quarters. We may begin with Hooke's theory of memory, my acquaintance with which I owe to a paper by the late Bernard Singer (Singer, 1976), on which the following discussion is largely based.

1 Robert Hooke's Theory of Memory

Hooke's theory of memory resembles modern Psychological theorizing far more closely than do its philosophical treatments in Descartes, Hobbes and Locke. He explicitly attempts to formulate a model of the phenomenon in terms of contemporary 'scientific' knowledge in a way directly ancestral to the use of physical phenomena as a basis for Psychological modelling by modern Psychologists. Memory is treated primarily as a natural object of enquiry, with theological issues in a firmly subordinate place. Published in 1705 as *An Hypothetical Explication of Memory; how the Organs made use of by the Mind in its Operation may be mechanically understood*, it was first presented as a lecture at the Royal Society in June and July 1682. In presenting this, let us note, Hooke made a clear disavowal that it was in any way meant to represent the Royal Society's position, stressing that he was offering a purely personal, speculative account. Schaffer (1987) provides a full description of the immediate intellectual climate in which it was produced. Hooke felt it necessary, then, to distance his treatment of memory from orthodox Natural Philosophical research. Even so, his intrusion into pneumatology got him into hot water with Henry More.

The paper incorporates a number of 'scientific' images and is couched in terms which reflect the emerging 'passive matter' concept of mechanism. It is radically materialist in conception; there is a material organ of Memory, or 'Repository of Ideas', Ideas themselves are resolutely 'corporeal', being formed by the soul from the motions supplied by the senses, and deposited in this repository. A material meaning is given to the notion of 'Attention', which has previously been explained 'only by giving the same Notion by some other ways of Expression, which it may be are as little intelligible' (Hooke, 1705; p. 140). He continues:

> My Notion of it is this, that the Soul in the Action of Attention does really give some material Part of the Repository into such a Shape, and gives it some such a Motion as is from the Senses conveyed thither; which being so formed and qualified, is inserted into and enclosed in the common Repository, and there for a time

> preserved and retained, and so becomes an Organ, upon which the Soul working, finds the Ideas of past Actions, as if the Action were present. (*ibid.*)

Both repository and ideas are formed from the material of the brain (Singer, p. 118). The model which finally emerges is of a chain of ideas coiled up in the repository which is rooted to the soul at one end, this being situated at a place where there is a 'a matter similar to . . . phosphorescent material' capable of retaining impressions, but for longer than ordinary phosphorescent material can retain light. Our sense of Time is generated by the length of the Chain of Ideas. Bells, strings and vases are invoked as materials capable of retaining sound. Once thus materially formed, these ideas (calculated as numbering ten million over a lifetime) can be renewed by a Radiation of the Soul. In describing this latter, and the mechanism of forgetting, Hooke has recourse to a solar system model, a rare instance of comprehensive physiomorphic assimilation of the heliocentric cosmology:

> I conceive . . . that besides the natural Decay there may be of the Form and impress Motion of the Ideas, there may be also an Impediment to this Radiation of the Soul, by the Interposition of other Ideas between the Center and the Idea sought; much after the manner as the Earth interposing between the Moon and the Sun, hinders the Sun from radiating upon the Moon. And in such case the Idea may sometimes be thought to be lost, which yet may afterwards be found again when the Obstacle is removed. . . . Again, as in the *Radiation of the Sun, which is as it were a Representation of the Soul of the World*; the Radiation of the Soul is more powerful upon Ideas at a nearer than at a further distance; and their Reaction is also more powerful back again, and that in a duplicate proportion to their Distance reciprocal much the same with that of Light, which is the most spiritual Action of all we are sensible of in the World. (Hooke, pp. 144–145; Singer pp. 122–3; emphasis added)

He goes so far as to suggest that the 'Sphere of Radiation' of the Soul may not be limited to the Ideas in the Repository: '. . . it may have a much bigger Sphere of influencing Power, and thereby may extend it, not only to all and every Point of the Body enlivened and preserved by it; but possibly it may extend even out of the Body, and that to some considerable Distance, and thereby not only influence other Bodies, but be influenced by them also' (Hooke, p. 147; B. Singer pp. 123–4).

We have here a complex conversion of the Natural Philosopher's mechanical and heliocentric physical world cosmology (incorporating *en route* such specific phenomena as phosphorescent materials, chains and eclipses) into a psychophysiological system. It enables Hooke to tackle such topics as the nature of ideas, time-perception, attention, forgetting, perception (and even perhaps, in view of the last-mentioned point, ESP!) in far more concrete detail than had been customary among philosophers. Hooke's theory appears to be a thoroughly materialist counterattack against the Neo-Platonist Henry More who held memory to be wholly contained in the incorporeal soul (Singer, pp. 126–8). Warily though he knows he has to tread, he is cautiously rejecting the view that psychological phenomena should be forever out of bounds for natural philosophizing. Even so, the precise nature of the soul's 'Radiations' remains quite obscure, they can be comprehended only by analogy with light itself, and the soul becomes the body's Sun, just as much as Louis XIV had, as Sun King, become France's. The influences of this work on Locke (and vice versa) are difficult to unravel, for each writer was – or could have been – aware of the other's work (drafts of the *Essay* circulating long before its publication, and Locke perhaps attending Hooke's lectures). Singer notes 'striking similarities' between them especially on time-perception and the perception of moments, but also notes their difference in approach: 'Locke makes his observations primarily in relation to philosophical problems whereas Hooke is concerned often to examine the limitations of man compared to scientific instruments and the consequent possibilities of assisting in overcoming these restrictions' (Singer, p. 125).

Memory had been treated by various English writers before – Bacon, Glanville, Digby and Margaret Cavendish among them – but none in so technical and Psychological a fashion. Yet what is most significant here about Hooke's theory is that it did not initiate any tradition of Psychological research. Rather, it took its place in the more immediate theological debates about the nature of spirit in which the Natural Philosophers were engaged. It rests in glorious isolation as a one-off piece of proto-Psychological theorizing of a kind for which the intellectual climate was quite unripe.

2 John Bulwer

John Bulwer, a physician about whom little is known, published four books, all relevant to us: *Philocophus* (1648), *Chirologia, or the Natural Language of the Hand* (1644), *Pathomyotomia* (1649) and *Anthropometamorphosis: Man Transformed; or, The Artificiall Changeling* (1653). The first is an attempt at developing a gestural language for the deaf and dumb and was dedicated to Sir Edward Gostwicke whom he had treated for this condition, (though as the *Dictionary of National Bibliography* contributor observes, surprisingly he did not consider finger gestures). This anticipated a similar scheme by Wilkins's associate John Wallis, presented to the Royal Society in 1662[44]. The second was not, as might often have been assumed, a text on palmistry. In it Bulwer claims that gestures of the hand are a universal language, 'the only speech and generall language of Humane Nature' (A6), 'and all these motions and habits of the *Hand* are purely naturall, not positive; nor in their senses remote from the true nature of the things that are implyed' (p. 3); and 'It speakes all languages, and as an *universall character of Reason*, is generally understood and knowne by all Nations, among the formall differences of their tongue . . . it may well be called the *Tongue and generall language of Humane Nature*' (p. 3). He sees gesture as primary (anticipating a point made by Gordon Hewes [1973]: that gestures anticipate or accompany speech, but do not follow it), even saying at one point that 'if words ensue upon the gesture, their addition serves but as a Comment for the fuller explication of the manuall Text of utterance' (p. 5). Animal rationality is vehemently defended (although a committed mechanist, he is thus far from Cartesian). From pages 8 to 10 we are given a solid list (in blackletter) of all the things we can do with our hands: 'sue, intreat, beseech, solicite, call, allure, intice, dismisse' etc.

The main body of the book contains a detailed survey of 62 hand gestures followed by two engraved tables illustrating 'The Alphabet of naturall expressions'. The gestures range from 'washing hands' motion (protestation of innocence) to 'to wag in a swinging gesture' (wantonness and effeminacy) and all the common beckoning, admonishing, pleading and affectionately expressive ones. From here he moves on to finger gestures, with a similar illustrative figure and a supplementary *Chironomia, or the Art of Manuall Rhetorique*.

The first thing to strike one in the present context is perhaps the universal character theme: Bulwer's belief that gestures are a natural, universal, rational language. But we must also recognize the work as a thoroughly naturalistic survey of non-verbal gestural communication, a pioneer kinesic monograph. *Pathomyotomia*, or a *Dissertation on the Significative Muscles of the Affections of the Minde* is perhaps the most intriguing of his works for a modern physiological Psychologist (albeit cheaply produced with, as he regrets, no illustrations). He attempts to survey the musculature underlying all expressive movements and gestures (particularly of the head and face):

> . . . in the semblances of those motions wrought in the parts by the behaviour of the Muscles, we may not only see, but as it were feel and touch the very inward motions of the Mind. (A4)

> . . . we will think it a thing worthy to be corrected with the whip of Ignorance if any rashly plunge himself into the Muscular Seas of corporal Anatomy, or of the outward man, without any mention of the Internall man, since the Soule only is the Opifex of all the movings of the Muscles, whose invisible Acts are made manifest by their operations in those parts into which they are inserted. (*ibid.*).

In the ensuing survey of our 'virgin Philosophie of Gesture', comparable to that of hand gestures in *Chirologia*, he leaves no gesture unexamined, including wrinklings of the nose. Nor can I resist quoting from the prefatory poem 'To the daring Advancer of all Somaticall Science' by his friend Thomas Diconson:

> To Make Anatomy by Muscles wind
> The swiftest motions of the minged* Mind
> Natures high piece of Clockwork this You call,
> Reason the Spring winds up, the Muscles all
> Like wheels move this or that way, swift or sloe
> As the Affections Weight doth make them go.
>
> The last Yeare stil'd You Deafe & Dumbe man's friend
> Now Thy Design more deeper doth descend.
> I see Thy knowledge and invention flowes
> As far in man as Sense and Motion goes.

* 'minged': *OED* definition 3 is 'To remember. Also *refl.* to bethink oneself.' Here it is thus, presumably, roughly synonymous with 'self-aware'.

The general tenor of *Pathomyotomia* anticipates modern Psychology far more closely than that of Descartes's work. Bulwer is not concerned with the philosophical question of the soul's relationship with the body, being content to accept that whatever the nature of the soul, its 'motions' are knowable only by the outward expression, but neither is he a physiological reductionist. He is simply fascinated, in all his works, with the universal language of expressive behaviour and its biological basis. On the soul–body relationship he penetrates no further into philosophy proper than noting that 'the force of the Soule residing in the Braine, moves the *Muscles* by the *Nerves*, as with Reines, for the *Will* is like the Rider, the *Nerves* to Reines and the *Muscles* to the Horse' (p. 14). Nor does he appear to have any theological axe to grind. Historians of Psychology have no excuse for overlooking *Pathomyotomia*, it is the very first work to receive a (respectful) footnote citation in Darwin's *Expression of the Emotions in Man and Animals* (1889, 2nd edn, p. 1); the footnote even continues with a reference to a work by D. Hack Tuke in which *Chirologia* is praised.[45]

Finally, in *Anthropometamorphosis* Bulwer surveys the ways humans have distorted and altered their bodies. This is more polemical, an 'Enditement' against all nations 'whereby they are *arraigned* at the Tribunall of Nature, as guilty of High-Treason, in Abasing, Counterfeiting, Defacing and Clipping her Coine, instampt with her Image and Superscription on the Body of Man' (Epistle Dedicatory, p. 2). Drawing copiously on the proto-anthropological literature and contemporary travellers' reports he exhaustively describes (with amusing woodcut illustrations), among other things, cranial distortions, hair fashion, 'auricular fashions', 'Lip-gallantry', 'Beard-haters', 'Face moulders', 'Pap-fashions', and 'Strange inventive contradictions . . . in ordering of Privie parts'. He provides a naturalistic explanation of the acephalic 'blemmys' and ends by moralistically surveying the 'Pedigree of the English Gallant' to prove that modern fashions at home are as bad as the exotic foreign ones just described.

Bulwer's surviving works suggest a distinctly secular and empirical curiosity about human communication and appearance, and a preparedness to apply this practically. All we know about him is that he was a physician, presumably in Bedfordshire (where the Gostwickes had their seat); the *DNB* provides no dates of birth or death. While he obviously accepts a 'mechanical' physiology, his affiliations are to Bacon rather than Descartes. He notes that *Pathomyotomia* remedies a defect observed in *The Advancement of Learning* (presumably in the passage on physiognomy 'which discovers the dispositions of the mind by the lineaments of the body' [EW IV, p. 376]; *Anthropometamorphosis* also echoes Bacon's attack on 'Cosmetics' (*ibid.* p. 394)). A more thoroughgoing and sophisticated 'physiological Psychology' than Bulwer's, however, was soon to appear.

3 Thomas Willis

The major seventeenth-century English forerunner of physiological Psychology was Thomas Willis. Willis, unlike Descartes or Hobbes, was a practising physiological virtuoso of the first order, who conducted his investigation of the anatomy of the brain with the aid of Richard Lower. He is in no doubt that

> within the Womb of the Brain all the Conceptions, Ideas, Forces and Powers whatsoever both of the Rational and Sensitive Soul are framed; and having gotten a species and form are produced into act. (1684, p. 64)

Willis's explanatory mechanisms extend way beyond (though they include) Cartesian atomistic inertial impacts of particles, and are drawn from chemistry rather than mechanics. Although he ubiquitously invokes 'Animal Spirits' (for which Mayow attacked him) his 1683 *Two Discourses concerning the Soul of Brutes, which is that of the Vital and Sensitive of Man* offers a chemical explanation of these in terms of fire:

> For truly, Fire, if we would describe it according to its Essence, signifies an heap of most subtil Contiguous particles and existing in a swift motion, and with a continued generation of some, renewed by the falling off of others; which indeed consumes both its motion and substance; for that its Food, on which it continually feeds, is perpetually supply'd from the subject matter, which is Sulphur or some other nitrous thing in the Air . . . (1683, p. 5)

(As Fox [1987] notes, this work is also entitled a 'Psychelogie or Doctrine of the Soul' – one of the isolated seventeenth-century occurrences of variants of the term 'psychology'.) From this Willis develops a chemical explanation of the creation of Animal Spirits, in which the process of fermentation was central: 'the business of extracting the animal Spirits is performed even as a Chymical Elixir'. Allen Debus (1977) quotes a remarkable passage from his paper 'Of Fermentation', in which

> 'the Brain with a Scull over it and the appending Nerves, represent the little Head or Glassie Alembic, with a Spunge laid upon it . . . for truly the Blood when Rarified by Heat, is carried from the Chimny of the Heart, to the Head even as the Spirit of Wine boyling in the Cucurbit, and being resolved into Vapour, is elevated into the Alembic.

And much more in the same vein.

The psychological functions of the various parts of the brain are proposed, and metaphors of many kinds are deployed to express their operation. One further passage must suffice here; in his explanation of 'the Senses' –

> . . . as often as the exterior part of the Soul being struck, a Sensible impression, as it were the Optick Species, or as an undulation or moving of waters, is carried more inward, bending towards the chamfered bodies, a perception or inward sense of the Sensation outwardly had or received, arises. If that this impression, being carried further, passes through the *callous Body*, Imagination follows the Sense: Then if the same fluctuation of Spirits is struck against the *Cortex* of the Brain, as its utmost banks, it impresses on it the image or character of the sensible Object, which, when it is afterwards reflected or beat back, raises up the memory of the same thing. (1684, p. 91)

– Willis was, as Debus (1977) shows, rooted in the Paracelsian 'iatrochemical' tradition (Bulwer, by contrast, opposed Paracelsians), resting in large part on a conception of chemical phenomena which still incorporated many alchemical notions (e.g. active and passive principles represented by 'spirit, sulfur, salt' and 'water, earth' respectively)[46].

While it would wrong to call Willis a psychologist, his variety of 'physiological Psychology' does, as far as I can see, approach its modern version far more closely than that of Descartes. This is most apparent in its evidently non-reductionist character. While Descartes is concerned with demoting a wide range of psychological phenomena (notably those which are most fallible, variable and sense-dependent) for doctrinally loaded philosophical purposes, leaving the soul with an attenuated but purer role, Willis is interested in trying to envisage physiological processes sufficiently complex to match the complexities of phenomenological experience itself. He is unconcerned, by and large, with metaphysical matters, and even if the soul as such must, in the final analysis, be left out of the equation, he does not exclusively reserve for it any subset of psychological functions as Descartes did. Willis's works are extensive and difficult, and although he is justly renowned among historians of medicine, a full analysis of his psychological thought lies in the future. My own – relatively brief – forays into his writing suggest that Willis is a transitional figure of considerable importance in whose works a diverse number of themes are interwoven. His medical approach was eclectic and he was a member of the Oxford circle of 'virtuosi' which included Wilkins, Wallis, Boyle and Seth Ward.

As physicians and anatomists Bulwer and Willis knew far more about physiology than Hobbes or Descartes, and if one wishes to find genuine seventeenth-century anticipations of physiological Psychology (as well as of the study of non-verbal communication) the forgotten Bulwer and Willis, hitherto monopolized by historians of medicine, are far better candidates than either.

4 Edward Tyson (1649–1708)

If 'psychology' was ever to become a natural object of enquiry within the scientific enterprise, humans as such had to come to be seen as part of, instead of apart from, the natural world. Religion inhibited acceptance of this until the mid nineteenth century. One text which played a distant part in putting the issue on the agenda was Tyson's *Orang-Outang, sive Homo Sylvestris: or the Anatomy of a Pygmie compared with that of a monkey, an ape, and a man* (1699). (His 'Pygmie' was in fact a chimpanzee.) While I in no way wish to claim that this text is Psychology (though it does contain some anthropology), I do see a role for it in the long process of acceptance of humans as subjects of scientific study. There was nothing new about studying anatomy – Vesalius was over a century and a half in the past – but there was something new in Tyson's comparison of human and primate anatomy, raising as it did the issue of the biological boundaries of the human. Tyson acknowledges the intermediate position of his 'Pygmie' between human and non-human: 'The Animal of which I have given the Anatomy, coming nearest to Mankind, seems the Nexus of the Animal and Rational' (p. 3) He enumerates 48 anatomical points in which it 'more resembled Man than Apes and Monkeys do' and 34 in which it 'more resembled Ape and Monkeykind' (pp. 92–95). In an appended 'Philological Essay' on the 'Cynocephali, the Satyrs and Sphinges of the Ancients' he rigorously demystifies these reported bizarre varieties of humanity and assigns them to the monkeys and apes ('Cynocephali' patently being baboons). As to the brain:

> . . . since therefore in all respects the *Brain* of our *Pygmie* does so exactly resemble a *Man*'s, I might here make the same Reflection the *Parisians* did upon the *Organs of Speech, That there is no reason to think that Agents do perform such and such Actions, because they are found with Organs proper thereunto*: for then our *Pygmie* might really be a *Man*. . . . [i]n truth *Man* is part a *Brute*, part an *Angel*; and is that *Link* in the *Creation*, that joyns them both together. (p. 55; original emphasis)

Although Tyson was no Psychologist, his *Anatomy of a Pygmie* constitutes a clear step towards the incorporation of *Homo sapiens* into the zoological framework (taken further by Linnaeus) and its eventual treatment as an object of naturalistic enquiry. Perhaps he would be better seen as a proto-physical anthropologist, but that is anachronistically to adopt contemporary discipline boundaries of increasingly uncertain status.

5 The Moon Illusion[47]

The 'Moon Illusion' – its apparently greater size when on the horizon than well above it, although when measured the angle subtended remains the same (thirty minutes) – had taxed philosophers since Antiquity and continued to do so during the seventeenth century (see H.E. and G.M. Ross [1976] on Ptolemy's account). Their explanations were critically reviewed by William Molyneux in the *Philosophical Transactions of the Royal Society* (repr. in Lowthorp, 1705). Two kinds of explanation were attempted;

both Hobbes and Gassendi had proposed physical explanations (as had an unnamed 'French Abbé'); Descartes, however, offered a psychological explanation and a variant of this by Dr Wall follows immediately on Molyneux's communication. In addition, Riccioli, in his *Treatise on Refraction*, claimed that he and a Father Grimaldi had found that both Sun and Moon, when on the horizon, really did subtend greater angles (of 'almost a degree' and forty minutes respectively). Hobbes's typically geometrical explanation was quite clever: the 'sphere' on which we see celestial objects has the centre of the Earth as its centre, but we observe them from the surface, not the centre, of the Earth, a displacement which (as an accompanying figure showed) elongates our view of objects nearer the horizon. Molyneux astutely sweeps this ingenious theory aside by proving that in reality the scale of things is so vast that such an effect would be 'beyond the possibility of the discovery of Sense'. Gassendi's theory was physiological – when the Moon is near the horizon, its light had to pass through 'a more foggy Air, casts a weaker Light, and consequently forces not the Eye so much as when brighter; and therefore the Pupil does more Inlarge it self, thereby transmitting a larger Projection on the Retina'. Molyneux has little truck with this fallacy that the size of the 'Aperture of the Pupil' affects retinal image size and refutes it at length, using two figures. The Riccioli and Grimaldi finding is dismissed out of hand – Molyneux himself had taken the relevant measurements using a six foot telescope with a 'fine lattice' of single human hairs on the inward side of the 'Eye Glass'.

Descartes's more psychological explanation was that when the Moon is on the horizon, the interposition of other objects enables us to make an estimate of its size and because it seems nearer the 'Tops of Trees, or Chimneys, or Houses', we are deceived into thinking that it is bigger. 'These Thoughts, my-thinks, are much below the Accustomed Accuracy of the Noble Des Cartes', observes Molyneux (whom we met earlier as a translator of the *Meditations*), because merely looking at the Moon through a tree or behind a rooftop is insufficient to cause the illusion, which is just as powerful when it is seen rising 'from an Horizon determined by a smooth sea'. The theory then proposed by Dr Wall reverses the logic of Descartes's account. For Descartes, size increases because we think the Moon has come closer. For Wall, it increases because we have come to appreciate how far away it really is. The 'Imagination of the

Eye' uses supposed distance, not only the angle subtended at the retina, in estimating object size. When the Moon is high in the sky we have no way of estimating supposed distance, but when it is on the horizon 'there is a Prospect of Hills, and Vallies, and Plains, and Woods, and Rivers, and variety of Fields and Inclosures between it and us; which present to our Imagination a great Distance capable of receiving all these'. He makes an effort to meet the kind of objection posed by Molyneux – that the illusion is as strong without such objects: 'the Memory suggests to us a view as large as is the visible horizon'. The Wall theory is not too far removed from that now generally accepted, in which the bowl of the sky as phenomenally perceived is, for 'hard-wired' neurological reasons, not a hemisphere but a saucer; thus the horizon does indeed look further away than the zenith, and an object subtending the same angle in both positions will look bigger in the former.

Both Descartes and Wall (the latter more subtly) propose psychological as opposed to physiological, astronomical or geometrical explanations of the phenomenon. They are both able to treat the Moon Illusion as an object of Natural Philosophical enquiry even though their theories have no clearly testable consquences. There are in fact no general 'Psychological' theories of perception of a testable kind being produced in the seventeenth century as opposed to speculative philosophical analyses of the ontological status of perceptions and their relationship to their objects. Nobody assembles a catalogue of types of visual illusion or analyses of the kinds of cue used for estimating distance and size – cues familiar to all the painters of the time. Indeed, if any period was in a position to pursue pioneering investigations of visual perception it was the seventeenth century, since such investigations had already been successfully accomplished by the Renaissance artists, and the Dutch masters were yet at work. Instead we get tangled, theologically loaded philosophical disputes about whether images are in the brain or the soul.

The reason why the Moon Illusion was an exception is given away, perhaps, by the 'General Head' under which it appears in Lowthorp's 1705 abridgement of the Transactions: Astronomy. It is a long-known, discrete phenomenon directly involving one of the central objects of astronomical interest, the Moon, and thus Natural Philosophers have no qualms about discussing it. In doing so they momentarily, and unwittingly, become engaged in Psychology. The Natural Philosophical study of perception was otherwise conducted under the rubrics either of Optics (stimulated primarily by the need to understand the behaviour of lenses and the nature of light) or physiology (see Crombie, 1964; Hatfield and Epstein, 1979 for reviews of this, including classical and medieval perceptual theories). I do concede, though, that perception is one topic on which a continuous tradition of enquiry clearly exists in some sense, even if a Psychological, as opposed to physiological or technically optical, orientation is somewhat rare. On Optics, certainly, the literature was copious, but rarely figures in history of Psychology. A major contribution here was Molyneux's *A Treatise of Dioptricks* (1692), in which, among other things, he cracks (albeit falteringly) the pseudo-problem of why we see things the right way up in spite of the retinal image being inverted (Boring, 1942). This work laid the basis for Berkeley's subsequent *New Theory of Vision* (1709). Molyneux, in discussion with Locke, also raised what has become known as 'Molyneux's question': whether a person blind from birth would, on acquiring sight, be able to identify shapes, hitherto known only by touch, by sight alone. He claimed not, and Locke agreed 'with this thinking gentleman, whom I am proud to call my friend' (*Essay*, II, Bk IX, Sect. 8, where 'Mr. Molineux's' question is discussed). By virtue of his name, Molyneux has sometimes been thought French; he was in fact Irish, to be sure.

6 Marin Cureau de la Chambre (1594–1669)

Perhaps the most remarkably neglected of seventeenth-century writers on psychological matters is Marin Cureau de la Chambre, physician to Richelieu, putative psychotherapist or counsellor to Mazarin, and personnel selection advisor to the Sun King himself. Our information regarding de la Chambre comes from a 1968 paper by Solomon Diamond reviewing his achievements and claims to attention by historians of the discipline. Diamond was unable to find any modern secondary literature on him, nor was he able to get hold of more than the first two volumes of his five volume work *Les Caractères des Passions* (1648–62). While content in the main to identify the numerous points in which de la Chambre can be spotted anticipating modern doctrines (e.g. a tripartite classification of the passions as derived from love, courage and fear, which is like Karen Horney's, and a belief in the non-localization of storage of memory) Diamond marshals sufficient evidence to convince us that the nature of de la Chambre's psychological concerns was a mixture of the literary and 'scientific' as opposed to philosophical or theological. It also transpires that Descarte's *Passions de l'Ame* was largely a response to de la Chambre's work. His writings were widely read by his contemporaries (including four translations into English between 1650 and 1665) and he was admired as a stylist. As a physician, though, he is able to write with authority on possible psychophysiological mechanisms. I also cannot help noting that 'he appeals to the nature of light in his argument that mind has the virtue of assuming the qualities of any object it embraces, as light takes the form and color of a crystal vase' (Diamond, 1968, p. 42).

Diamond ascribes de la Chambre's neglect to the fact that he never aspired 'to be more than a fashionable writer' (p. 53), and the passages quoted certainly possess a 'literary essay' quality. Even so, one wonders if this explanation is sufficient. In spite of Diamond's paper, de la Chambre fails to appear in recent histories such as Leahey (1987) or Hearnshaw (1987). Again it appears that cultural eminence as a philosopher is a *sine qua non* for counting as important in the history of Psychology in this period. De la Chambre's interests ranged from a general *Système de l'Ame* (1664) through emotions and emotional expression, animal thought and memory to diagnosis of character (including physiognomy). Even more than those writers we have been looking at previously in this section, de la Chambre looks, at any rate, like someone with interests matching those of a modern Psychologist. Diamond's paper confirms this. May we not construe his neglect as evidence that in France, as in Britain, a tradition of Psychological enquiry simply could not take root in Natural Philosophy this early?

The number of anticipatory texts and writers could be enlarged considerably from those – somewhat arbitrarily – selected here, notably in the fields of education, rhetoric, characterology, courtesy books, and anthropology, plus unique texts like Huarte's *Tryall of Wits*[48]. But they were not numerous. As a group they are highly diverse, while they rarely initiated any subsequently continuous body of research or enquiry (educational writings being perhaps an exception). It is only to be expected that Natural Philosophers and their associates of this period would from time to time turn their attention to specific 'psychological' matters of a discrete kind, and in so doing their investigations may legitimately be considered as anticipating, in spirit, contemporary Psychological studies of the same topics. But the genealogy of these can rarely be traced back continuously to such forebears. On the contrary it is only when the modern research tradition has become established that its more antiquarian-minded practitioners – seeking, like scientific *nouveaux riches*, for a respectable ancestry – discover these distant and largely forgotten texts from which they can then delightedly claim an honourable descent. Such anticipations did not, taken *en masse*, constitute a coherent proto-Psychology in the discipline sense. Little connection was seen between them at the time, and no moves were made to draw them together.

VIII SPINOZA AND LEIBNIZ

No review of seventeenth-century psychological thought can ignore the work of Spinoza and Leibniz. In the case of Leibniz, if not Spinoza, there is no doubt that he played an important role in introducing several concepts which, however falteringly they were pursued for the following century and a half, eventually became central to several major Psychological theories, particularly in the nineteenth century. And in Boring's view, 'the development of thought was continuous and the lines of influence are clear' (1950, p. 168). Again, the question to be asked is how far these concepts as originally formulated, possessed the Psychological character they later assumed.

1 Benjamin Baruch Spinoza (1632–77)

Spinoza, Bertrand Russell tells us, 'is the noblest and most lovable of the great philosophers'. He continues:

> Intellectually, some others have surpassed him, but ethically he is supreme. As a natural consequence, he was considered, during his lifetime and for a century after his death, a man of appalling wickedness. (Russell, 1946, p. 552)

An extended case for Spinoza's significance for Psychology is made by Klein (1970, ch. 13). His 'double-aspect monism' solution to the mind–body problem ran directly counter to Descartes's dualism, and implied a thoroughgoing unity between the psychological and the physical. Klein's case is built on the identification of a series of 'anticipations' of modern Psychological theories and findings: Spinoza's account of emotions anticipates the James/Lange theory, he anticipates the Freudian unconscious in observing that 'men are unconscious of the causes of their desires'; while other quotes demonstrate anticipations of Adler's feelings of inferiority and need for acceptance within a group and, more systematically, McDougall's 'hormic' Psychology (while Klein admits the total absence of references to him by McDougall). He also evinces a modern type concern with mental hygiene and mental health.

Undoubtedly it is justifiable to see Spinoza as peculiarly 'modern' and prescient both in his metaphysics and in the psychological doctrines he derives therefrom. But this very modernity, which had to wait a century before anyone else was modern enough to appreciate it, and his long notoriety as a wicked atheist, tell against ascribing to him any immediate historical role in the development of psychological ideas. This may well be regretted; his theory of the emotions as all derivative from Joy, Sorrow and Desire, and the extensive exploration of the nature of the effects and operations of these emotions (Parts III and IV of the *Ethics*) contain much perennially valuable wisdom, and would that his high aspirations for science had been more deeply realized:

> I wish to direct all sciences in one direction or to one end, namely, to attain the greatest possible human perfection: and thus everything in the sciences that does not promote this endeavour must be rejected as useless. (*On the Correction of the Understanding*, para. 3, p. 231, 1959 edn)

But the unpublished manuscript of *On the Correction of the Understanding* was not even discovered until nearly a hundred years after his death. His motivation, even more strongly than Descartes's, was religious, and he spent his life ascetically in the service of his spiritual quest. His editor, T.S. Gregory, writes against the common accusation of atheism or pantheism:

> Spinoza's *Ethics* is the voice of a mystical devotion so relentless, a sanctity so pure, that such misconception of it serves only to reveal the scope of its *amor intellectualis Dei*, as if one should complain that the sky was empty because it was cloudless. (1959 edn, p. vii)

It is no mean testimony to Spinoza that Bertrand Russell, a man as anti-mystical in temperament as one could imagine – and as cantankerous too – seems almost to revere Spinoza's ethical system above all others in the Western philosophical canon, as 'a help towards sanity and an antidote to the paralysis of utter despair' (1946, p. 562).

That Spinoza's philosophy is wise, subtle, enduring and prescient is not in question. Our concern though is whether he played a role in the history of Psychological thought and, more specifically, whether he succeeded in introducing any new psychological ideas. On currently available evidence, the answer on both counts has to be negative. Current disciplinary historians have certainly failed to show otherwise; Leahey (1987) finds an anticipation of B.F. Skinner; Murphy and Kovach (1972) note his monism, the 'strangely modern cast' of his ideas and belief in unconscious processes, then concede that his ideas had no appeal to his contemporaries. Hearnshaw's position is a little contradictory in that, having castigated Gardner Murphy and R.I. Watson for their (correct in our view) cursory treatment of Spinoza as having little influence, he then says:

> The fact is that many of Spinoza's ideas were far in advance of their time, and only in the twentieth century have they ceased to seem bizarre and unacceptable. (Hearnshaw, 1987, p. 72)

– which rather concedes their point. The only qualification to this general picture of Spinoza's lack of influence is Freud's admission in a letter of 1931: 'My dependence on the teachings of Spinoza I do admit most willingly. I had no reason to mention his name directly, as I got my presumptions *not from studying him, but from the atmosphere he created*' (quoted by Hearnshaw, *ibid.* p. 75; emphasis added). Otherwise Hearnshaw's relatively extended account of Spinoza, like Klein's, demonstrates only how far Spinoza was 'ahead of his time'.

2 Gottfried Wilhelm Leibniz (1646–1716)

Leibniz presents an unusually difficult case for historians of Psychology (and, let it be said, for intellectual historians generally) to construe. His philosophical concerns spanned logic, physics, metaphysics, theology, mathematics and law. His ideas are contained in an extremely fragmented corpus of writings, many never published in his lifetime. While this fragmentation itself causes problems, it is the arcane nature of much of his thought which presents the greatest hurdle to modern readers. Leibniz, striving simultaneously to redeem scholasticism and advance the new scientific world-view, to transcend the mind–matter distinction in a way which concedes to both phenomenalists and materialists their best insights, and to dissolve the free will–determinism problem, holds a unique position in Western thought. For Ernst Cassirer (1934) he was the pivotal figure around whom European Enlightenment philosophy subsequently revolved.

Leibniz is often classified as a 'Rationalist', but it is now admitted that the label fails adequately to capture the subtleties of his position. As another thinker 'ahead of his time', Leibniz's only equal is perhaps Leonardo da Vinci; inventor of the modern form of the infinitesimal calculus, binary logic and topology, a more radical relativist in some senses than Einstein (G.M. Ross, 1984), an inveterate technological speculator and political internationalist. Like Wilkins – albeit from a different direction – he aspired to devising a 'Universal Character' within which it would be impossible to formulate false propositions, though for him it would be based on mathematics. He strenuously opposed the crudities of contemporary French mechanism, and eventually Newton's too. In many of these areas his contribution is unambiguous and circumscribed, but not when it comes to the metaphysical-cum-logical system within which he attempted to integrate his thought, incorporating the 'monadology', the 'principle of sufficient reason', and the 'identity of indiscernibles'. In tackling Leibniz's system, most historians of Psychology – forgivably, in this case – have relied primarily on secondary texts, and I think it is fair to say that apart from professional Leibniz experts, most of us have been unable to make head or tail of it. We have diligently cobbled together a more or less credible précis and then moved on to his impact and influence. Some have been bold enough to sweep the problem aside:

> The theory of monads is extremely difficult and according to some

> writers self-contradictory (Russell, 1900) or untenable (Hacking, 1972); however, it is not necessary to understand the monadology to appreciate Leibniz's psychology. (D.J. Murray, 1983, p. 167)

This implies that a coherent subset of ideas identifiable as 'Leibniz's psychology' can be teased from the less coherent mass of his overall metaphysical system. This seems doubtful. But let us first look at the psychological ideas which Leibniz introduced.

Traditionally the most salient of these are held to be his notions of unconscious perception [*petites perceptions*] and apperception, together with his view of individual development as determined by an unfolding inner dynamic. To these we might add, even more remarkably, an anticipation of modern Cognitive Psychology's computational account of thought processes. Is the descent of these into modern Psychology, then, as continuous as Boring claimed? Can they, in fact, be detached from the overall structure of Leibniz's system to constitute part of a separate 'Psychology'?

With regard to the first question, there is no serious doubt that it was Leibniz who firmly established the concept of unconscious mental processes in the Western – particularly German – philosophical repertoire, although other roots may also be traced (see, for example, Bakan [1975] on its background in Jewish thought). We may also query how far its later presence in Psychology is due not directly to Leibniz but to eighteenth-century physiologists such as Whytt (see below, p. 199) who needed concepts of 'sensibility' and 'irritability' which, while in a sense mentalistic, did not imply consciousness. 'Apperception' unambiguously originates with Leibniz and can be traced directly via Kant, Herbart, Lazarus and Steinthal, and Lotze to Wundt (see Lange, 1907, Part III). Its meaning gradually changes at each step, from something akin to self-conscious perceptual awareness to – in Wundt – a term more or less synonymous with 'attention'. The broad image of individual development proceeding as an unfolding of some endogenous scheme was a powerful one affecting much continental cosmological thought in the eighteenth century, particularly the shift from a static to a dynamic view of the universe as proceeding *towards* perfection (see below, p. 176). While contributing to the conceptual climate in which evolutionary theory flourished in the nineteenth century, it was, in contrast to Darwinism, teleological. In Psychology it culminates, fused with materalist evolutionism, in twentieth-century Freudian and Piagetian thought.

The link between Leibniz's 'computational' account of cognition and modern versions is far less clear – there is a thread of such speculation, associated with attempts at building calculating machines, predating Leibniz (see G.M. Ross, 1984) and continuing via figures such as Babbage, Boole and Jevons who were not in any specifically Leibnizian tradition (see Kassler, 1984 for the early history of calculating machines in this context). Leibniz may well be said to have anticipated cognitive Psychology, but he was hardly its founder. Only the concept of 'apperception', never popular in Anglophone Psychology except among followers of German schools of thought, is completely Leibnizian – and that fell rapidly into disuse after 1900. On the other hand Leibniz's wider impact on the terms in which subsequent continental Psychological thought was conducted was considerable, especially as mediated by his follower Christian Wolff (1679–1754). While admitting an initiatory role for Leibniz, we still need to assess how far his uses of these concepts corresponded to their later Psychological uses.

The answer to this second question is not difficult – all these concepts derive their Leibnizian meanings from their places in his system as a whole, and if any philosophical system has been genuinely original and unique it was this one. The concept of the unconscious, or unconscious*ness*, may serve to illustrate this. The most accessible account is in his *New Essays on the Human Understanding* (a riposte to Locke not published until 1765). He begins unexceptionably enough by observing:

> . . . there are a thousand signs which make us think that there are at all times an infinite number of *perceptions* in us, though without apperception and without reflexion; that is to say changes in the soul itself which we do not apperceive because their impressions are either too small and too numerous, or too unified, so that they have nothing sufficiently distinctive in themselves, though in combination with others they do not fail to have their effect and to make themselves felt, at least confusedly, in the mass. (1973 edn, p. 155)

This is illustrated by the oft-cited examples of habituation to the sound of a mill or a waterfall, and the fusion of noises of individual waves in the general sound of the 'roar or noise which strikes us when we are on the shore'. There is nothing especially obscure about this, but in the following paragraph these unconscious *petites perceptions* begin to acquire a deeper significance:

> They it is that constitute the indefinable something, those tastes, those images of the qualities of the senses, clear in the mass but confused in the parts, those impressions which surrounding bodies make on us, which include the infinite, that link which connects every being with all the rest of the universe. (*ibid.*, p. 156)

It is these 'insensible perceptions' which actually characterize the individual, connecting 'his previous states' with his present one; they 'can be known by a superior spirit, even though the individual himself may not be conscious of them'; and moreover:

> But they . . . also provide the means of rediscovering this recollection at need through periodic developments which may one day occur. This is why, because of them, death can only be a sleep, and cannot even go on being that, since, in animals, the perceptions only cease to be sufficiently distinguished and become reduced to a state of confusion which suspends animation, but which cannot last forever – not to speak here of man, who must have in this great privileges in order to retain his personality. (*ibid.*, p. 157)

Not until Jung in his most metaphysical moments would the unconscious again be so infused with cosmic portents. The Leibnizian unconscious is incomprehensible unless we take into account its place in his 'monadology', his philosophical-cum-cosmological system as a whole, only then can we fathom what is meant by a passage such as 'the perceptions only cease to be sufficiently distinguished and become reduced to a state of confusion which suspends animation'. It is these unconscious perceptions, after all, which, he tells us, explain:

> that wonderful pre-established harmony of soul and body, and indeed of all monads or simple substances, which takes the place of the untenable theory of the influence of the one on the other . . . (*ibid.*)

Simply to pluck out the opening, uncontroversial, phenomenological observation that we are affected by sensations of which we are unaware as a profound insight separable from what follows is surely to distort what unconsciousness means here. In Leibniz's exposition this opening observation, in itself relatively superficial, serves merely as an entrée into far more profound issues.

But to unravel the entire 'monadology' coherently is the tallest of orders. The 'pre-established harmony' or 'mind–body parallelism' position which Leibniz espouses is, *prima facie*, among the least appealing of doctrines on this perennial issue, and the one which it is hardest to explain convincingly within the constraints of a non-specialist text. Yet, as we have just seen, Leibniz's 'unconscious' is an integral part of his system, supporting the parallelist doctrine. The notion of the 'monad' is even more resistant to succinct exposition, fusing the properties of atom, geometrical point, and unit of consciousness. To understand it requires a study of Leibniz's writings on logic as well as his metaphysics. And overarching the whole intellectual edifice there remains a theological goal, congruent with his political-diplomatic aspirations to heal the Catholic–Protestant breach.

If the 'unconscious' cannot be detached from its context, neither can any other of Leibniz's influential psychological ideas; each turns out, on inspection, to derive its meaning from its role within the whole philosophical system. This dependency goes beyond that which we now appreciate holds between any scientific concept and its theoretical context. We are not dealing here with a *scientific* theory, wherein the relevant meanings of terms may be articulated by some operational procedures; we are dealing with a self-contained and non-empirically based cosmology. Freud's 'unconscious' may be different in meaning to Jung's or Helmholtz's, but such differences can be specified within the context of a broader framework – namely, that they arise within would-be 'scientific' accounts of the psychological generated according to some implicit (however hazy) common criteria. They are moves in a common game of 'scientific theorizing'. In Leibniz, by contrast, they are generated as moves in a quite different game – the game of metaphysically constructing a complete, rational, cosmological system; and this is a game which Enlightenment scientists and their successors came to eschew as incompatible with their own.

Even Klein, who provides one of the best synopses of Leibniz's psychological thought, has obvious difficulty in presenting his role in other than retrospective and very general terms: his view of the mind as active, his holistic 'organic' orientation and the notion of an unconscious level to mental life. But none of these bears disciplinary fruit until the nineteenth century after over a century of collective rumination by German philosophers. Thus Leibniz's admitted influence on Psychology cannot be construed apart from its complex mediation via later thinkers, and nor does it signify that he himself was in any sense a 'Psychologist'.

IX SEVENTEENTH CENTURY PSYCHOLOGY: A REVISED VERSION

Changes in our conceptions of ourselves occur as responses to changes in our experience of the world around us, of which the social world constitutes the major, but not the only, part. When novelty of experience extends throughout a culture, so the very terms in which psychological discourse is conducted change. Such novelties of experience continuously befell the inhabitants of Europe throughout the seventeenth century. Civil War, the Thirty Years War, regicide, new ideas and new discoveries, changes in the social order and changes in the economic system – the encounter with the novel was unrelenting. It is against this background that developments in psychological ideas must ultimately be understood. In 1601 Philemon Holland translated Pliny's *Natural History*, and in it we find this description of the brain:

> And in truth, it is the fort and castle of all the sences, into it all the veines from the heart do tend: in it they all do likewise end. It is the very highest keep, watchtower, and sentinell of the mind: it is the helme and rudder of intelligence and understanding. (Book II, xxxvii, p. 333)

A little later, as we saw above, Bacon depicts the soul as a sovereign prince whose affairs are being managed by a bureaucracy of the faculties and senses. By 1684 the imagery has changed yet further:

> Having hitherto continued the former Tract of the oblong Marrow, which as it were the Kings High-way, leades from the Brain, as the Metropolis, into many Provinces of the nervous stock, by private recesses and cross-ways, it follows now that we view the other City of the animal Kingdom. The situation of this being remote enough from the former, its kind of structure is also different from it; yea it seems that there are granted to this, as to a free and municipal City, certain Priviledges and a peculiar Jurisdiction. (Willis, 1684, p. 90)

The castle yields to Renaissance bureaucracy, and this in turn to the 'metropolis' and the 'free and municipal City'. Behind this change lies much more than simply an increase in anatomical knowledge, for each metaphor, suitably elaborated, could have continued to serve as well. It signifies, rather, a change in the worlds in which the writers are living.

The impact of novelty is not always immediate, however, especially novelties of human behaviour. Here there is always the problem of how one talks about it. As Hodgen (1964) has demonstrated in her study of early anthropology, accounts of alien cultures persisted in assimilating foreign religious and cultural institutions into European terms, partly for the want of any alternative vocabulary. An admittedly early example is Richard Eden on Calcutta, who tells us (translating Muenster): 'the King hath in his Chappell the image of this devyl Deumi, sytting with a diademe or crowne on his head, much lyke unto the myter which the Romayne Bishoppes weare' (1553) (Hodgen, p. 195). As she says, 'when abroad, their eyes saw no more than their minds, shaped at home, were prepared to accept' (p. 184). Differences were defined negatively, by what 'savages' or 'heathens' lacked, actually perceiving the genuinely novel and creating a language in which to refer to it was an achievement which, in the field of anthropology, arguably took several centuries. And it was achieved primarily by incorporating into English the actual terms used by members of those cultures – something English was particularly good at, for reasons previously mentioned. English was pre-adapted to being an ideal imperialist language. The point of more immediate concern is that encounters with the novel are significant only if they are experienced as such. Encountering foreign cultures was, paradoxically, not an area where this was particularly evident; Renaissance travellers were already freighted with a vast repertoire of stereotypes and images, dating back to Antiquity, regarding what they might expect to meet. Notwithstanding the efforts of Bulwer and Tyson, even as late as 1724 the 'blemmys', with its face on its chest, appears in a plate (from a French work) depicting North American Indians (having presumably emigrated from Libya, where Isidore of Seville had placed them over a millennium previously)[49]. The impact of encounters with alien cultures was initially more profoundly felt at a theological level than a psychological one, raising as it did questions about the origins of such peoples and the state of their souls: How exactly did the sons of Noah succeed in peopling the Earth? How could a just God eternally damn peoples who had never heard the gospel? The significance of such discoveries for us therefore lies in their input into (a) the intensifying climate of doctrinal doubt and controversy, undermining old cosmological and theological certainties; and (b) the general European development of the 'civilization' versus 'savagery' polarity into a fundamental construct – the source, Daniel Defert (1982) claims, of the nature–culture distinction itself in Western social thought. The impact of novelty on reflexive discourse need not, therefore, be direct or immediate, and in the period under discussion it was frequently neither.

In this chapter I have been trying to do two things: first, I have been attempting to clear the ground for a revised approach to the role of the seventeenth century in the history of Psychological thought. All the major orthodoxies on this matter appear to be seriously flawed, at least in their present forms, by a retrospective ascription to the major philosophers of the period of interests, aims and attitudes analogous to those of contemporary Psychologists, their major failing being a methodological one. On the contrary, it appears that their prevailing interests were either theological or political, and that their statements on psychological matters were invariably manoeuvres within the theological-cum-political arena or normative moral discourse. Even the 'mechanization of the mind', a ubiquitous theme in orthodox histories, turns out to have been a very much more left-handed affair than is generally appreciated, and its pioneers to have been other than those normally named. If the usual account is rejected, then an alternative must needs be proposed.

My second task, then, has been to suggest directions in which an alternative account could be developed. To this end I have identified a number of facets to the overall process of psychological change during this period which in turn affected the nature of psychological discourse: (a) the 'epistemization' of the mind adumbrated in Bacon and culminating in Locke; (b) the 'mechanization' of psychological language mediated via the use of novel 'scientific' concepts by physiologists; (c) the move towards rational analytic styles of discourse which entailed an 'atomistic' concept of mental phenomena as reducible to quasi-corpuscular 'ideas' and 'sensations'; (d) the move (of which the previous change was part) from faith to reason-orientated discourse and the aspiration, in Britain at least, towards the creation of a 'Rational Religion'; and finally (e) the evolution of the concept of the 'private' – of the authenticity and value of the individual's own vision of the world, and their responses to it.

From this point of view, no single central tap-root of Psychology is present in the seventeenth century, but there is a range of one-off, discrete anticipations of specific realms of Psychological enquiry, both within and outside the texts in the orthodox canon. These nearly always failed to initiate continuous traditions of enquiry and contributed little to the development of the modern enquiries they anticipated (with the possible exception of theories of perception). With Locke the ball appears to be firmly in the philosopher's court, and as we will see the following century saw a great efflorescence of philosophical texts on the nature of mind.

Ideally, the next step would be a detailed linguistic investigation into the changing terms in which reflexive discourse was conducted over the century from Bacon to Locke. Modern Psychology emerged from – and is a particular form of – reflexive discourse, but the latter is universal and a superordinate category. My tentative hypothesis regarding this historical phase – the end of the seventeenth century – is that the World Language novelties being forged by Natural Philosophy were becoming too technical for physiomorphic assimilation in the usual way by the linguistic community as a whole. The reflexive exploration of these innovations as images of the psychological came to require an expertise comparable to that of the Natural Philosophers themselves. (Hooke's theory of memory is a particularly illuminating case here.) But such a reflexive exploration was inhibited by deeply held assumptions about the nature of language – an acceptance of the spirit, if not the 'character', of Wilkins's strange masterpiece. The only available route was via physiology. By the beginning of the eighteenth century, then, we have a situation where the central philosophical issue has become epistemology and a distinctively philosophical *method* of rational analysis has emerged, separate from (if remaining related to) both theology and 'Natural Philosophy'. At the same time ordinary psychological language is being infiltrated with new terms derived from physiology, Natural

Philosophy, and Lockean philosophy. It is from this complex matrix that Psychology will eventually emerge, but neither in total nor in part does it yet constitute even a neonate discipline.

Psychological texts can be read in two ways: as examples of the discipline and as examples of its subject matter. The present chapter is not meant to imply that Bacon, Descartes, Hobbes and Locke should no longer be included in the history of Psychology, what it is recommending is a switch in their mode of construal from 'discipline' to 'subject matter'. That is to say, they are primarily significant as evidence for the earlier state of our subject matter rather than for the earlier state of our discipline. They – and their non-canonical contemporaries – are offering us their *reflections* on the human condition, and the directions from which they are conducting these reflections testify to the nature of contemporary psychology, in the subject matter sense, as do the terms in which they couch them. And whatever the truth about the origins of our Psychology in the seventeenth century, regarding our psychology there can be no doubt that the descent is continuous. To subordinate the history of Psychology to the history of psychology seems a more promising and genuinely Psychological project than continuing an antiquarian hunt for disciplinary origins and false starts (though that, too, is part of the story).

Our tentative 'revised version' of the seventeenth century sees its central movement as a shift in the prevailing cultural modes of reflexive discourse from the 'moral' and 'religious' to the 'rational' and epistemological. This change arises from two complementary features of the political, economic and cultural legacy of the previous century: the collapse of religious doctrinal unity and the emergence of a rigorously rational mode of discourse in the proto-scientific and mathematical work of such figures as Galileo, Kepler and Bacon. As religious dissension heightens, the virtuosi of reason across Europe seek increasingly radical intellectual (but also, they hoped, applicable) solutions to problems of religious doctrine and civil order, with the latter progressively taking priority over the former. This is very different from the quest for solutions to problems of individual deviance which Rose (1987) sees as central to the discipline's emergence in the nineteenth century. In Britain, as Natural Philosophy becomes a cultural force after the Restoration, religious modes of discourse come under increasing pressure from rational and 'mechanistic' modes, a compromise eventually being reached in Latitudinarian Rational Religion in the 1690s. This involves a psychological recentring in the 'understanding' as opposed to faith or belief, a move reinforced by the emergence of the 'private'.

Translated to the European mainland at the end of the century, the secular English approach triggers a vehemently anti-clerical and anti-establishment philosophical movement in France, where Catholic orthodoxy remained supreme and uncompromised. The English compromise solution left British philosophers for the most part well within the pale until the last years of the eighteenth century, while in France they adapted Lockean philosophical doctrines to increasingly revolutionary and social utopian ends. Following Leibniz, a German philosophical Rationalist tradition will steadily develop in the eighteenth century, but proto-Psychological thought and innovations in psychological ideas were effectively confined to Britain, France and the Netherlands throughout the seventeenth century. Any further elucidation of this will require integrating a much broader range of historical scholarship and primary texts than I have been able to undertake here.

Finally, for Psychology this period is significant (a) in seeing the first major conceptual struggles regarding basic psychological concepts such as Mind, Idea, Sensation, Soul, Passion and the like; (b) in seeing the first faltering moves towards the formulation of its present subject matter as a unified field of natural enquiry; and (c) in seeing the first, albeit scattered, examples of the kinds of enquiry we now term Psychological. By contrast, 'the mechanization of mind' and similar familiar ways of encapsulating the period would now appear to be fundamentally misleading.

PART TWO Psychological Ideas in the Eighteenth Century

. . . from the principles of the secular sciences to the foundations of religious revelation, from metaphysics to matters of taste, from music to morals, from the scholastic disputes of theologians to matters of trade, from the laws of prices to those of peoples, from natural law to the arbitrary laws of nations . . . everything has been discussed and analyzed, or at least mentioned.

Jean Le Rond d'Alembert [1759]

Introduction

If the seventeenth century story moves the foci of reflexive discourse from faith to knowledge, theology to philosophical analysis, and soul to body, the eighteenth continues the momentum towards a more unified 'Science of Man'; although even by 1800 it still lacked any clear disciplinary embodiment. Hume, in 1739, parcelled out the field between Logic, Morals, Criticism and Politics, in which were 'comprehended almost every thing which it can any way import us to be acquainted with, or which can tend either to the improvement or ornament of the human mind' (*A Treatise of Human Nature*, p. xx) (and note the absence of physiology from this list). These are, conventionally, all humanities rather than sciences. At the century's end there did emerge two – now scorned – embryonic Psychological disciplines of continental origin, Lavater's physiognomy and Gall's phrenology, while an infant discipline of anthropology had also, by then, become established. But as Fox (1987) demonstrates, the contexts in which psychological issues were addressed were numerous and intersecting: 'physics and natural philosophy, metaphysics, moral philosophy, logic, pneumatology, physiology, medicine, literature, aesthetics and criticism' (p. 12) – a list to which he promptly adds rhetoric, education and pharmacology. Partly for this reason, the problem of retrospectively projecting contemporary categories becomes even more acute than in the seventeenth century, but partly, too, because the apparently increasing modernity of the vocabulary is treacherously deceptive (not least with respect to 'psychology').

This variety of contexts also highlights a more immediate problem: a full unravelling of the web of eighteenth-century psychological thought seems to require a daunting level of multidisciplinary historical expertise. The previous century is just about manageable, and in the ensuing one the salient developments are visible enough to provide some relatively secure landmarks from the outset. In the eighteenth century, however, we are challenged, in Britain alone, to range from Johnson's *Dictionary* to Whytt's physiology, from

Hume to Pope, from madness to political philosophy, from Sterne to Priestley, not forgetting the changing nature of marriage, if we are to do our theme justice. Since such an exercise would require a multidecker work of Victorian proportions, what follows must be read as no more than a preliminary survey.

Beneath this heterogeneous surface there remains the linguistic issue of how psychological ideas are to be generated within a Natural Philosophical context. It was argued in Chapter 1 that a major inhibiting factor for the emergence of Psychology, a 'Science of Mind', was the dominance of the Hobbes–Wilkins concept of language. This issue provides us with a basis for analysing, in a deeper, more generalized way, the continued failure of eighteenth-century thinkers to create such a discipline. The first chapter of this part is thus devoted to language rather than, as would usually be the case, to philosophy.

Another point of entry is the notion of 'Natural Law'. Philosophers had long talked of God ruling by 'laws of nature', but the use of the term to refer to a specific, empirically determined, regularity discovered by a 'scientist' (Hooke, in fact) seems to date from 1678[1]. But by the middle of the next century, 'the concept of a physical law of nature had become one of those most basic of all concepts, which apparently require no metaphysical justification for their use and which are therefore employed with complete confidence'[2]. The aspiration to apply this central Natural Philosophical concept to the human realm exercised thinkers across Europe, and in Britain had been an explicit element in the 'Natural Religion' orthodoxy (based on elaborated versions of the 'Argument from Design') formulated following the Williamite settlement by such figures as the Boyle lecturer William Derham[3]. Numerous treatises and philosophical disquisitions extended the concept of Natural Law not only to the operations of the mind itself but also to subjects as varied as aesthetics, ethics, the rise of civilization, madness, character, economics and education. From the physiological direction came pioneering studies of the nervous system and the senses. The theological dimension to such work continued to wane as the perceived adequacy of the 'Natural Law' framework of analysis increased (though Berkeley represents a counter-movement to this). Theological issues were nevertheless still prominent during the first third of the century and religious or moral philosophical aims continued even thereafter to underpin perhaps the majority of 'Psychological' discourse. In Britain in the 1790s religious anxieties returned in full force, profoundly affecting writings on education, for example (see Chapter 4), but in France the secularizing trend continued after the Revolution and into the Napoleonic period.

There were numerous underlying tensions. Accumulating knowledge in the physical sciences began to set constraints on proto-Psychological studies, while growing cross-cultural data gathered in the course of European imperial expansion pointed in a relativistic direction at odds with efforts to demonstrate the 'natural' and 'lawful' character of the European cultural status quo. The implications of such data could (as in Rousseau) be read as supporting conclusions radically subversive of the existing social order. Eventually the cerebral orientation towards matters psychological, which had dominated British and much European thought since Locke, collapsed in the face of Romanticism and German *Naturphilosophie* – and although the situation had been largely recouped by the 1830s, Romanticism had enormously enriched the agenda, and the blithe intellectual self-confidence of the doyens of the 'Age of Reason' was never recaptured. But though the existence of such self-confident doyens is not in question, it is questionable how real the 'Age of Reason' really was. Stock (1982) has argued for a persistently active 'irrationalist' literary tradition – or at least preoccupation with the 'holy and dæmonic' – in Britain from Glanville (1681) on witches to the Gothic novel and Blake. It is surely worth querying how far this label (along with 'Enlightenment') is itself a positivist retrojection of a lost golden age when Reason reigned supreme. It would be more judicious to accept that the cultural tension between the two sides was endemic and of long standing. While it is customary to identify a polarity between British 'Empiricists' and continental 'Rationalists' as emerging in eighteenth-century philosophy, this is obviously an oversimplification. Not only – as Norton (1981) has shown – were the leading British philosophers fundamentally indebted to Gassendi and Malebranche, but Cassirer (1934) portrays a complex and continuous Europe-wide renegotiation going on regarding epistemological fundamentals, a process with numerous dialectical twists and turns. Here we are only peripherally concerned with this.

How have historians of Psychology interpreted this period? In some respects the eighteenth century presents something of an embarrassment, for having announced the 'mechanization of mind' and the advent of an empirical approach to psychological issues at the end of the previous century, they are faced with the fact that no Psychological research of an experimental character, no (even quasi-scientific) discipline, and no unambiguously identifiable 'Psychologist' appear in the canon to follow up this supposed breakthrough. This is, though, an embarrassment but rarely confronted, and masked by presenting, once again, the pantheon of great and not-so-great philosophers – Berkeley, Condillac, Hartley, Hume, Hutcheson, Kant, La Mettrie, Leibniz, Reid, Stewart and Wolff – as jointly constituting some kind of coherent proto-Psychological lineage. Now certainly in many cases – notably those of Hume, Hutcheson, Hartley and the Scottish Enlightenment philosophers in Britain and La Mettrie, Condillac, Bonnet and Cabanis in France and Tetens in Germany – we are dealing with discourses far less removed from modern Psychological concerns than those of the previous century. It is also true that the Lockean image of mind and the more evolved Associationist and sensationalist philosophies which elaborated his 'new way of Ideas' served as the intellectual reference point for those treating of psychological matters; either they explored the applicability of this orientation in areas of human experience beyond epistemology (e.g. Edmund Burke and, more directly, Archibald Alison [1790] with regard to aesthetics[4]) or they sought to counter the more sceptical implications of such an approach (especially the Humean version). This latter could take the form of alternative 'common-sense' accounts, based nevertheless on varieties of empirical enquiry (Reid and Stewart) or, in the case of Germany, transcendental or rationalist philosophies (see Chapter 7 below). The question 'why no Psychology in the eighteenth century?' is, I acknowledge distinct from that of how the psychological was conceptualized at this time. The first is really a 'presentist' issue, but in the context of disciplinary history we are bound to ask why there is an almost complete absence (neurology barely excepted) of experimental research on psychological or behavioural matters. Not only are we entitled to ask – unless we arrive at an answer, we are likely to be handicapped in addressing the second question.

Technology alone was no barrier – many basic experiments on learning, perception and reaction time, or such techniques as questionnaires and observational diaries of child development, require no exotic technologies beyond those available in Georgian England (indeed, Honora Edgeworth *did* keep a child-development diary of sorts). The impression usually given is that this virtual absence is either due to philosophical arguments that the mind was inaccessible to such investigation, or that somehow it simply never occurred to anybody that it was necessary to go beyond common experience for empirical evidence to support 'Psychological' theories. The former, powerfully stated by Kant, has a degree of validity for the latter end of the century and remained influential until around the 1840s (even so, Britain's earliest Kant enthusiast, Samuel Taylor Coleridge, did not accept it). It is not significantly present as an argument before Kant and in Britain, at any rate, the dominant philosophies remained non-Kantian. On the contrary, the idea of a 'Science of Man' or 'Mind' was being widely propounded, and 'Psychology' was included in some texts (see Fox, 1987, p. 3) under the heading 'Physiology', which itself turns out to include most of the physical sciences including astronomy and 'chymistry'. (Such categorizations perhaps raise problems for the meaning of the category 'Science' in general in the eighteenth century, but that is by the by.) If Cavendish could weigh the Earth, the learning curve of a rat would have presented no difficulty. A better explanation is that writers on psychological matters at this time were simply not addressing the questions which lent themselves in any obvious way to systematic empirical research. They were not, *contra* Schultz (1975), asking the same kinds of questions as modern Psychologists but using different methods (nor, as Jaynes [1973] has it, are we dealing with 'a continuing discussion of the perennial and enduring problems of human and animal nature'). They were asking different questions. They might for example, like Burke, ask the question of how our ideas of the Sublime and the Beautiful originate – a question which both arises, and is to be answered, within the terms of the analytical philosophical Lockean 'paradigm'. Why, though, were their questions different?

A more recent, and plausible, explanation propounded by Nikolas Rose (1985, 1990a) (and implicit in Foucault-influenced texts such as Shotter [1990]), is that it was only during this period that a concept of self-contained, self-regulating, (or 'possessive' [Shotter]) individuality evolved, which provided the basis for a discipline focusing on the unitary individual conceptually detachable from social context. This is part and parcel of the rise of the modern bureaucratic state with its needs for surveillance, data-gathering and managerial control of the population. This in turn requires the formulation of categories for classifying or 'inscribing' individuality – and also techniques for reproducing, via socialization, this self-regulating personality. Such a new individuality contrasts with an earlier mode appropriate to a society where control was autocratically imposed by a more or less absolute ruler, and also with more 'socially embedded' modes of individuality characteristic of other cultures. (The Stock Exchange motto 'My Word is My Bond' perhaps typifies one contemporary expression of this shift.) The discipline of Psychology is thus seen as originating in needs to control the deviant, marginal and disruptive elements of the population (the criminal, the insane, 'idiots' and, in a different sense, children). While we should not reject such a thesis out of hand – indeed it provides an essential contextualizing dimension to the story – the mystery is not entirely solved by it. Not all Psychology, after all, is about social control, classification and monitoring of this kind (for example the study of memory and perception, and much of the study of emotion too). Given that the rhetorical advocacy of a Science of Man or of the Mind dates back at least to Bacon, and was prominent in the work of Enlightenment philosophers of all schools, its failure to materialize remains puzzling. What was hampering the creation of new 'Psychological' ideas and concepts? It is in order to clarify this that an examination of the language issue proves so crucial.

In considering the eighteenth century, we are examining what Kurt Danziger has called the 'prehistory' of Psychology, at the close of which we discern for the first time the possibility of something like a scientific Psychology being realized. But the trek towards it was laborious. To bring some semblance of order to the variety of concerns feeding into the repertoire of psychological ideas, I have organized this part into chapters dealing with the following topics. First, as I have explained, I consider the various concepts of language itself which determined the linguistic conditions governing the possibility of generating new 'Psychological' ideas within a scientific context. Only secondly do I turn to the impact of philosophy, generally given pride of place in (if not actually monopolizing) orthodox accounts. This chapter will include discussion of the impact of political and social philosophy (which eventually merge into anthropology). Thirdly, I look at a wider range of topics, including developments in physiology and medicine (especially psychiatry), attitudes to sex and educational thought, areas where 'human management' problems began to manifest themselves. Finally in this part, I will attempt to sum up the evidence that has been reviewed and suggest some of its implications for future history of Psychology research. In proceeding on to the nineteenth century, however, it will be necessary first to consider Mesmerism, Lavater's physiognomy and Gall's phrenology. In their various ways, each of these served the kind of cultural role which Psychology subsequently assumed. In their origins they are all eighteenth-century, but the impact of phrenology and Mesmerism was felt mainly in the nineteenth. Phrenology in particular is a complex and fairly long-lived phenomenon, and its evaluation carries us into the 1840s. Fuller discussion of the German philosophical tradition is reserved until Part Three to facilitate a more unified treatment of the developments centring around Kant.

2

The Vehicle of Conjecture: Ideas of Language from Locke to Tooke

> . . . nothing could more effectually contribute to the benefit and glory of this country, than to bring the English language to as great a degree of perfection, stability, and general use, as those of Greece and Rome.
>
> (Thomas Sheridan [1769], pp. 222–3)

> The language of mind . . . is not peculiar, not derived as the nomenclature of modern chemistry, in which names are impregnated with elements of their composition; but figurative or metaphorical, the vehicle of conjecture, and the ornament of hypotheses.
>
> (John Haslam [1819], p. 61)

That language was the hallmark of 'Man' and signified his proclivity for a social existence were commonplaces throughout our period. Its origins and nature, though, were riddles which engaged almost every serious thinker sooner or later[1]. In attempting to account for the nature of language, eighteenth-century thinkers produced a variety of theories, and voiced a variety of attitudes, regarding its relationship to thought, its origins, and its metaphysical significance. Our concern here focuses on but one aspect of this, the nature of what I am calling Psychological Language. Locke and his eighteenth-century successors were not unaware of a problem here, but a satisfactory solution continued to elude them. We may retrospectively identify four principal schools of linguistic thought in the period from 1700 to about 1830, although such an identification inevitably obscures the unique features of individual accounts – and the function of this classification is, I must stress, to be understood as limited to serving the exposition of the matter in hand. Indeed one of the peculiarly frustrating aspects of attempting to explore the issue is that while, as Land (1986) states, linguistic thought during this period was 'centrally concerned with the problem of the relation of language to mind' (p. 238), the origin of psychological concepts as such receives little direct attention. It is this very absence for which I am of course attempting to account. Furthermore, *contra* Chomsky, Land fails to find any 'clearcut distinction of empirical and rational theories of language in this period' (p. 195). The provisional, pragmatic nature of the ensuing classification is thus unavoidable.

The first of these, stemming from Locke and proceeding through the French philosopher Condillac and David Hartley to Horne Tooke, may be called the 'Materialist Sensationalist' school. The second, identified with those in philosophical reaction against Locke, includes Thomas Reid, Lord Monboddo and James Harris, and ends with a kind of recantation by Dugald Stewart. This I will call the 'Structuralist' school, in view of their belief in underlying innate principles of grammar. A third lineage, with its source in Condillac, may be termed the Romantic school, and goes through Rousseau and Herder to Coleridge. The fourth, 'Literary' school, includes Swift, Samuel Johnson and Thomas Sheridan.

I argue here that none of these produced an account of language congenial to the generation of novel psychological terms in a 'scientific' context. In its final transformations the Materialist Sensationalist approach did, however, serve to inspire a more nearly 'scientific' approach by the late Associationists (for example James Mill). The 'Structuralists' remained constrained within the limits of existing folk-psychological language, albeit elaborating and systematizing it. The Romantics, while expanding PL, did so outside the framework of a formal scientific discipline (though Coleridge, as we shall see, is an exception). The Literary school accepted PL innovation up to a point, but their programme was essentially a conservative one of disciplining what they saw as linguistic chaos and returning the tongue to earlier standards of stylistic rigour. All schools tended to accept the basic psychological uniformity and immutability of Mankind, although Romanticism began to move away from this. Given that their accounts of language are framed within the terms of this premiss, the absence of attention to PL innovation may seem unproblematic, this however is to put the cart before the horse, since one might expect linguistic investigation itself to raise the issue in its own right. The question is thus why none of their investigations did in fact do so, at least in the terms which interest us here.

1 Materialist Sensationalists

The initial Natural Philosophical view of language as it emerged from the writings of Hobbes, Wilkins and others in the seventeenth century was considered at some length in the previous chapter. In brief, it assumed that words corresponded in a direct fashion to the natural – we might say 'objective' – categories of phenomena in the world. As far as PL was concerned, it failed to recognize any special problems, tending to accept traditional classifications of psychological phenomena uncritically as naming natural categories in the same way as all other uses of language. Errors arose from the irresponsible use of figurative language, rhetorical mystification, failures to define words clearly in terms of the phenomena they signified, and so on. It was argued that this 'univalent' concept of meaning greatly inhibited PL change in the Natural Philosophy arena precisely because such change involves the figurative application to the psychological of novel terms and concepts, a process incompatible with the reforming vision of Hobbes and Wilkins.

This view of language was largely accepted by Locke, whose own vocabulary was fairly ascetic. Although Locke's *Essay* does not accept Wilkins's scheme for a universal grammar and 'character', it is pervaded by a concern with the potentially misleading properties of language and a rejection of metaphorical rhetoric (Bennington, 1987)[2]. Linguistic reform, Locke believes, may be effective only within philosophical discourse itself. Both Condillac and, later, Horne Tooke read the *Essay* as basically a linguistic treatise. On the issue concerning us here however, Locke readily acknowledged the metaphorical nature of psychological terms, but this evinced no anxiety in him regarding the status of psychological concepts. The key, oft quoted, passage occurs in Book III, Chapter 1, section 5, headed 'Words ultimately derived from such as signify sensible ideas':

> It may also lead us a little towards the original of all our notions and knowledge, if we remark how great a dependence our words

> have on common sensible ideas; and how those which are made use of to stand for actions and notions quite removed from sense, have their rise from thence, and from obvious sensible ideas are transferred to more abstruse significations, and made to stand for ideas that come not under the cognizance of our senses: v.g., [sic] to *imagine, apprehend, comprehend, adhere, conceive, instil, disgust, disturbance, tranquillity*, &c., are all words taken from the operations of sensible things, and applied to certain modes of thinking. *Spirit*, in its primary signification is breath; *angel*, a messenger: and I doubt not but, if we could trace them to their sources, we should find, in all languages, the names which stand for things that fall not under our senses to have had their first rise from sensible ideas. By which we may give some kind of guess what kind of notions they were, and whence derived, which filled their minds who were the first beginners of languages; and how nature, even in the naming of things, unawares suggested to men the originals and principles of all their knowledge.

On the face of it, this is remarkably close to the theoretical position underlying the present work. The problem arises in the final – admittedly rather opaque – clause, which seems to imply pre-existing 'originals and principles' which we came, naturally, to recognize as a result of a 'suggestion' by sensible ideas. As well as ascribing a core fixed character to mind, this basically passive image ignores the possibility that even in the present we may be encountering novel sensible ideas – ought, even, to seek them out – which would serve as input for the same process. The major difficulty with this account is that it conceives of the process as involving (a) the experience of a psychological event/phenomenon; (b) the identification of an analogous public phenomenon; (c) the use of the name of the latter to name the former – for which it is appropriate by virtue of its self-evident analogical resemblance. This obscures the possibility that the psychological is itself initially experienced in terms of the public, that there is an active, structuring process going on in which the psychological is being rendered meaningful as well as communicable by such equations. In Locke the psychological remains a realm separate from the linguistic (and the public) for language to refer *to*, not a realm created by language out of the public. The psychological stays, in some sense, formally fixed, even if its contents are derived from experience. As we saw in Chapter 1, Locke was far from accepting a *tabula rasa* account of the origins of Reason itself. Even less did he seem to spot that the entire language of sensible ideas is in principle capable of usage to 'stand for ideas that come not under our senses' (which includes all psychological ideas)[3].

The task, as Lockean philosophers saw it, became to carry the sensationalist analysis of the origin of ideas through to its limit, accounting for the origin of the most apparently abstract 'ideas of reflection', the categories referring to those mental operations themselves, which Locke had left unaccounted for. Even for those wishing to privilege words over ideas, ideas pre-existed the words for them. We use words to name ideas, and for non-sensible ideas we somehow analogically apply words coined to name sensible ones. For us this was something of a side-tracking from the main implication of the situation – namely, that if references to consciousness are structured in terms of available 'sensible ideas' then so, to all intents and purposes, must consciousness itself be so structured. How an idea can be said to exist before its naming is not clearly considered. Such a tack would not, however, have recommended itself to those Empiricist sensationalists set on producing ever more rigorous materialist accounts. For them, the theory that psychological terms can be explained reductively as rooted in 'sensible ideas', physical sensations operating mechanistically, was tantamount to a materialist theory of mind.

The figure who most eagerly seized the opportunity of pursuing this line of thought to its logical conclusion was E.B. de Condillac (*c.* 1715–80). In his *Essai sur l'origine des connaissances humaines* (1746; English translation 1756) Condillac proposed an account of language origins of a kind which in some respects remained popular until quite recently[4]. Language, he argued, begins in gesture and natural expressive cries, but owing to their inherent superiority the latter gradually supplant the former as the primary medium. Human reflexive consciousness itself, which depends on memory, comes into being only when expressive gestures and calls [*les signes naturels*] begin to constitute '*signes d'institution*' (primarily words) – conventional signs *chosen* to refer, arbitrarily, to ideas (these initially being images of things not present):

> . . . aussitôt qu'un homme commence à attacher des idées à des signes qu'il lui-même choisit, on voit se former en lui la mémoire. (1798 edn, p. 85)
>
> (. . . as soon as a man begins to attach ideas to signs he chooses himself, one sees memory forming within him.)

While claiming that reflection is born from imagination and memory – which, once active, stimulates further imagination and memory – Condillac acknowledges a problem of priority; for the creation of '*signes d'institution*' does not seem possible unless reflection is already operating, while at the same time reflection itself seems to depend on the existence of such signs (*ibid.*, pp. 90-91). But having identified this chicken and egg problem, he remains confessedly unable to resolve it.

Concrete vocabularies precede abstract ones, and grammar comes to replace reliance on variations in intonation (though this was still present, Condillac believed, in Chinese). Hence the older a language, the more closely it approaches song (*ibid.*, p. 345). One factor affecting all such speculation was the relatively contracted time-scale on which thinkers were operating. Even if they were now happy to take rigid fundamentalist calculations of 4004 BC as the date of Creation with a pinch of salt, few could countenance anything approaching six-figure estimates, at least for the age of the human race. In writing his *Essai* Condillac was quite explicit that he was offering a supplement to Locke's *Essay*. By giving concrete vocabularies temporal precedence over abstract ones he was rendering the metaphorical genesis of psychological concepts a fundamentally necessary property of language. And he intepretes this as a basically materialist account, all the qualities of the soul, he tells us, being nothing but the effect of various

> états d'action et de passion par où elle passe, ou des habitudes qu'elle contracte, lorsqu'elle agit ou pâtit à plusieurs réponses. (*ibid.*, p. 372)
>
> (states of action and passion through which it passes, or habits which it acquires, when it performs or experiences [*lit.* suffers – the point is to contrast active and passive modes] various responses.)

Condillac's focus on the origins of language had a further effect:

it made the study of etymology appear to be a route towards understanding the nature of the mind and thought. This initiated a tradition of what Dugald Stewart, with reference to Adam Smith's *Considerations concerning the First Formation of Languages*, would later term 'conjectural history'. By tracing terms back to their origins we would be obtaining access to the modes of thought of our distant ancestors, enabling us to trace the way in which these modes changed over time (a move, note, which begins to undermine the belief in human nature's universal character and immutability). Such an assumption remained powerful throughout the rest of the century, receiving a serious challenge only in the 1820s, when Dugald Stewart, departing from Reid's views on language, attacking Horne Tooke (and perhaps taking on board Monboddo's position), argued that philological matters had no direct relevance to philosophical ones[5]. Ignoring Stewart, several eminent nineteenth-century linguists – the most influential being Max Müller – continued to view etymology as a study of thought[6].

Condillac's impact was ambiguous; on the one hand it marked a further expansion of Lockean materialist sensationalism (which Condillac had also espoused in his *Traité des Sensations* [English translation 1754], his famous thought-experiment of progressively endowing a statue with the various senses, starting with smell). On the other, as we will see, he also provided a starting point for the very different Romantic school. Three years after Condillac's *Essai*, a home-grown elaboration of the Lockean account of language appeared as part of Hartley's *Observations on Man* (1749), with particular emphasis on its associative character. This section of the *Observations* has attracted little attention, being overshadowed by his 'vibratiuncles' in histories of Psychology, but curiously. it is not noticed by Aarsleff (1983) either. Although Hartley adopts a 'party line' Associationist account, there are hints of difficulties; at one point he feels forced to admit: 'the Author perceives himself to be still a mere Novice in these Speculations; and it is difficult to explain Words to the Bottom by Words; perhaps impossible' (1749, p. 277). Even so, there is no significant departure from the notion that words are attached to 'Ideas' in a basically straightforward associationist fashion: 'Words and phrases must excite Ideas in us by Association, and they excite Ideas in us by no other means' (p. 268). Words exist at four levels, which represent the successive stages of their acquisition: as 'impressions' made on the ear, as 'actions of the organs of speech', as 'impressions made upon the eye by characters', and as actions of the hand in writing (*ibid.*). The child learns the meaning of the word 'Nurse' by associating the sound with the picture of the nurse upon the retina (p. 270) and

> . . . an Idea, or nascent Perception, of the Sweetness of the Nurse's Milk will rise up in that Part of the Child's Brain which corresponds to the Nerves of Taste, upon his hearing her Name. (p. 272)

Nevertheless, the process is not in reality quite so atomistic as this:

> . . . both Children and Adults learn the Ideas belonging to whole Sentences many times in a summary Way, and not by adding together the Ideas of the several Words in the Sentence. And where-ever Words occur, which, seperately taken, have no proper Ideas, their Use can be learnt in no other way but this. Now Pronouns, Particles and many other Words, are of this Kind. (p. 274)

Turning to psychological terms, Hartley sees no real difference in the acquisition process:

> . . . the Words that relate to the several Passions of Love, Hatred, Fear, Anger, etc being applied to the Child at the times when he is under the Influence of these Passions, get the Power of raising the Miniatures or Ideas of these Passions, and also of the usual associated circumstances . . . (p. 275)
>
> However, it is to be noted, that the Words denoting the Passions do not, for the most part, raise up in us any Degree of the Passions themselves, but only the Ideas of the associated Circumstances. (p. 276)

A word like 'dog' supposedly 'raises up' a 'Miniature', a picture-like representation of the class of objects to which it has become associated, but in the case of words denoting 'Passions', this is lacking – the word 'Love' does not raise up in us a miniature representational state of love, but only of the external circumstances to which we have learned to associate the term. Hartley does not recognize that this line of analysis, if pursued, would undermine the Associationist 'picture-theory' of meaning itself on which his whole concept of language rests. Nor does he recognize, as Peter Browne did (see below, pp. 137–139), that the very notion of having 'ideas' of psychological operations is paradoxical for a sensationalist epistemology. Rather, Hartley glosses over the issue somewhat hastily:

> The Names of intellectual and moral Qualities and Operations such as Fancy, Memory . . . stand for a Description of the Qualities and Operations; and therefore, if dwelt upon, excite such Ideas as these Descriptions in all their particular circumstances do. But the common Sentences, which these Words enter, pass over the Mind too quick, for the most part, to allow of such a Delay. (p. 276)

While this is almost within hailing distance of a Rylean 'dispositional' account of such terms, Hartley feels himself losing his bearings and makes the confession of his 'mere Novice' status quoted earlier. He now tries classifying words into those 'such as have Ideas only' (names of 'simple sensible Qualities', basically Locke's 'Ideas of Sensation'), those with both Ideas and Definitions (names of 'Natural Bodies' exciting 'aggregates of Sensible Ideas, and also geometrical figures), those with definitions only (e.g. 'Algebraic Quantities' such as 'Roots, Powers, Surds', and most 'abstract general terms'), and finally words with neither Ideas or Definitions such as the 'Particles'; 'the', 'of', 'to', 'for', 'but', etc. Of the third category, those with definitions only, he notes that some of these have 'mental emotions' 'apt to attend them' which may be considered as Ideas, and gives Gratitude, Mercy, Cruelty and Treachery as examples. It is nevertheless significant that Hartley feels bound to reject the view that *all* words are directly rooted in Sensible Ideas, but presumably the terms used in defining those in this third category would eventually lead one back to this source. From then on he reverts to a true Hobbesian model of language as a 'Species of Algebra'.

He further holds that if we made a dictionary in which words were precisely explained, we might eventually, 'with Care and Candour', 'come to understand one another' (p. 285). Clear echoes of Wilkins here, as in the ensuing reference to such a dictionary being 'a real as well as a nominal one' extended 'to things themselves'. Hartley, though, is less worried by figurative language, even if it can conceal 'Disparities' and magnify 'Resemblances' (pp. 296–7). He notes the way in which words shift from being figurative to literal over time (p. 292) and has no difficulty explaining this by association. The essentially figurative character of PL remains, even so, unappreciated.

Two things are immediately apparent from Hartley's discussion of language: first, the Hobbes/Wilkins orthodoxy remains basically intact with its 'picture theory' of meaning, notion of language as algebraic, belief in the prophylactic value of univalent definitions and the possibility of reforming language to ensure mutual understanding. Hartley also shared Wilkins's concern with written character (though not to the same obsessional pitch), advocating the virtues of John Byrom's shorthand system (not actually published until 1767). Secondly though, Hartley is far less confident and iconoclastic, and has pondered the way language actually operates sufficiently deeply to see difficulties being raised for this orthodoxy, even if he tends to evade rather than solve them. His is, in any case, a more comprehensive and philosophically sensitive account of language than either Hobbes or Wilkins actually provided. As far as the origin of language is concerned, Hartley was far less innovative than Condillac, retaining a belief in its Divine creation. The traditional religious view was that speech was Divine in origin; God had endowed Adam with this faculty and this unique legacy had been handed down ever since, though with the disruption of Babel the original pure Adamic language had been lost. Hartley actually buys only half this story: God taught Adam names by the 'use of the visible Appearances or Actions, or perhaps of the Several Cries of the Brute Creatures' (p. 297), but this language was narrow, applicable only to visible things, Adam was not 'capable of deep Speculations' (p. 298). This corresponds to the 'concrete'–'abstract' succession in Condillac, but is left unexplored. On this basis modern language could nevertheless develop: 'the Growth and Variations of a Language somewhat resemble the Increase of Money at Interest upon Interest' (*ibid.*).

The fortunes of this account of language go into decline from the 1750s on, as the Scottish 'Common Sense' school, and to a lesser degree Romanticism, come to dominate British philosophy and linguistic thought at Associationism's expense. In 1786, however, they were dramatically revived – in linguistics if not, immediately, in associationist philosophy at large – by Volume I of Horne Tooke's *Επεα Πτεροεντα, or the Diversions of Purley*, Volume II following in 1805, and a second edition of Volume I in 1798 (see

Aarsleff, 1983, on which the following account of Tooke is based). This work, in the form of a rambling trialogue, attempted a radical reduction of thought to language. This was Locke's true message, his *Essay* being not really on 'Understanding' but on language. For Tooke the function of language is accepted as being the communication of ideas, but a problem arises in matching the speed of communication to that of thought. Words are initially the signs of things (i.e. are all nouns or verbs, although Tooke's account of verbs apparently remained undeveloped). In order to speed verbal communication a new set of words, signs of other words, is developed, from which come all the other parts of speech: pronouns, prepositions, conjunctions, adjectives, etc. To carry this argument Tooke pitched into speculative etymology with unprecedented enthusiasm, deriving words such as *by, up, then,* etc., from nouns. His image of the origin of language begins with a fairly conventional gestural-origins story: gestures are gradually accompanied by interjections, vocal gestures, and these eventually become arbitrary signs: 'The dominion of Speech is erected upon the downfall of Interjections' (quoted in Aarsleff, *op. cit.*, p. 23). In this achievement humans finally gain reflective control over their mental processes, which otherwise proceed mechanistically. The mind is therefore entirely passive except in so far as we use language, and language itself is explicable materialistically as the outcome of nature, need and instinct; no divine or mysterious principle need be invoked to account for it. Ironically, the development of language has been a two-edged sword, for whilst it enhances communicative efficiency, the proliferation of abbreviations and abstractions by which this has been achieved has cut us off from its original clarity of expression, rendering us prey to metaphysical confusion.

In a way the mind disappears altogether in Tooke's account, its study replaced by the study of language. As far as PL is concerned the picture is pessimistic, because innovations in this area can be construed only as moving us yet deeper into the swamps of mystification. For Psychology, though, it served one useful purpose. Its appearance happened to coincide with a boom in interest in chemistry in the wake of Lavoisier, Priestley and Dalton. Tooke's method of etymological analysis for identifying elementary forms of language seemed to correspond very closely with that now employed by the chemists, being analytical yet not, like physics, mathematical. He was thus seen as opening up the possibility of studying the mind (via language) in a manner far closer to that of the natural sciences than had been possible hitherto. It was this which revived the torpid Associationist tradition, helping to convert it from philosophy into 'Mental Science' – a move in which the leading figures were to be Thomas Brown (though 'Associationist' sits a little awkwardly upon him) and James Mill.

Tooke's immediate impact was dramatic and he remained in high esteem until the 1830s, arguably stultifying British philology by comparison with that arising in Germany. He inspired a number of absurd works, such as Walter Whiter's three-volume *Etymologicon Universale* or *Universal Etymological Dictionary* (1822–25) and *Etymologicum Magnum* (1800), characterized, says Aarsleff, by a 'complete absence of even the most rudimentary common sense' (1983, p. 79) and Samuel Henshall's *Etymological Organic Reasoner* (1807), the author being in the eyes of one contemporary, 'an irrecoverable madman' (Aarsleff, *ibid.*, p. 77). Even Alexander Murray, whose *A History of the European Languages* (1823) was not without considerable merit, ventured to identify nine original short words from which all others ultimately derived, all implying 'power, motion, force, ideas united in every untutored mind' (quoted in Aarsleff, *ibid.*, p. 83)[7]. The great achievement of Sir William Jones – who, in 1786, demonstrated the kinship between Sanskrit and European languages – failed to bear immediate fruit in Britain, largely because of Tooke's steamrollering speculative approach to etymology.

In spite of the absurdities he inspired, and the damage he inflicted on British linguistics, Horne Tooke nevertheless marked a crucial turning point for Psychology:

> Here is the key to Tooke's persistent influence. Impressed by the success of Newtonian science, his age was eagerly trying to convert mental philosophy into a branch of natural philosophy, encouraged by the simple schemata of Hartley's association of ideas, Priestley's and Bentham's pleasure–pain principle, and etymology with its exploration of the 'causes of language'. (Aarsleff, 1983, p. 88)

A materialist Science of Mind again seems to be a distinct possibility, and people such as James Mill take up the challenge to realize it. Yet actual innovations in PL, genuinely novel Psychological ideas, remain inhibited, for the strategy now adopted is a kind of reductive deconstruction of the existing folk-psychology vocabulary into component quasi-atomic sensations or perceptions. Although terms such as *idea, sensation, feeling*, and the like may acquire a more technical character in this context, we search there in vain for the truly new[8].

2 The 'Structuralist' school

British philosophical reaction against Locke and his followers came most forcefully from Thomas Reid's 'Common Sense' school and other Scottish Enlightenment thinkers. These are discussed in more detail in Chapter 3, our concern here being restricted to their view of language. The central issue on which they differ is their belief that the mind contains certain innate, spiritual, active faculties which, defying further analysis, must be taken as given. In this context, language presents Reid with some difficulties. He is aware of the uniqueness of the individual's consciousness and the precariousness of mutual comprehension based on the use of psychological terms:

> There is no greater impediment to the advancement of knowledge than the ambiguity of words. ((*Essays on the Intellectual Powers of Man*, ed. Sir William Hamilton, p. 219)

But he also wishes to claim that the meanings of these terms are at once self-evident and indefinable:

> There is no subject in which there is more frequent occasion to use words that cannot be defined, than in treating of the powers and operations of the mind. The simplest operations of our minds must all be expressed by words of this kind. No man can explain, by a logical definition, what it is to *think*, to *apprehend*, to *believe*, to *will*, to *desire* . . . every man can form a clear and distinct notion of them; but they cannot be logically defined. (*ibid.*, p. 220)

On linguistic innovation in the mental realm, Reid is distinctly edgy:

> The language of philosophers, with regard to the original faculties of the mind, is so adapted to the prevailing system, that it cannot fit any other, like a coat that fits the man for whom it was made,

> and thus shows him to advantage, which yet will sit very awkward upon one of different make, although perhaps as handsome and well proportioned. It is hardly possible to make any innovation in our philosophy concerning the mind and its operations, without using new words and phrases, or giving a different meaning to those that are received – a liberty which, even when necessary, creates prejudice and misconstruction, and which must await the sanction of time to authorize it, for innovations in language, like those in religion and government, are always suspected and disliked by the many, till use hath made them familiar, and prescription given them a title.
> (*Inquiry into the Human Mind,* [1764] ed. Hamilton, pp. 98–99)

As Land (1986) observes, Reid's view of language shifted, under the influence of James Harris's work, from a more or less Lockean position in the *Inquiries* to a more stucturalist account in the *Essays*, in which the concern is with universals of linguistic structure. The upshot, in the opinion of some commentators (e.g. Grave, 1965), was that Reid ended by groping towards a rather modern pragmatic view of language. If so, such gropings progressed little before Stewart, with whom they finally ground to a halt. The commoner formulation was that words were the signs of ideas in a quite direct fashion, and were thus in some sense a picture of our thoughts. Since it was axiomatic that there was no fundamental difference between people concerning the nature of mind – that we all shared the same faculties, sensations, perceptions, etc – the study of language was underpinned by a quest for a 'universal grammar'.

This quest has an honourable ancestry, and was anticipated particularly by the French Port-Royal philosophers of the previous century, as well as by Leibniz, but we cannot enter here into this perennial linguistic theme (see Land, 1986). The implication for us is that such an approach promises to reveal the universal structure of the human mind via the study of grammar. Unlike the Condillac tradition, this is concerned not with language origins but with a more 'synchronous' (as it would now be termed) form of analysis. Nor, like the Lockean tradition approach, does it attempt to reduce psychological language to a language of quasi-material sensations, or to convert psychological issues into linguistic ones, but sees in linguistics a route towards psychological knowledge of a universal kind. For such thinkers the origins of language may still be considered as in some degree Divine, and certainly unaccountable for mechanistically. (The issue, in any case, raises questions about the universality axiom.) Language is a qualitatively unique human faculty with no precedent. The best example of a British text of this kind is perhaps the Aristotelian James Harris's *Hermes or a Philosophical Enquiry concerning Language and Universal Grammar* (1751). Influential in its time but generally considered mediocre by modern linguists, this can be taken, according to Land (*op. cit.*) as exemplifying the state of philosophical grammar in this period. An important feature is Harris's rejection of the Wilkins idea of language as a picture of the world. Words are symbols, not 'imitations':

> But now, while our Minds lie inveloped and hid, and the Body (like a Veil) conceals every thing but itself, we are necessarily compelled, when we communicate our Thoughts, to pass them to each other, *through a Medium which is corporeal* . . . If therefore we were to converse, not by *Symbols* but by *Imitations*, as far as things are characterized by Figure and Colour, our Imitation would be necessarily thro' Figure and Colour also . . . The like may be said of all the other Senses . . . We see then how *complicated* such Imitation would prove. (p.335)
> Hence we may perceive a Reason, *why there never was a Language, nor indeed can possibly be framed one, to express the Properties and real Essences of things, as a Mirrour exhibits their Figures and their Colours.* (p. 336) (original emphasis)

Now a language expressing the 'Properties and real Essences of things' was just what Wilkins had striven for, as well as being the goal of more mystical thinkers who believed in an original pure Adamic tongue of exactly this kind.

Words, for Harris, symbolize general ideas 'such as are common to many individuals' (p. 340), and he makes a gesture towards the Romantic position (see below) by noting that among the causes of linguistic diversity are 'the distinguishing Character and Genius of every nation' (p. 374). The book's rationale, given in the Preface, makes it clear that Harris sees the value of his work as extending beyond simple linguistics – for example, in studying the linguistic 'Form' of the syllogism:

> In viewing the MIND during its process in these syllogistic employments, we may come to know, in part, what kind of Being it is; since

> Mind like other Powers, can be only known from its Operations. (p. xiii; original emphasis omitted)

A further major work which has to be mentioned is James Burnett, Lord Monboddo's, vast six-volume *Dissertation on the Origin and Progress of Language* (1773–92), particularly Volume I. Monboddo's central thesis is that language is highly artificial, a human invention for expressing ideas through sounds. Nor, as generally held, is it essential to social life – he believes the orang utan to be a kind of human, enjoying a social existence, which lacks this capacity even though it possesses the organs of speech (he also believed that people were born with tails, severed by midwives at birth, an eighteenth-century Highland Freudian fantasy we will pursue no further). The capacity for language, if not language itself, remained, though, Divine in origin. This theme of artificiality was pursued also in James Beattie's *Essay on the Nature and Immutability of Truth* (1770) where, from imitative origins, it reaches a state of cumbersomeness which can be alleviated only by artificially invented rules of grammar and the like. Language remained 'inspired' even so (see Aarsleff 1983, pp. 37–41). Land (1986) credits Monboddo, for all his eccentricities, with making the crucial separation between the philosophy of mind and the study of the formal structures of languages on which modern linguistics depends, the science of language begins here, he says, 'with this separation of the study of language from the study of mind' (p. 162).

Adam Smith's *Considerations concerning the First Formation of Languages*, an appendix to the *Theory of Moral Sentiments* from the second edition onwards, is a little essay elaborating the idea that starting from proper names for single objects, these were extended to become class names, and thence the need for relation-terms, etc. He speculatively traces the logical sequence for the appearance of each new grammatical category and form of syntax. Brief though the essay is, Christie (1987) discerns in it a particularly complex understanding of the principles determining the evolution of grammar and the consequences of linguistic changes at this level (see also Land, 1986, for an extended analysis of Smith's linguistics). He notes a continuing, though not essential, dislike of figurative language in Smith, even though Smith's theory of the evolution of grammar is in terms of a basically figurative process (e.g. proper names become class names by extending the proper name as we do when we call an orator a Cicero – or, to give a modern example, a very clever person an Einstein). The development of language takes us progressively further from Nature and into abstraction and metaphysics, since each stage in this development involves a simplification of some kind in order to render language manageable in the face of expanding vocabularies, and so on. As Christie puts it:

> Smith's history of language becomes a history of the division of referential labour and its effects upon the nature of language. (p. 221)

Language becomes a 'machine' for understanding the world, and the principles governing its development are the same as those governing the improvement of machines. This is not something Smith likes, in fact; he clearly prefers the older inflected languages to modern ones, both on aesthetic grounds and for their superior fidelity to Nature, even though he has no notion of an original superior, pure language. As far as psychological concepts are concerned, these receive no special attention from Smith, although their concrete origin is implicit, and metaphysical concepts as a whole are viewed ambivalently.

Their difference from the Lockeans lies most centrally in the refusal of these Scottish Enlightenment thinkers (or James Harris) to accept any 'naturalistic' explanations of language which would seem to undermine the primacy and prior reality of active mental operations as *presently identified.* Resemblances occur, perhaps inevitably, between, say, Adam Smith's sequence and those proposed by the Lockeans when discussing the order in which various features of language appeared. Nearly everyone agrees that concrete concepts, words naming things, were some kind of starting point, but etymology and analyses of language origins as a natural phenomenon are not the major part of their armoury. They prefer speculative social history and formal logic to epistemological and philological arguments. The significance of language is that it represents thoughts and general ideas – even if, in Harris's case, this representation is 'symbolic' rather than 'imitative'. Words *represent* ideas in some way, they do not merely *name* them as they do for the Lockeans. Conceptual innovation regarding the psychological is again hamstrung; the folk-psychological classifications of the faculties and basic mental operations correspond to realities, albeit hidden ones. Such expressions as 'operations of the mind' and 'intellectual powers' are somewhat novel and presumably had a scientific ring for contemporary readers, but basically the task is to unravel, catalogue and classify this conceptual corpus in a quasi-botanical fashion, in terms of the various superordinate kinds of 'power' (e.g. Natural versus Acquired Powers, Active vs Passive Powers etc., see below, pp. 168–169)[9]. As for the Associationists dealt with previously, this may endow existing PL with more finely honed technical nuances, but it does not encourage active exploration of novel models or the introduction of neologisms.

The Reid tradition eventually decouples itself from linguistic speculations in the work of Dugald Stewart, usually considered a faithful proselyte of Reid. Stewart reverts in a sense to the Hobbes–Wilkins position regarding the treachery of metaphor, as in the following passage:

> The moment that the terms *attention, imagination, abstraction* . . . *deliberation*, are pronounced, a great step towards their interpretation is made in the mind of every person of common understanding; and although this analogical reference to the Material World adds greatly to the difficulty of analyzing, with philosophical rigour, the various faculties and principles of our nature, yet it cannot be denied, that it facilitates, to a wonderful degree, the mutual communications of mankind concerning them, in so far as such communications are necessary in the ordinary business of life. (Stewart, *Philosophical Essays*, Essay V, ch. 1, 1818 [1810], p. 206)

Aarsleff (1983) also quotes him as saying '[the] common analogical phraseology concerning mind [is] mistaken for its genuine philosophical theory' (pp.107–8)[10] and further suggesting that

> it is by the exclusive use of some favourite figure, that careless thinkers are gradually led to mistake a simile or distant analogy for a legitimate theory. (Aarsleff, *ibid.*, p. 108)[11]

But despite superficial resemblances to the Hobbes–Wilkins position, in Essay V, Chapter 1, of his *Philosophical Essays* Stewart comes closer than anyone else we have considered to spotting the real problem. Unlike them, he is not attempting to extirpate figurative usages from the language. His recommendation elsewhere (*ibid.*, ch. 3, p. 234) is to vary the metaphors so as to keep their status evident and because different people comprehend different 'figures' (Aarsleff, 1983, p. 108). From this it is a short distance, even if Stewart does not walk it, to acknowledging the possibility of actively generating novel metaphors and figures as a way of construing the psychological in new ways. His understanding of language use, though, can be pretty astute:

> The fact is, that, in cases of this sort, [i.e. involving 'notions which are abstract and complex'] the function of language is not so much to *convey* knowledge (according to the common phrase) from one mind to another, as to bring two minds into *the same train of thinking*; and to confine them, as nearly as possible, to the same track. (Stewart, op. cit. p. 211)

Stewart denies the notion, common to both Reid (if not all 'structuralists') and Horne Tooke, that to study language is to study the mind, and attacks Tooke's belief that etymology lays bare the nature of human thought. While it may not be entirely false to say that 'Language is the express image of thought', this itself is a figurative expression not to be taken, as Reid often does, too literally or rigorously (*ibid.*, pp. 207–8). For Stewart etymology provided 'an interesting, and not unprofitable employment' which afforded the philologer 'amusing and harmless gratification' (p. 213) but was as void of philosophical import as tracing the Latin origins of the word *pecunia* would be for helping us to understand 'the political effects of the national debt' (*ibid.*, p. 214). In saying this he prematurely ejected some elements of infancy along with the bathwater, for the relevance of etymology to Psychology is not quite so clearly absent as he thought. Rather it needs to be kept in the picture if the general message about the metaphorical or figurative character of PL is to be borne in mind and the errors of mistaking metaphor for theory avoided. In his own words, 'This has too often been overlooked by writers on the Human Mind' (*ibid.*, p. 208). Where I obviously part company with Stewart is in his acceptance that prolonged use renders such figurative expressions 'virtually equivalent to literal and specific appellations' (p. 212) rather than pursuing the theoretical implications of the situation to their logical conclusion as leading to a physiomorphic metatheory, itself Psychological (he would have said philosophical) in kind.

3 The Romantic school

While Condillac himself was an adamant Lockean, his story about the origins of human language and thought provided inspiration for those who would take an altogether different tack. Rousseau, for example, in his 1755 *Essai sur l'origine des langues*, while accepting much of Condillac's account of language emerging from gestures and cries, makes the final stage of converting these forms into language proper more of a voluntaristic act than a natural process (Monboddo would have agreed) and, contrary to Condillac, imagines the first languages to have possessed a natural vitality and vivacity, a passion, lost as reason and writing came to dominate over poetry and the spoken word (though Condillac, as mentioned above, did hold them to be more song-like, since they utilized intonation instead of grammar). The turning point for Romantic theories of language came in 1772 with publication of a prizewinning 1769 essay for the Prussian Academy by J.G. Herder, *Abhandlung über den Ursprung der Sprache*[12]. This stressed, with a force absent hitherto, the intimacy – mutual dependency even – of speech and thought. Neither could be granted primacy (in this exploiting Condillac's impasse regarding the priorities of reflection and language). From the great flux of experience our ancestors first separated out, as distinct and recurrent components, certain natural sounds – and this act of thinking immediately involved usage of that very sound to name the being so identified (e.g. a species of animal). Each advance in thinking, in identifying the discrete phenomena of the world, was accompanied and facilitated by an enlargement of the vocabulary, grammar and abstraction emerging in due course.

Herder, who later translated part of Monboddo's mighty opus into German, increasingly saw the significance of language as lying in its intimate connection with the spiritual, psychological character of its speakers. It becomes a collective creative expression of the national soul. While all human languages had a common origin, national languages thus represent different national spirits, different collective identities of the profoundest kind which forever elude translation. This harmonized well with both Romanticism and the growing political nationalism of the late eighteenth and nineteenth centuries; a patriotic linguistics surfaces in which the respective merits of languages are vehemently contested, and the supposed purity of a nation's language is something to be jealously guarded. There were earlier hints of this of course, but Herder's essay provided a firmer intellectual base and inspiration for such thinking. Herder can also, as Robins (1967) suggests, be seen as distantly anticipating modern Whorfian theories about the dependence of thought on language. By inspiring German linguists to seek the roots of their national spirit in their language, by endowing tedious philological labours with an exciting spiritual rationale, Herder laid the basis for German pre-eminence in the field in the following century, in the work of the Grimm brothers, Wilhelm von Humboldt, and Bopp.

In Britain Romanticism's impact on language study, Coleridge aside, was far weaker, although writers like Monboddo were expressing ideas which were not entirely dissimilar. It is only in Coleridge that British Romanticism finds a philosophical, as opposed to poetic or artistic, voice[13]. Coleridge's doctrines on language, however, are sufficiently distinct to require separate consideration (see below, pp. 128–130). If we cannot identify a clear linguistic impact of Romanticism in Britain, we can nevertheless see the impact of Romanticism as a literary movement. The lyrics and impenetrable prophetic books of William Blake, the poetry of Wordsworth and Coleridge and of the triumvirate of Shelley, Byron and Keats, amounted to a revolution in the poetic use of language. Here, after the 'Age of Reason', came the 'return of the repressed': an upsurge of the emotional and intuitive, a revaluation of the irrational, an urgent spiritual striving and openness to new experience. This undoubtedly revitalized psychological language, created new forms for articulating, evoking and evaluating subjective experience, and permanently affected British consciousness, though its impact on PL vocabulary as such is (again excepting Coleridge) less clear. Poets, Shelley proclaimed, were the unacknowledged legislators of the world. The Romantic poets certainly had as powerful an impact in legislating the terms of psychological discourse as their philosophical contemporaries, but their kind of psychological language would long remain quite incompatible with the kind of Psychological language scientists would seek to create.

4 The Literary school

As the eighteenth century opened, literary figures such as Swift, no less than Wilkins, felt the urgent need for some official reformation and standardization of the language, which they believed to be declining rapidly in quality (e.g. Swift's *A Proposal for Correcting, Improving and Ascertaining the English Tongue*, 1712). These other critics of contemporary language share little of Wilkins's aspirations for an objective universal language; they are vexed, rather, by what they see as a stylistic falling off, a vulgarization of the language, a flood of neologisms and a plague of undisciplined usage. This sorry state of affairs is dated to the outbreak of the Civil War, since when religious fanatics and decadent Restoration courtiers have successively sullied that purity which the tongue acquired under Elizabeth and her two Stuart successors (with some qualifications in the case of James I). Their concerns are aesthetic and moral, not epistemological. The exception is Mandeville, who has no wish to reform anything, and sees language as an instrument of social manipulation (see below, p. 178), but his was a minority voice with which few dared to agree.

Thomas Sheridan's *British Education* (1756) is discussed at length below (see pp. 219–224), but must be mentioned briefly here as perhaps the most extreme version of this standpoint. Almost certainly taking his cue from some passing observations in Swift's *Proposal*, Sheridan proceeds to fulminate against the anarchic condition of the language and diagnoses the situation as due to a decline in oratory, his aim being to turn English into the third great classical language after Latin and Greek.

Among the most significant mid-century texts on language were Dr Johnson's dedicatory Plan (To the Earl of Chesterfield) and Preface to his *Dictionary*, which appeared in 1755. It is important that we consider these here, since Johnson's cultural influence was of no mean magnitude. (And Thomas Sheridan cited him – along with Swift – incessantly.) Though short, the Preface marks a new level of consciousness regarding the problems of studying language. In characteristically lugubrious and apologetic fashion Johnson catalogues the difficulties besetting a lexicographer: etymology, spelling, definition and selection assail the dictionary compiler with problems of many kinds. Although we need not enumerate them here, what Johnson achieves by detailing the hurdles and pitfalls besetting his laborious task is to confront us with the sheer scale of any attempt at single-handedly mastering an entire language. He is more thoroughly acquainted in a practical sense with the empirical realities of language as a phenomenon than any of his predecessors, at least in English. His final attitude is a complex one: he shares the common aspiration of stabilizing and improving the language and the view that it has been in decline since the Restoration (hence choosing to draw his examples of usage primarily from the 'Golden Age' spanning writers from Sir Philip Sidney, whose *Arcadia* appeared in 1590, to Milton), at the same time he has to concede the ultimate futility of trying to stop the language from changing. At best its degeneration can be slowed, or particular stylistic delinquencies discouraged. He, like many contemporaries, also believes English to be in state of parlous disorder:

> I found our speech copious without order, and energetic without rule: wherever I turned my view, there was perplexity to be disentangled, and confusion to be regulated; choice was to be made out of boundless variety without any established principles of selection. (1818 edn, Preface, p. 181)

The result is that the Dictionary is, in intention, both descriptive and prescriptive[14]: 'The chief intent of it is to preserve the purity, and ascertain the meaning of the *English* idiom. (1818 edn, Plan, p. 163). But our language

> did not descend to us in a state of uniformity and perfection, but was produced by necessity, and enlarged by accident, and is therefore composed of dissimilar parts, thrown together by negligence, by affectation, by learning, or by ignorance. (Plan, p. 170)

Johnson's bind is best captured, however, in these two paragraphs from the Plan, with the Natural Philosophical imagery of the first perhaps echoing Wilkins's aspirations and the second the worldly wisdom of one who has really immersed himself in language as it is, rather than as it ought to be:

> Thus, my Lord [i.e. Chesterfield] will our language be laid down, distinct in its minutest subdivisions, and resolved into its elemental principles. And who upon this survey can forbear to wish, that these fundamental atoms of our speech might obtain the firmness

> and immutability of the primogenital and constituent particles of matter, that they might retain their substance while they alter their appearance, and be varied and compounded, yet not destroyed. . . . But this is a privilege which words are scarcely to expect; for, like their author, when they are not gaining strength, they are generally losing it. Though art may sometimes prolong their duration, it will rarely give them perpetuity; and their changes will be almost always informing us, that language is the work of man, of a being from whom permanence and stability cannot be derived. (Plan, p. 171)

But eight pages later he is again hoping that his will be

> . . . a dictionary by which the pronunciation of our language may be fixed, and its attainment facilitated; by which its purity may be preserved, its use ascertained, and its duration lengthened. (Plan, p. 179)

Johnson eschews philosophical issues, being content to accept that 'words are but the signs of ideas' (Preface, p. 185). Yet when he comes to consider 'a class of verbs' of 'vague and indeterminate signification' which includes '*bear, break, come, cast, full, get, give, do, put, set, go, run, make, take, turn, throw*', a more modern, dynamic, collective vision momentarily breaks through:

> . . . it must be remembered, that while our language is yet living, and variable by the caprice of every one that speaks it, these words are hourly shifting their relations, and can no more be ascertained in a dictionary, than a grove in the agitation of a storm, can be accurately delineated from its picture in the water. (Preface, p. 192)

Though *ad nauseam* quotation is a temptation for all who would touch on Johnson, the last sentences of the Preface contain the pith of the Stoic posture with which he finally launched his great *Dictionary*:

> I have protracted my work till most of those whom I wished to please have sunk into the grave, and success and miscarriage are empty sounds. I therefore dismiss it with frigid tranquility [*sic*], having little to fear or hope from censure or from praise. (Preface, p. 207)

(I love 'frigid tranquility'.) In retrospect how curious, but also how natural, it is that Johnson and his contemporaries, in a period when written English was possibly at the peak of controlled stylistic self-consciousness, were unprecedentedly anxious about its anarchy.

In the *Dictionary* itself, and also in his other writings, Johnson provides us with clear evidence of the incorporation of Natural Philosophical WL into PL[15].

5 Coleridge

Although Coleridge can be dealt with but sketchily here, he is an especially significant figure for the history of Psychology. After an early espousal of Hartley he became enthralled by contemporary German philosophy, particularly by Schelling's *Naturphilosophie* and Kant. While his strivings were towards an integration of the insights of all competing philosophical schools and physiological knowledge, he never succeeded in fully elaborating his 'system' in a single work.[16] His writings were the major conduit by which the ideas of Kant and Schelling were first brought to the attention of British thinkers, although they largely fell upon stony ground. Unlike the others whom we have discussed, he actively generates new psychological expressions and holds these to be scientific in character, rejecting Kant's disproof of the possibility of a science of the mind ('In Psychology Kant is but suspicious Authority', he says in his notebooks). And yet, in contrast with Psychology as it eventually emerged, Coleridge appreciates the *constitutive* (as opposed to descriptive) character of PL, and PL innovations. He is the first figure we have met whose deliberately contrived neologisms (occasionally recoveries of terms long obsolete or 'desynonymizations' of existing usages of a word – this itself being his word for it) remain with us; *psychology* itself largely owes its modern English usage to his keen espousal of the term (as does *aesthetic*), while *associative, narcissism, psycho-somatic*[17] *phobia, neuropathology* and – very nearly – *collective unconscious* all originate with him (Barfield, 1974; McKusick, 1986). In his notebooks he even used the term 'psycho-analytical'. (Other words ascribed to him include *teleological, relative* and *phenomenal*).

Like Horne Tooke, though in a different spirit, Coleridge believes in the value of etymology as reconnecting us with the original perceptual meaning of a term – this providing the key to all its subsequent meanings. A naturally occurring process of 'desynonymization' continually serves to elaborate and extend the resources of language. While Coleridge is deeply influenced by Tooke, whose etymological speculations he profoundly respects, for him this reconnection is not a matter of mere intellectual interest but denotes a central spiritual, metaphysical truth – it means that language is the vehicle of creative power mediating between the human soul and God. He is in fact reinvoking the Johannine *Λογος* – The Word – eventually accepting the idea that Hebrew was the original language, and that modern languages originated, if not with Adam, from the sons of Noah (see McKusick, *op. cit.*, pp. 127–8).

While heading in such mystical directions may, on the face of it, appear to augur ill for Coleridge's linguistic thought, it entails in the event a quite advanced appreciation of the role of language in creating and/or exploring the psychological realm. For Coleridge, by mastering the etymological origins of psychological terms, by becoming conscious of their literal perceptual meanings, one is then equipped to transcend this purely sensuous level and acquire and identify truly abstract ideas. Greek and Latin serve as the fountainheads of such linguistic innovation, providing resources to which we can continue to turn. His linguistic thought is motivated throughout by a desire to reconcile the insights of Tooke's sensationalism with those of German Idealism, and in attempting this he identifies, particularly in grammar, features of language which represent and manifest inbuilt, universal properties of the mind comparable to Kantian *a priori* categories. There is thus an almost Chomskyan dimension to Coleridge's account of language structure, as well as linkage with the Scottish position.

Many of Coleridge's neologisms did not catch on – '*esemplastic*', for example, which he wished to use, instead of *imagination*, to refer to what he believed was our most important capacity, that of creatively bringing ideas into genuine unity (as opposed to 'fancy' which merely played with associations). In *Biographia Literaria* Chapter X, he even seems to claim the credit for 're-introducing' the words 'subjective' and 'objective'[18]. Coleridge is of relevance to us here for two main reasons: first, he does successfully launch some new psychological concepts, but second, in examining how he achieves this rule-proving exception role, we are drawn to identify in his view of language precisely those facilitating components which are lacking elsewhere. If modern Psychology has turned a perennial blind eye to the physiomorphic character of PL,

Coleridge was well aware of it; but rather than construing it as a failing, he saw the situation in profoundly spiritual terms, as an aspect of the creative power of the *Λογος*. The philosophical and religious – as distinct from poetic – writings of Coleridge seem to have long remained marginalized, notwithstanding the tremendous impact he had on his contemporaries, John Stuart Mill pairing him with Jeremy Bentham as one of 'the two great seminal minds of England in their age': 'Every Englishman of the present day is by implication either a Benthamite or a Coleridgian'. His ideas on language were in flux for a long time and are scattered through *The Friend, Biographia Literaria* and *Aids to Reflection*, as well as his copious notebooks and other manuscripts only now being disinterred and published. Needless to say, disciplinary historians (other than Hearnshaw [1964][19]) seem hardly to acknowledge his existence.

Conclusion

As we will see when we discuss Political Philosophy, the idea that societies evolved over time in an orderly progressive fashion inevitably led to speculation about the origins of social institutions and the primeval condition of the species – a trend which would ultimately help to subvert the notion of an immutable universal 'human nature'. For eighteenth-century writers, no longer merely engaging in Hobbesian thought-experiments about Man in a State of Nature, the question had become a quasi-empirical one. By turning to the records of Antiquity and reports of contemporary voyagers among 'savages', it was hoped, a more direct light could be shed on human origins. (The influence of Natural History, a booming and popular area of Natural Philosophy was an important factor here, as Wood [1990] has shown, particularly as far as Scottish Enlightenment philosophers were concerned.) One component of this, of course, was the origin of language itself. By 1800 few seriously believed any longer that Hebrew was the original language, or in any way specially related to it. Alongside this historical approach to language, which emphasized etymology and speculative histories of grammar, were those, like Harris, who remained interested in 'universal grammar' and analysed language in more 'synchronic' ways.

In conclusion, then, by 1800 language had come to be recognized as a complex – indeed, mysterious – phenomenon, regardless of the theoretical standpoint of the individual thinker. In 1700, language (though not without a mystical side for some) was generally considered amenable to a dose of straightforward analysis, its flaws easily diagnosed and remedies immediately identifiable – either by implementing Wilkins-style programmes of reform or by the diktat of a refined state-appointed committee such as Swift's *Proposal* urged on the Earl of Oxford. Few challenged simple picture-theories of meaning, or doubted associationist accounts of its acquisition, and only Mandeville appears to have questioned the notion that its primary function was the communication of ideas (see below, p. 178). Culturally, the prevailing concerns of the early-eighteenth-century Augustans were with style and systematization. Johnson – who, more than any other person, actually struggled to bring order to English and to defend aesthetic standards of usage – finally realized that it was an impossible task, though he was consoled by the thought that he had at least tried. By 1800 the notion that words were uncomplicated signs of ideas in the speaker's head could no longer be uncritically sustained, whether one followed Reid or Herder or Tooke. In France, Degerando now scorned the notion of creating a universal language: '*ce projet est absolument chimérique*' (1800, III, p. 551). There is a broad sense that language is as much a determinant of thought as determined by it, that it has a kind of life of its own. For Reid its basic categories cannot be challenged, for Herder it is the vehicle of a national as well as an individual consciousness, for Tooke all has become arbitrary and language *is* thought. For the Romantic poets it becomes magic, a creative force, in the words Blake gives to Los in *Jerusalem*:

> I Must Create a System or be enslav'd by another Man's;
> I will not Reason and Compare: my business is to Create.

Words regain their own invocatory, prophetic, bardic power. Language has again become a route for exploring the psyche, not merely a (potentially transparent) representation of thoughts. In Britain it is only in Coleridge that a balance between this Romantic image of language and a belief in the possibility of scientific Psychology is really achieved.

If there is a single idea, word, or rhetorical slogan which

encapsulates the psychological change wrought by the eighteenth century, it is 'humanity', connoting both an aspiration and a realization; and implicated in this is language itself, shifting from ego's instrument to medium of shared subjectivity. But conversely, it is the sharing of subjectivity between egos typically of a far more self-conscious, autonomous and differentiated variety than those who had been happy with the simpler formulation of language as a vehicle of the speaker's thoughts. It is this very differentiation which renders the role of sharing subjectivity so apparent: to the extent that subjectivities are the same, sharing is implicit. (Is this why, until mid century at least, philosophers can appeal so routinely to the introspective testimony of their readers as evidence?) This is neither to put too rosy a gloss on 'humanitarianism', nor to ignore the web of power relations being covertly negotiated and reordered in the way Foucault and his successors have shown. But I am unsure how far the new autonomous individuality (a) was/is an illusion; (b) represented an independent psychological development; or (c) was actually being constituted by the very discourses which articulated it and rendered it self-conscious. In other words: (a) Had people simply been unaware of the extent of their autonomy and self-containedness; (b) Did they really, but initially unconsciously, become more autonomous and self-contained (as a function of changed cultural conditions); or (c) Did they unwittingly render themselves more autonomous and self-contained in the very act of engaging in increasingly sophisticated reflexive discourse?

Deconstructionist critics of Psychology would, I imagine, prefer the second, since it is this mode of individuality which is diagnosed as being central to the discipline's current failure (Parker and Shotter, 1990), while to locate the change purely in the discourse might decouple it from the ensemble of socioeconomic developments within which the discipline emerged. But this is perhaps a false dichotomy, since such discourses are part and parcel of this very ensemble. Assuming that it occurred, the way the advent of this new mode of individuality was mediated clearly requires further research[20]. The lesson of the present chapter in this respect is that in so far as the linguistic level is involved, its contribution would not have been in terms of vocabulary, since all linguistic positions (bar Coleridge's) were implicitly uncongenial to innovations in Psychological Language; where it may have contributed, by contrast, is in covertly transforming the way in which language itself was conceptualized. Even though no consensus is reached, by the early nineteenth century thinkers of all kinds have become aware (if hazily) that there is a *communication problem*, and this must entail in its turn a consciousness of variance in interpersonal – or inter-ego – distance. Isolated despair and Romantic soul-fusion become the complementary poles of turn-of-the-century consciousness.

If we are to find any genuine PL innovation within a disciplinary setting during the eighteenth century we have, as will be shown in Chapter 7, to turn to the German academic philosophy of Wolff, Baumgarten and Tetens. Before Kant himself, however, this was relatively little known in Britain, and uncongenial to pre-revolutionary French *philosophes*. Within this tradition, as we shall see, a more sophisticated technical vocabulary for discussing psychological matters evolved, which in the following century gave German thinkers a head start in creating a would-be scientific discipline of Psychology. Indeed in Tetens they came close to creating one in the 1770s. Their failure to do so remains, I think, due in part, at least, to their at first incipient, and later manifest, endorsement of Romantic ideals regarding the irreducibility of the spiritual to the material, and the view of the nature of PL this entailed.

3
Sensible Reasoning: Philosophical Moves towards Psychology

> Philosophy has always insisted upon this: thinking its other. Its other: that which limits it, and from which it derives its essence, its definition, its production.
>
> (Jacques Derrida [1982])

1 The Impact of Empiricism and Associationism

As an opening note of clarification: Empiricism refers to the doctrine that knowledge is obtained via the senses and cannot be acquired by reasoning alone. It is conventional to oppose this to Rationalism, the belief that rigorous reasoning can yield knowledge unaided. This requires some elaboration. Empiricism may more properly be described as seeing no role for reason except in relation to sensory information. The origins of reasoning itself remained notoriously recalcitrant to Empiricist explanation. Rationalism, on the other hand, places the weight on the other foot: reason (or the mind) ultimately frames the kinds of meaning which sensory information can have, this logically requiring the presence of some pre-existing modes of meaning. A dispute, essentially concerning the respective roles of reason and the senses, has often been caricatured as one about their 'importance'. Clearly no philosopher of merit ever believed that either was expendable. Associationism is a more specific epistemological doctrine tracing knowledge to *quasi-atomistic* sensations, 'ideas of sensation' or sensory 'impressions' which are then linked, according to certain laws, to yield all other 'ideas' (however abstract) and mental phenomena (though with qualifications in respect to some of the last). Associationism has been seen as the 'Psychological' face of Empiricism. But while the most eminent British Empiricists (Locke, Berkeley, Hume, Hartley and James Mill) were indeed also

Associationists, many Scottish Enlightenment thinkers (notably Thomas Reid) were anti-Associationist while remaining committed to Empiricism. The doctrine of a sensory origin of knowledge need not imply that this comes ultimately in the form of quasi-atomic units, or that knowledge consists of discrete entities called 'ideas'. British attacks on Locke are by and large aimed at his doctrine of 'ideas' – which later became known as Associationism – rather than on Empiricism *per se* (though opponents such as Broughton may sometimes attack him using Rationalist techniques), while even his strongest continental opponents, such as Wolff and Kant, viewed Empiricism as inadequate rather than fallacious.

(i) The Opposition

The issue on which battle first commenced in the aftermath of Locke's *Essay* was, on the face of it, a continuation of earlier concerns: the nature of the soul and whether thought could conceivably be a property of matter. In retrospect this controversy, ending with the effective elimination of the immortal soul as a topic of serious philosophical discussion and a victory for the 'thinking matter' school, may be seen as the point where the conceptual decks were finally cleared and an empirical 'Science of Mind' at last became conceptually feasible, in principle if not in practice.

In 1702 a work by William Coward appeared, under the pseudonym 'Estibius Psychalethes', entitled *Second Thoughts Concerning Human Soul.* In this it was scandalously argued that the notion of an immaterial soul was erroneous. The 'Notion of a separate Self-existent Being, call'd *Human Soul* is Vain, Frivolous and Idle' and has no scriptural basis. Rather, the term 'Soul' was synonymous with 'Life' – referring to a life-principle or 'Anima' which was indeed of Divine origin, but in no sense a substance or entity in its own right (his position was thus 'Vitalist' rather than fully materialist in the modern sense). No rational man can have a sufficient ground for believing in the existence of an immortal soul, a belief of heathen origin which had descended via ignorant early Christians and the corrupt Roman Catholic Church. Life, 'or Motion with Sensation, is sufficient to denominate and make . . . Man'. The following year the House of Commons ordered the book to be burned (the same fate as had befallen John Toland's *Christianity not Mysterious* in 1697). Replies to Coward were fairly numerous, one of the best among them being John Broughton's *Psychologia or, an Account of the Nature of the Rational Soul* (1703).

Broughton's calibre as a philosopher was, it must be acknowledged, far higher than Coward's, and his real targets were Locke and the 'moderns' generally. He sided with Descartes and Malebranche on the existence of an unextended Immaterial Substance, Spirit or Soul, and espoused a strong 'passive matter' position. His main argument hinged on the difference between 'Substance' and 'Accidents' (or properties) – all properties are properties *of* a substance of some kind. We can know a Substance only via its Accidents and 'from the difference we find in the Nature of Accidents, we must conclude a like difference in the Nature of those Substances to which they belong' (p. 10). From this he can move on to argue that the properties of 'Cogitation' and 'Extension' are so radically different and 'repugnant' in kind that their unity in a single Substance is inconceivable:

> Let him . . . frame as clear and distinct an idea as he can of each of them seperately; and then let him endeavour what he can to conjoyn them; let him try to mark out an *Inch of Reason* or an *Ell of Contemplation*; which wou'd be as easy to do, were the two Properties consistent, as to conceive a *reasoning Inch* or *contemplative Ell of Matter*; for wherever two Properties are united in one Substance, they may be *reciprocally predicated: Thus I can conceive an extended Whiteness* as well as a *white Extension*. (*ibid.*, p. 25)

Broughton saw in the doctrine of thinking matter the threat of atheism and 'Universal Corporealism' and in *Psychologia* he bravely attempted to stem the Lockean tide, though he failed to counter convincingly the full case Locke had mounted, in Book III of the *Essay*, against the possibility of our knowing anything about the real essence of substances. But while clearly theological in intent, Broughton's method is now plainly philosophical; there are no appeals to scriptural authority, no attempts to carry the day with theological rhetoric and *ad hominem* arguments – it is, however, 'Rationalist' rather than 'Empiricist' in technique. Indeed, as he states at the outset, his aim is to 'build upon the Foundation of Reason' a firm case for the Immortality of the Soul as an 'Article of Natural Religion', 'Natural Religion' being founded in turn upon 'Natural Reason'. Had it simply been Broughton versus Coward and those like him[1], the Lockeans would have had a major struggle to carry the day. History is, proverbially, written by the victors. In histories of Psychology the rise of Associationism is too often depicted as happening without serious philosophical opposition until Reid in the 1760s. In fact Locke's opponents could on occasion mount sophisticated and philosophically insightful attacks. But in doing so they had already conceded the most important point – they had accepted the terms of secular debate within a now firmly established mode of philosophical discourse (although the two sides may differ in how they are weighted towards *a prioristic* argument or appeals to evidence). Even more evidently, they had to adopt the 'way of Ideas' – Lockean vocabulary and the Lockean model had become the point of departure, and even in opposing it his early adversaries felt compelled to use the technical language of 'Ideas', 'Sensations', 'Reflection', etc., in which it had found expression.

Of these early opponents one of the most powerful was Peter Browne, Anglican Bishop of Cork, whose two major works were *The Procedure, Extent, and Limits of Human Understanding* (1728) and *Things Divine and Supernatural Conceived by Analogy with Things Natural and Human* (1733). That the first is pitched against Locke is signalled in its very title, but Toland's *Christianity not Mysterious* (1696) was an additional target. Browne's final aim is to prove that we can have knowledge of the Immaterial Divine world, but this task is for the most part reserved for the second work. Browne directs his initial attack at Locke's doctrine of 'Ideas of Reflection', and very general use of the term 'Idea'. He reserves the term 'Idea' for 'what stands in the Mind for an Image or Representation of something which is not in it . . .' (1728, p. 65), it 'should be limited and confined to our simple Sensations only, and to the various Alterations and Combinations of them by the pure Intellect of our Mind' (*ibid.*, p. 63). These are conceptually distinct from the 'Operations of the Mind', the '*Actions* and *Workings* of the Intellect upon *Ideas*, first lodged in the Imagination for that purpose' (*ibid.*, p. 65). The term 'Ideas of Reflection' is absurd, for 'we have an immediate *Consciousness* of the Operations themselves being already within us, and essentially belonging to our Make and Frame' (*ibid.*, p. 66). But consciousness of such workings still requires 'some precedent Idea in the Imagination for it to work on' (*ibid.*, p. 67). He thus differentiates between two kinds of knowledge: that of external objects, 'which we have . . . by their internal Ideas' (*ibid.*, p. 72) and that of the Operations and Workings of the Intellect, which does not consist of Ideas but is better referred to by words such as 'Notion, or Conception, or Apprehension, or Consciousness' (*ibid.*). In arguing thus he is following up Berkeley's earlier critique of Locke's notion of 'Abstract Ideas' (see below, pp. 144–149), but abandoning his radical Idealism.

It is especially notable that Browne appears intuitively to have anticipated the impossibility of defining psychological terms by associating them to private internal events – an insight underlying his insistence on the different logical status of Ideas, derived from sensation, and 'Notions and Conceptions' regarding the 'Intellect's Consciousness of its own Operations'. He even produces a proto-Wittgensteinian argument that we do not have an idea of pain (*ibid.*, p. 71). But the following passage from Book III, Chapter 5 is surely quite remarkable:

> That there can be no such things as *Ideas* of the Operations of the Mind by *Reflection*, is most evident; for granting (what we have seen is evidently false) that the Mind could take a View of its Operations by *Turning* in upon itself, then there would be no want of *Ideas* to discern them by. An Idea is some representation of an *External Object* in the Mind; it stands *For* the Object, and supplies its absence; and there would be no *Need* of any Representation, if the Object itself were there: But the Operations of the Mind are all *within* it self; and in order to prove Ideas of Reflection, you must suppose either that these Operations are their *Own* Ideas; or that the Objects themselves are overlooked, and their *Ideas* only made the Objects of the Intellect. . . . To say that the Operations Themselves, and the Ideas of these Operations are in the Mind *Together* at the same time, is most absurd, as being *Superfluous*, and altogether without any necessity in Nature, which doth nothing in vain. Upon this Supposition it would be utterly impossible for the most acute Logician to determine which of the two were the *Object* of our *Understanding*. (*ibid.*, pp. 413–14; original emphasis)

This subtle move enables Browne to sustain a dualist position, while acknowledging the epistemological necessity for Ideas of Sensation and the 'essential union of the pure Spirit with our material Frame' (*ibid.*, p. 148) – this union itself being what he wishes to call Soul (Ψυχη). In his later book he develops the notion that knowledge of the Divine and Supernatural may be gained by 'Analogy', which he differentiates from Metaphor. Whereas Metaphor 'consists only in an *Appearing* or *Imaginary* Resemblance and Correspondency', Analogy is founded on an '*Actual Similitude* and Real Correspondency in the very *Nature* of Things' (1733, p. 3). We need not pursue this further here (although it should be noted that it was on this issue, the nature of our knowledge of God, that Browne and Berkeley clashed, *Things Divine and Supernatural* . . . containing an extended reply to Berkeley's attack upon him in *Alciphron* [1732]). Browne's phrase 'Operations of the Mind', and his view of these as primary naturally implanted principles, anticipates Reid's later Common Sense philosophy. Though Browne's is clearly the finer intellect, Reid's greater historical significance has made him the better remembered.

With few exceptions, the contents of *The Procedure* . . . (23 out of 29 chapters) are concerned with epistemology and the status of reflexive knowledge. It concedes a large amount of the Lockean account (e.g. in opposing 'innate ideas', and the processes whereby Ideas of Sensation are combined) and in some respects penetrates more deeply into the logical difficulties in reflexively conceptualizing the mind's own workings. Browne is clearly influenced by Berkeley, but evidently unwilling to accept his Immaterialism.

Passing mention must also be made here of what professed itself to be 'the first Attempt that hath been made on the Subject' of consciousness: Zachary Mayne's *Two Dissertations Concerning Sense and the Imagination with an Essay on Consciousness* (1728). Mayne strove to prove that humans differed fundamentally from 'Brutes' by showing that Human Intellect is radically different from mere perception and imagination and is, furthermore, essentially the same as Consciousness; Consciousness is the Self: '*Consciousness* denominates *Self*, and *Self* may rightly be defined, *That which is Conscious*' (*ibid.*, p. 149). He acknowledges that although we have a 'sense of consciousness' we cannot proceed beyond this without getting involved in an infinite regress (*ibid.*, p. 165). While it cannot be said that Mayne was a particularly good philosopher, his extended discussion of the relationship between Self and Consciousness may perhaps be read as foreshadowing the impending changes in the nature of selfhood in the latter part of the century.

A final instance of reaction against Locke is Ashley Cooper (Lord Shaftesbury), who was actually tutored by Locke. Finding

Locke's atomism and materialism repugnant he was drawn towards the Cambridge Neo-Platonist tradition, his first published work being an edition of Whichcote's Sermons. Philosophically he is most important for his analysis of the basis of morality and ethics in *An Inquiry Concerning Virtue or Merit*, which first appeared in an unprepossessing, unauthorized edition in 1699. In developing his ideas Cooper became, as far as religion was concerned, more radical than Locke ever admitted to being, espousing Deism which, while believing in God, rejected the doctrines of the Trinity, Salvation and direct Divine intervention in the world. The completed version of the *Inquiry* which appeared in 1711 (as part of the three-volume collection of his writings known as the *Characteristics*) shared only about half the text with the original edition (Walford, Intro. to 1977 edn). The thrust of this work is that Virtue is an objective reality irreducible to utilitarian and egoistic terms. Often seen as a harbinger of Romanticism, Ashley Cooper's writings present a wholeheartedly benign and optimistic vision of human nature, while his belief in a 'moral instinct' was enthusiastically adopted by later Scottish philosophers as a central tenet in their efforts to devise naturalistic accounts of human society (see below, pp. 181–188). In rendering Virtue natural and objective Cooper made a move which the ensuing century found especially appealing, since it offered a confident, urbane and secularized but non-reductionist account of morality, serviceable as a defence against religious 'enthusiasm' and Hobbesian atheism alike. In expounding his moral philosophy Cooper provides a full account of the 'Oeconomy of the Passions', which he divides into the 'natural' which lead to the good of the 'Publick', 'Self-Affections', which benefit 'the Private'; and 'unnatural Affections', which do neither. This can be left aside here, however, since Hutcheson's account (discussed below, pp. 142–144) derived from Cooper's, and was more influential. His significance in the present context is that his anti-Lockeanism is not motivated by a desire to defend the religious status quo or Cartesian Rationalist metaphysics, but is directed, rather, against both reductionist materialism (with its implicit moral relativism) and irrational religious dogma. His goal is an image of human nature at once spiritually refined and secular, rational yet emotionally sensitive[2]. One figure who responded very positively to Cooper was Francis Hutcheson, in whom, however, we see a move back towards the Lockean approach.

Before considering Hutcheson we need to make two final points about Locke's theologically motivated opponents. First, they are as much participants in the transformation of psychological discourse as those they were attacking – this is evidenced even at the superficial level of their titles: the first work in which a variant of 'psychology' is the title (Broughton's *Psychologia*) and arguably the first English essay on consciousness *per se* (Mayne, 1728). Secondly, if the name of the historical game were merely 'spot the anticipation', the texts of this neglected group of philosopher/theologians might prove as rich a site as those of their 'progressive' opponents. Browne in particular verges at times on Wittgensteinian insights[3].

(ii) The Lockeans

The constituency to which Locke's thought most immediately appealed was an intelligentsia (often Scottish and Irish) *au fait* with developments in Natural Philosophy and weary of theology. Among the most eminent of these was Francis Hutcheson (an Irish Presbyterian minister's son who in 1730 became Professor of Moral Philosophy at Glasgow). From a very different position Bishop George Berkeley (also Irish, of course) was able to convert Lockean Empiricism into a radically Idealistic form – a move which, if theologically motivated, was also a philosophically legitimate exploitation of some latent implications of Locke's analysis. The first phase of British Lockean thought culminates in the work of David Hartley and David Hume in the 1740s. By this time the character of the discourse had shifted from that of a meta-commentary on 'Understanding', which, as I argued in Chapter 1, was the position of the *Essay*. It was now merging into Natural Philosophy rather than transcending it, and its goal had become to identify the Natural Laws by which the mind worked (Hume) and even to integrate these with a now prevalent mechanistic physiology (Hartley). We must, however, be cautious; Hume's radically sceptical *A Treatise of Human Nature* (1739) hardly broke like a thunderclap upon the contemporary intellectual scene; as Graham (1908) put it: 'Anxiously he awaited the effect on the world; he listened eagerly for the explosion his theories were to create. Alas! "it fell" as he says, "still-born from the press". Instead of a storm, it raised not a ripple. A few obscure reviews noticed its arrival; that was all, for the English mind was utterly indifferent to philosophy' (p. 37). It is apposite to note here that the centre of gravity for philosophical and psychological thought in Britain shifted to Edinburgh, Glasgow and Aberdeen for the majority of the eighteenth century. From Hutcheson in the 1720s via Hume, Reid, Adam Smith, Lord Kames, Lord Monboddo, James Beattie and Adam Ferguson to Dugald Stewart at the century's close, 'Scottish Enlightenment' thinkers constitute the dominant force in British philosophy, even if they do not entirely monopolize it. The cultural factors behind this cannot be pursued here.

A look at Hutcheson may illuminate the beginnings of the transformation from meta-commentary to quasi-Natural Philosophy.

(a) Francis Hutcheson (1694–1747)

Francis Hutcheson, an ardent (if religiously orthodox) fan of Ashley Cooper, whilst accepting much of Cooper's analysis, largely adopts the Lockean conceptual framework – seeking to elaborate and expand rather than reject it. Hutcheson is generally seen as a prime mover in the 'new spirit of enlightenment in the Scottish universities' which evolved into what is known as the 'Scottish Enlightenment'[4]. (This movement will be commanding much of our attention in due course.) Hutcheson's major philosophical texts for present purposes are *An Essay on the Nature and Conduct of the Passions and Affections with Illustrations on the Moral Sense* (1728) and *An Inquiry into the Original of our Ideas of Beauty and Virtue: in Two Treatises* (1725). If we turn to the *Essay*, a failure to see any need for experiment beyond appeal to common experience is immediately apparent in the introductory claim that

> to discover Truth on those subjects, nothing more is necessary than a little *Attention to what passes in our own Hearts*, and consequently every Man may come to Certainty in these points, without much Art or Knowledge of other Matters (1728, pp. v–vi; original emphasis)

Hutcheson's immediate concern is to attack the claim that all our 'Desires' and 'Affections' 'proceed from *Self-Love*' (p. vi), an aim which underlies his subsequent elaboration of the notion that we possess a 'Moral Sense'. So far he is closely following the Cooper line. In order to carry this moral philosophical argument, however, he utilizes the Lockean account, proposing an investigation 'into the several kinds of *internal Perceptions*' (pp. x–xi). For Hutcheson

'External Senses' are but one of five classes of senses, the others being (a) 'Pleasant Perceptions' – those arising from '*regular, harmonious, uniform* Objects, as also from *Grandeur* and *Novelty*' (a theme he pursued in *An Inquiry into the Original of our Ideas of Beauty and Virtue*); (b) 'Public Sense', defined as 'our Determination to be pleased with the *Happiness* of others, and to be uneasy at their *Misery*'; (c) Moral Sense, 'by which we perceive *Virtue* and *Vice* in our selves and others'; and finally (d) 'Sense of Honour', our sensitivity to the 'Approbation' and 'Gratitude of others' and to their '*Dislike, Condemnation* or *Resentment* of Injuries done by us'. In short, he expands the notion of 'Sense' beyond the usual five senses to 'every Determination of our Minds to receive Ideas independently on our Will, and to have Perceptions of Pleasure and Pain' (p. 4). By so expanding our sensory repertoire he can 'naturalize', as perceivable objects or quasi-sensory properties, such things as Beauty, Honour and Virtue. He thus reconciles a 'Naturalistic' Moral Philosophy with a basically Lockean epistemology. His subsequent complex analysis of the nature of 'Desires and Aversions' need not detain us long, what is significant as an indication of the drift of philosophical thought towards closer integration with Natural Philosophy is its culmination in an account of 'the manner of acting from calm Desire, with Analogy to the *Laws of Motion*'.

First he differentiates between 'Natural Good and Evil', Absolute and Relative Good and Evil, and Universal, Particular and Private Good and Evil, plus 'Compound' good events and objects and Mixed objects and events. Then he proceeds to formulate twenty 'Axioms or natural Laws of *calm Desire*'. This directly anticipates the Benthamite Utilitarian 'hedonistic calculus' of nearly a century later. In the 1728 edition for example, axiom 7 states that 'In computing the Quantities of Good or Evil, which we pursue or shun, either for ourselves or others, when the *Durations* are equal, the Moment is as the *Intensiveness*: and when the *Intensiveness* of pleasure is the same, or equal, the Moment is as the Duration' (p. 39). In the *Inquiry* Hutcheson had actually offered a fully algebraicized version of this, although he abandoned it (for reasons which are unclear) in the fourth edition of 1738[5].

His analysis of what we term 'emotion' goes beyond those of Descartes and Malebranche (whom he admires but also criticizes). In particular he wishes to differentiate the 'pure Affections' of

'Desire and Aversion' from the 'Passions' themselves. The former arise 'necessarily from Apprehension of Good and Evil', the latter are 'violent *confused* Sensations, connected with *bodily Motions*', while an additional category, 'Instinct', is distinct from both Desire and Sensation. It is difficult to do justice here to Hutcheson's systematic survey of the 'Affections and Passions'. Clearly he now sees psychological matters as being amenable to a kind of scientific treatment, and psychological phenomena – the Affections and Passions at least – as being 'directed' by 'mechanick laws' (1728, p. 203). While remaining centred in moral philosophical issues, he eschews theological argument almost completely, seeking instead to ground morality in a Lockean style philosophical argument based on the twin foundations of a 'little Attention to what passes in our own hearts' and logic. In Hutcheson we thus encounter a complicated fusion of a traditional concern with morality (which Locke had seemed to subvert), Lockean philosophical method, and Natural Philosophical style. Although a couple of works emulating Hutcheson's mathematical approach appeared in the first half of the century[6], Reid's scorn effectively stifled its serious development until Jeremy Bentham's *An Introduction to the Principles of Morals and Legislation* (1789; see below, pp. 188–192).

(b) Bishop George Berkeley (1684–1753)[7]

The first major philosophical response to Locke came from Berkeley, perhaps the most difficult and subtle of his immediate followers. It is, however, an ambivalent response, for while advancing the Empiricist philosophy in several important respects (especially in strengthening the case for the primacy of perception as the ultimate source of knowledge), he also sought, like the anti-Lockeans, to avert the religious scepticism which Locke's philosophy seemed (in spite of Locke's own protestations) to promote. Psychology has had some difficulty in finding him an appropriate niche. His work on perception would place him neatly in a progressivist story, but his Idealism is contrary to the spirit of down-to-earth Empiricist realism allegedly characteristic of the British tradition and rendering it so dear to the discipline. Even so, he is a founder of that very tradition. A 'Psychological' study of perception had, as we have seen, begun to emerge in the late seventeenth century as a topic of empirical Natural Philosophical enquiry (the most important work being Molyneux's). There are several reasons why this should be the first psychological topic to have been uncontroversially captured within the orbit of Natural Philosophy. Foremost is the sheer intimacy of the connection between empirical research as such and visual perception, with the associated recognition of the eye as an optical instrument apparently operating on the same principles as the new optical instruments available to the Natural Philosophers. Secondly, perception inevitably becomes a focal issue in any epistemological debate concerning the relationship between what is seen and what is really there. Thus it is a topic where philosophy and science converge, and can serve to mediate between their several concerns.

Berkeley's *An Essay towards a New Theory of Vision* (1709) is a calculated prelude to the philosophical works which were to succeed it and which, their author rightly foresaw, would prove highly contentious. Berkeley expounds here what became the main tenet of Associationist accounts of perception: our perception of the world as containing stable objects within a three-dimensional space is a product of experiential, basically Associationist, learning. Initially we see only constantly changing coloured patches, we then learn to assign meanings to these as representing stable objects and as cues of distance and movement. Eventually the mind, 'by the mediation of visible ideas' (using 'idea' in the Lockean sense), 'doth perceive or apprehend the distance, magnitude, and situation of tangible objects' (para. 121). This learning process involves such achievements as associating movements of the eye with the proximity of the objects being looked at (para. 16). He also returns to the Moon Illusion (paras. 67–78), offering his own explanation[8]. Much consideration is given to evidence regarding the perceptual experience of the congenitally blind on first acquiring sight ('Molyneux's Question') – evidence apparently endorsing his theory. Beneath all this is an epistemological message: all knowledge is sensory in origin. The work did not though initiate a tradition of Psychological research into perception, the only other eighteenth-century English text of any importance on the subject being William Porterfield's *A Treatise on the Eye, the Manner and Phaenomena of Vision* (1759, 2 vols), which according to Boring, 'made . . . no new historically important discovery and urged no new significant view' (1942, p. 122) but served mainly to summarize comprehensively the existing state of knowledge. It would not be until Johannes Müller a century later that the subject would be significantly advanced beyond Berkeley's position. Porterfield did, however, differ (erroneously) from Berkeley regarding the cause of the fact that there is a single field of binocular vision (Boring, *ibid.*, p. 123). Whatever his immediate impact and longer term motives, Berkeley has certainly provided us, in *An Essay towards a New Theory of Vision*, with a genuinely Psychological text.

But motives are none the less relevant if we are to assess the overall meaning of Berkeley's philosophy as developed in the subsequent *Treatise Concerning the Principles of Human Knowledge* (1710) and *Three Dialogues between Hylas and Philonous* (1713). Once again a primary theological motivation is greatly in evidence. Berkeley was deeply concerned to demonstrate how, ultimately, belief in God rationally ensues from pursuing to their logical conclusion what initially appear to be the principles of scepticism. Behind this, though, one discerns an attempt to articulate a very personal mode of experiencing the world as immanently sustained by a Divine principle – indeed, it appears to me that his personal orientation was dominated by what I have elsewhere called the 'Signal mode'[9]. This latter interpretation requires some justification, but first a brief summary of Berkeley's philosophical position is necessary.

Berkeley's starting point is an attack on Locke's concept of 'abstract ideas'. Warnock argues that this was far more than a technical quibble[10]. He had astutely spotted that Locke's argument that we can possess or 'frame' abstract ideas (such as 'triangle') was rooted in a mistaken understanding of the nature of language. Locke held that we were able to derive from our experience of actual triangles an abstract idea of triangularity which was – to cite his oft-quoted list – 'neither oblique nor rectangle, neither equilateral, equicrural nor scalenon; but all and none of these at once' (*Essay*, IV. 7. §9). Berkeley, rightly, found this absurd; Locke's error was his belief that words (such as 'triangle') named ideas. On the contrary, such general words do not name single abstract ideas but are 'made the sign . . . of several particular ideas'. Their constancy of meaning is sustained by their *definition*, in which the features which differentiate particular instances are omitted: 'It is one thing to keep a name constantly to the same *definition*, and another to make it stand everywhere for the same *idea*: the one is necessary, the other useless and impracticable' (1710, 1962 edn, Introduction, p. 58).

This provides the conceptual entry into the 'Idealist' or 'Immaterialist' case elaborated so skilfully in the bodies of Berkeley's two main philosophical works. Abstract ideas being impossible, he can develop a far more thoroughgoing sensationalist epistemology than Locke's. He can abandon the 'primary and secondary qualities' distinction, since the notion of 'matter' on which it rests is, as an abstract idea, incoherent. Matter gone, we are left with perceptions themselves, which exist in the mind, hence everything exists in some sense 'in the mind'; 'Esse is percippi' – to be is to be perceived. This famous slogan must, I think, be understood, as Warnock suggests, in the context of his linguistically based rejection of abstract ideas; it is ultimately a definition of how we use the abstract term 'exist'. Berkeley is actually far from wanting to end up in the solipsistic position of arguing that everything exists only in his own mind; indeed he holds that his philosophy salvages commonsense from the mystifications of his matter- or 'substance'- fixated philosophical predecessors.

Whilst everything exists only in so far as it is perceived, the fact remains that, unlike the things which I can imagine, the furniture of the apparently external universe is independent of my will, and the phenomena therein are amazingly regular and harmonious in their occurrence and relationships. Since the 'esse is percippi' principle is logically sound, we must, Berkeley concludes, accept that everything is sustained by God's omnipotent perception. The relationships we identify as causal in truth have no necessary connection but are signs of Divinely maintained 'Natural Laws'. Berkeley's argument for the immanence of Divine perception as the ontological basis of the universe is no mere supplementary saving hypothesis, but the object of the whole philosophical exercise in which he has been engaged. The world presented itself to this devout Bishop of Cloyne as a direct message or sign from God. This was no simple 'argument from design' but a fundamental metaphysical necessity:

> . . . whithersoever we direct our view we do at all times and in all places perceive manifest tokens of the Divinity; everything we see, hear, feel, or anywise perceive by sense, being a sign or affect of the power of God . . . (1710, para. 148)

In Berkeley's 'Immaterialism' the concept of 'matter' has no place, and with its elimination we can cease to worry about the relationship between matter and spirit which had so perplexed philosophers hitherto. To Berkeley it was obvious: the universe was an entirely spiritual entity, 'matter' a sophistical, incomprehensible hypothesis. We should give him the credit for honestly reporting on his experience of the universe, and take him at his word, but this requires a somewhat greater effort of hermeneutic imagination than he has generally been afforded. It demands that we see the world as animated by an active Divinity, a world in which every object is a Divine utterance, a 'manifest token' of the Spirit of its Creator. Like the Zen master's 'satori', nothing is changed but everything is somehow transformed. In Berkeley we have, perhaps, a 'mystic' temperament seeking expression within the intellectual framework of an anti-mystic age. To return to the 'Signal mode' to which I referred above: I have argued[11] that this involves construing phenomena as messages or signals – it would be difficult to find a clearer expression of the world-view of someone in whom this mode is dominant than the passage just quoted.

Leahey (1987) sees Berkeley as possessing a twofold significance for Psychology. First, in his work on vision and generally introspective method he finds the roots of later nineteenth-century Structuralism: 'Berkeley thus set Titchener's empirical problems' (*ibid.*, p. 110). Second, he argues that Berkeley asserted 'the fundamental tenet of positivism that underlies radical behaviorism: If something cannot be perceived, it is a metaphysical relic to be expunged from science' (*ibid.*). This, for Leahey, makes Berkeley Skinner's ancestor. Neither claim strikes me as rigorously sustainable. Berkeley's account of perception was indeed influential, but by the mid nineteenth century it had filtered through so many intervening (mostly German) minds that a direct ancestry is hardly justifiable beyond the general point that he was the first systematically to make a case for perception being learned (and Kant's opposing case had also, by then, to be addressed). His introspective method was philosophically orthodox for the period and, being in no way experimental in the modern sense, quite different from that of Wundt and Titchener[12]. As far as Berkeley as a proto-positivist is concerned, this really stretches retrospective labelling to the point of absurdity. Not only is there no line of direct intellectual descent from Berkeley to modern positivism, but his acceptance of the reality of 'spirit' and rejection of 'matter' as the 'metaphysical relic' signifies a diametrically opposite interpretation of the primacy of perception.

Berkeley's contribution to Psychology's history is, we must conclude, relatively peripheral. It is confined, in fact, to his theory of vision, a theory originally formulated to further a philosophical, epistemological argument. His immediate successors (with a few exceptions such as Hume and, I suspect, Peter Browne) found his Idealism and 'Immaterialism' impossible to take seriously, generally construing it overcrudely as solipsistic. While philosophers in addressing his arguments have since come to appreciate their power and ingenuity, his role has always been that of someone to be argued *against* rather than someone to follow. There have been precious few avowed Berkeleyans. He was, by contemporary consensus, a lovely man, and remained so dear to the American heart that they named a Californian university after him. And in the quadrangle of his own Trinity College, Dublin, one can still see the tree, which according to the famous limerick, ceases to exist when no one is looking at it.

The next major figure in the orthodox canon with a claim to be considered as a proto-Psychologist is David Hartley, and his claim is somewhat better founded.

(c) David Hartley (1705–57) and J. O. de La Mettrie (1709–51)

We have already seen how the notion of humans as machines, so often cited as the seventeenth century's major contribution to Psychological thought, was confused by the variety of concepts of 'mechanism' in circulation. The kind of 'mechanistic' image which became popular in Britain in the early years of the eighteenth century seems to have owed more to the variegated version represented by Willis's physiology than to the simpler Cartesian model. However, the philosophical works so far considered have largely been conducted in quite different terms. Although Hutcheson can, as we saw, talk of 'mechanick Laws', there has as yet been little integration between the Lockean tradition of analytical philosophical method and the empirical work of mechanistic physiologists. Indeed, Boyle and Willis came in for much pillorying by writers such as Swift and Mandeville[13]. The fusion of the two kinds of discourse – philosophical and 'scientific' – begins to occur only in the 1740's. Hartley's *Observations on Man* (1749; facsimile reprint 1966) and La Mettrie's *L'Homme machine* (1745) translated as *Man a Machine* (Dublin – 1749,

London – 1750) are the most important works representing this development.

David Hartley's *Observations on Man, His Frame, His Duty, and His Expectations.*
The outcome of over a decade of writing and rumination by its author[14], this is the first fully elaborated attempt at integrating Newtonian physics with Associationist philosophy to produce a comprehensive Natural Philosophical account of mind. The long-term impact of the work was considerable; Joseph Priestley, Samuel Taylor Coleridge and the Mills accorded it enormous respect and acknowledged its influence on their own philosophical development (Coleridge actually named his first son David Hartley – but his second Berkeley!). Its wholehearted commitment to the grounding of discourse about the nature of 'Man' in physiological knowledge has earned Hartley the high esteem of historians of Psychology since Rand (1923); indeed Webb (1988) goes so far as to say that 'it is commonly acknowledged' to have 'set psychology on the course it has followed to the present day' (p. 202). Here, surely, we have a clear attempt, albeit crude, at producing a physiological Psychology (or perhaps a Psychophysiology), at least in Part One of the work. Huguelet, in his introduction to the 1966 facsimile edition, fully endorses Rand and Boring in claiming that

> Hartley became the first philosopher to relate the bodily frame, with all its complicated apparatus of sense-organs and nerves, to all phenomena of sensation, imagination, memory, understanding, affection, and will . . . (p. ix)

The impact of the work was relatively slow until Joseph Priestley issued an abridged edition in 1775 (which left out the very physiological speculations for which Hartley is now praised). Hartley, a doctor born in Bath, identifies two major influences: first, and more immediate, Gay's *Dissertation Concerning the Fundamental Principle of Virtue or Morality* (1731)[15], an Associationist account of ethics in the Hutcheson tradition, and second, but more profound, Newton's account of sensation as given in the *Opticks* (1704).

The work is in two parts, the first containing Hartley's influential 'Psychological' doctrines, the second an account of how these support and strengthen religion[16]. Hartley's first task is to demonstrate how the Lockean philosophical doctrine of Association and the Newtonian physical doctrine that sensation takes the form of 'vibrations' are complementary:

> The Doctrine of *Vibrations* may appear at first *Sight* to have no Connexion with that of *Association*; however if these Doctrines be found in fact to contain the Laws of the Bodily and Mental Powers respectively, they must be related to each other since the Body and Mind are. One may expect that *Vibrations* should infer *Associations* as their Effect, and *Association* point to *Vibrations* as its Cause. (p. 6)

This doctrine of 'Vibrations' has, understandably, attracted most attention from historians as representing a pioneering attempt at firmly grounding the psychological in the physical, and does indeed read as a distant anticipation of Hebb's 'reverberating cell-assemblies' of exactly two centuries later (Hebb, 1949). 'The white medullary Substance of the Brain' is both 'the immediate Instrument of Sensation and Motion' and 'the immediate Instrument, by which Ideas are presented to the Mind: Or in other Words, whatever Changes are made in this Substance, corresponding Changes are made in our Ideas, and vice-versa' (p. 8). An often repeated impression or cluster of impressions will bring about a permanent representation of itself in the brain in the form of a small residual vibration or 'vibratiuncle'. He even notes that 'Electricity is also connected in various Ways with the Doctrine of Vibrations' (p. 28).

Hartley's elaboration of the doctrine of vibrations is more complex than many secondary sources indicate, for he finds himself in a position of having to differentiate between vibrations of the particles of the medullary substance and those of the Newtonian 'aether' pervading their interstices[17]. Vibrations can also differ in four ways: Degree, Kind, Place and Line of Direction (p. 30). This would generate eight dimensions of variance, but Hartley does not pursue these systematically. Significantly, he abandons the idea of fluid-like 'Animal Spirits' running through tubular nerves; nerves are, as Newton says, 'rather solid Capillaments', not Booerhaave's 'small *tubuli*'. He also has to find a solution to the relationship between physical vibrations and mental phenomena consistent with the orthodox religious rejection of the view that 'Matter can be endued with the Power of Sensation' – the old 'thinking matter' issue which had been in the arena since Hobbes. In dealing with this he is drawn to a position on the mind–body relationship in which some find echoes of Malebranche's 'Occasionalism'. The following passage is certainly rather contorted:

> If we suppose an infinitesimal elementary Body to be intermediate between the Soul and the gross Body, which appears to be no improbable Supposition, then the Changes in our Sensations, Ideas, and Motions, may correspond to the Changes made in the medullary Substance, only as far as these correspond to the Changes made in the elementary Body. And if these last Changes have some other Source besides the Vibrations in the medullary Substance, some peculiar original Properties, for Instance, of the elementary Body, then Vibrations will not be adequate Exponents of Sensations, Ideas and Motions. Other Suppositions to the same Purpose might be made; and, upon the Whole, I conjecture, that though the First and Second Propositions are true, in a very useful practical sense, yet they are not so in an ultimate and precise one. (p. 34)

Finally, at the end of Part One, he tackles the Free-Will Problem, which he resolves less than satisfactorily by differentiating between a 'philosophical sense' (in which Free Will is incompatible with the deterministic 'Mechanism of our Natures') and a 'popular and practical sense' (in which Free Will, as 'the Power of doing what a Person desires or wills to do' is unaffected)[18].

Hartley's major achievement, then, was an account of psychological phenomena in which neither the physiological nor the philosophical level of analysis is given priority. He cannot really resolve the issue of how the two are related, but Part One of the *Observations* approximates more closely to the concerns of modern classics of theoretical Psychology (such as James's *Principles of Psychology*, Koffka's *Principles of Gestalt Psychology* or Hebb's *Organization of Behavior*) than any other eighteenth-century work. In this respect, as Danziger (1983) observes, Hartley is at the end of a tradition in physiological theorizing rather than a pioneer; but his contemporary Robert Whytt would soon inaugurate an approach which emancipated physiology, especially neurophysiology, from the shackles of the mind–body issue (see below, pp. 197–199).

A second, more immediately influential contribution derived from Hartley's desire to reconcile a basically hedonistic Associationist model with a Christian ethical system. In order to do this he identifies a sevenfold hierarchy of Pleasures and Pains. At the bottom are those of Sensation, directly originating in the Impressions made on the external senses. Then come Imagination (where the Pain or Pleasure derives from deformity or beauty), Ambition (opinions of others about us), Self-interest (related to our possession of the means of security), Sympathy (Pain and Pleasure of our fellow creatures), 'Theopathy' ('The Affections excited in us by the Contemplation of the Deity') and Moral Sense (originating from Moral Beauty and Deformity). This schema made a considerable impression on later Utilitarians, and was, so far as I know, genuinely original. Hartley's Associationism itself was fairly orthodox, although his terminology differs slightly from Hume's and Locke's (Impressions on the senses cause Sensations, these yield Ideas of Sensation which are simple, and the association of these in turn generates complex Intellectual Ideas); for Hartley (anticipating James Mill in this) the sole associative principle appears to be contiguity, in either time or space. His account of language has already been discussed in Chapter 2.

Hartley's purely philosophical merits are of a lower order than those of Berkeley and Hume. On the other hand, since he was a practising physician this is offset by a fuller appreciation of contemporary physiology and Newtonian methodological principles (to which he strives to adhere). Ironically, the balance Hartley struck could not be maintained by his immediate successors, and Priestley himself, as already noted, omitted the crucial sections on the doctrine of vibrations from his own edition of the *Observations*. The white medullary substance of the brain fails to figure in the ruminations of any of the Scottish philosophers except to be derided by Thomas Brown (see below, pp. 353–4), while the physiologists, fully occupied with conceptualizing the nature of organic life, progressively lose interest in grand philosophizing. His high symbolic significance for modern physiological psychologists must on balance be judged as at variance with his very limited impact on Enlightenment physiological thought. Hartley's influence is carried primarily through a somewhat heterogeneous range of philosophical, rather than physiological, thinkers, from the Romantic Coleridge to the more mundane Mills, each able to find in him doctrines congenial to their own.

J.O. de La Mettrie's *Man a Machine*
This is a more consciously iconoclastic and polemical work than Hartley's, infused with French anti-clericalism. La Mettrie assails 'lame philosophers', 'and above all, the divines' for holding forth 'without modesty, on a subject they have never been qualified to examine thoroughly', i.e. 'the labyrinth of Man' (1750 edn, p. 5). In terms reminiscent of Coward's he attacks the notion of the soul – 'nothing but an empty term, of which we have no idea' (*ibid.*, p. 55), and offers a thoroughgoing materialist account:

> The least principle of motion being granted, then animated bodies will have all that's requisite to make them move, feel, think, repent, in a word, enough to lead them into all the physical and moral consequences which depend thereon. (*ibid.*, p. 55)

> . . . man is but an animal made up of a number of springs, which are all put in motion by each other; as yet we cannot tell to which part of the human structure nature first set her hand. . . . [t]he soul is only the first principle of motion, or a sensible material part of the brain, which we may certainly look upon as the original spring of the whole machine, which influences the rest, and appears to have been first formed, so that all the other springs seem to derive their motions thence . . . (*ibid.*, p. 66)

The body is like a clock and 'fresh chyle', which leads to 'fermentation' of the blood, is the pendulum. In La Mettrie, as in Hartley, vibration plays a part, for there is a 'vibrating principle' in all organized bodies (*ibid.*, p. 69). La Mettrie is confident enough in his mastery of physiology to attack figures as eminent as Boerhaave, Stahl and Willis, for whom the soul is envisaged as somehow suffused throughout the body (though he holds Willis in high esteem otherwise). For La Mettrie, as for Coward earlier, soul equals motion. As for 'thought' (or consciousness):

> So far . . . am I from thinking that thought is inconsistent with organized matter, that I look upon it to be a property as much belonging thereto, as electricity, impenetrability, extension &c. (*ibid.*, p. 77)

This mechanistic vision, he claims, is in the true Cartesian spirit, offering perhaps the first example of a 'revisionist' reading of

Descartes intended to make him the fount of rigorous anti-clerical materialism:

> For in short, tho' he descants upon the two different substances; *yet it appears very plain, that this is only a stroke of policy, a piece of finesse, to make the Divines swallow the poison which was conceal'd in that analogy*, of which they alone were ignorant, whilst everybody else could not help being struck with it. (*ibid.*, pp. 75–6; emphasis added)

It was argued in the previous chapter that, on the contrary, 'it appears very plain' that Descartes's motives were quite the reverse. With La Mettrie we begin to see the 'scientist' waxing confident over the legitimacy of 'Man' as part of the territory of science, and prepared to scorn theology's claims on the grounds of scientific ignorance. On the other hand, there is nothing in La Mettrie's account which suggests an interest in empirical psychological or behavioural, as opposed to physiological, enquiry. The fame of *Man a Machine* owes much to its character as a rhetorical manifesto, in detail its doctrines generally have less novelty than is often claimed.

As the century progressed, another philosophical voice began to gain an increasingly wide audience – that of the greatest of Locke's heirs, David Hume.

(d) David Hume (1711–76)[19]

Hume's *Treatise of Human Nature* (1739–40) is, by almost universal consent, a work of the very highest calibre as philosophy and, in parts, literature. From optimistic beginnings he is led inexorably to deeply sceptical conclusions, which he never baulks at drawing. In this work, written in Hume's early twenties, British Associationism attains its finest formulation, and some of the arguments he raises (for example, about the concept of 'cause' and the relationship between reason and emotion) continue to exercise philosophers. Its initial lack of success led him to publish a shorter account: *Enquiry Concerning the Human Understanding*, in 1748. In 1751 the *Enquiry Concerning the Principles of Morals* appeared. He then turned to history and politics (his *History of England* [1754–62] being his most important non-philosophical work). In 1779, *Dialogues Concerning Natural Religion* was posthumously published (written initially in the early 1750s; Hume revised it around 1761 and again just before his death in 1776). This last includes his refutation of the 'Argument from Design', a refutation which remains sound although it failed to make much immediate impact in the ensuing heyday of Paleyite Natural Theology[20]. At the risk of imbalancing the text, Hume demands a rather more extensive account than those discussed so far. Book I of the *Treatise* in particular is, I think, a crucial expression of the condition of the psychological substructure of the period (if that is not too grandiose a way of putting it). That is far from meaning it is 'typical' – quite the contrary, it ruthlessly seeks to articulate those implications of the contemporary *mentalité* which are typically being evaded.

The difference between Hume's *Treatise* and Locke's *Essay* is more profound than at first appears. It would be easy to read Hume as offering a polished up, more systematized version of the same philosophical position, but there is a major difference in underlying intention between them. Locke, as we have seen, was attempting to delimit the range of human understanding in the context of a complex contemporary politico-theological debate; he was not offering a putatively scientific Psychological theory. Hume, by contrast, appears to be doing just this, quite explicitly, and although his epistemological conclusions have had the most enduring impact on philosophical thought, his Psychological concerns are comprehensive. It is 'Human Nature', not 'Human Understanding', which figures in his title – while in full it reads *A Treatise of Human Nature: being an attempt to introduce the experimental Method of Reasoning into Moral Subjects.* (But there could be few better examples of the difficulties involved in elucidating eighteenth-century 'Psychological' thought than this. What is 'the experimental Method of Reasoning? And what did he mean by a 'Moral Subject'?)

By the time Hume was writing a weariness with inconsequential and clamorous philosophical debate had begun to settle on the English, if not Scottish and Irish, scene. As Hume saw it:

> Amidst all this bustle 'tis not reason, which carries the prize, but eloquence; and no man needs despair of gaining proselytes to the most extravagant hypothesis, who has art enough to represent it in any favourable colours. The victory is not gained by the men at arms, who manage the pike and the sword; but by the trumpeters, drummers, and musicians of the army. (1964 edn, p. xviii; all quotations are from this reprint of L.A. Selby-Bigge's 1888 edn)

Yet all the sciences 'are in some measure dependent on the science of MAN' (p. xix) and 'we ourselves are not only the beings, that reason, but also one of the objects, concerning which we reason' (*ibid.*):

> In pretending therefore to explain the principles of human nature, we in effect propose a compleat system of the sciences, built on a foundation almost entirely new, and the only one upon which they can stand with any security. (p. xx)

While this sounds not too far from Locke in so far as a conceptual underpinning of the sciences is his goal, his tone a page later is more akin to that of modern Pychology:

> For to me it seems evident, that the essence of mind being equally unknown to us with that of external bodies, it must be equally impossible to form any notion of its powers and qualities otherwise than from careful and exact experiments, and observation of those particular effects, which result from its different circumstances and situations. (p. xxi)

But what, for Hume, is a 'careful and exact experiment'? He tells us we must go about 'tracing up our experiments to the utmost . . . explaining all effects from the simplest and fewest causes' (*ibid.*). Later, he notes that 'Moral Philosophy' has

> . . . this peculiar disadvantage, which is not found in natural [philosophy], that in collecting its experiments, it cannot make them purposely, with premeditation, and after such a manner as to satisfy itself concerning every particular difficulty which may arise. (pp. xxii–xxiii)

And thus

> We must therefore glean up our experiments in this science from a cautious observation of human life, and take them as they appear in the common course of the world, by men's behaviour in company, in affairs, and in their pleasures. Where experiments of this kind are judiciously collected and compared, we may hope to establish on them a science, which will not be inferior in certainty, and will be much superior in utility to any other of human comprehension. (p. xxiii)

Clearly, Hume's term 'experiment' differs considerably from modern usage, referring to the gathering of the data of experience, reflective introspective exercises, and what we now term 'natural experiments' rather than methodically systematized surveys or active manipulation of experimental variables by an 'experiment*er*'. It is the imperative to restrict our data to that of experiential observation (as opposed to abstract speculation and sophistry) which is central, and this rather general Empiricist imperative, rather than any specific method of empirical investigation, defines, for the eighteenth century, what it is to be engaged in science. Phrases such as 'the Science of Man' do not, therefore, signal the presence of Psychology or anthropology in any modern sense. Nevertheless, with Hume we have reached some kind of halfway point at which the insistence is (a) that philosophy itself should be empirical; and (b) that in being so philosophy itself constitutes a 'Science of Man'.

In the event, however, Hume fails to fulfil these Introductory ambitions, but finds himself driven into an extreme epistemological – even existential – scepticism. He begins confidently enough differentiating 'impressions' (which include sensations, 'passions and emotions' 'as they make their first appearance in the soul') from 'ideas', which are copies left in the mind after an impression ceases[21]. Each may be simple or complex, and impressions may be those of Sensation or of 'Reflexion', the latter deriving from existing ideas which can arouse 'new impressions of desire and aversion, hope and fear' (p. 8). At this point he makes the – to us – curious assertion (curious, that is, if we wish to classify him as a psychologist): 'The examination of our sensations belongs more to anatomists and natural philosophers than to moral; and therefore shall not at present be enter'd upon' (*ibid.*). Is he or is he not, then, seeing himself as a 'natural philosopher' ? Well – yes and no; his ambiguity regarding how far 'Moral Philosophy' is an integral part of the Natural Philosophical programme or a parallel enterprise to be modelled on, but kept separate from, the latter is precisely what is significant. I shall return to this again later.

With these preliminaries out of the way, he can enter into the 'association of ideas' and the principles governing this process. As Locke had striven to show how all our 'Ideas' were built up from 'simple ideas of sensation', so Hume builds them up from 'simple ideas' being connected by the three 'qualities' of 'Resemblance,

Contiguity in time or place, and Cause and Effect' (p. 11). In these, all complex ideas 'divisible into Relations, Modes and Substances' have their source. This presents no real difficulty until he returns in – Book I, Part 3, Section ii – to the idea of cause and effect: the central 'relation' on which scientific knowledge hinges. Unlike Berkeley, Hume cannot expain this as some kind of Divine illusion; rather, it turns out, on his analysis, to originate in 'contiguity' – A causes B because B is spatially and temporally contiguous with A: 'I find . . . that whatever objects are consider'd as causes or effects, are *contiguous . . . We may therefore consider the relation of* CONTIGUITY *as essential to that of causation*' (p. 75; original capitals and emphasis):

> Having thus discover'd or suppos'd the two relations of *contiguity* and *succession* to be essential to causes and effects, I find I am stopt short, and can proceed no farther in considering any single instance of cause and effect. (p. 76)

The potential subversiveness of this position does not strike home immediately; it is only later (in I. 3. xiv: 'Of the idea of necessary connexion') that Hume confronts its sceptical implications. Causation – 'necessary connexion' – is a quality of 'perceptions, not of objects' (p. 166). It is 'internally felt by the soul, and not perceived externally in bodies' (*ibid.*). This leads him to a final redefinition of 'cause' which, by virtue of the impact it has had on all subsequent epistemological debate, we must state in full:

> A CAUSE is an object precedent and contiguous to another, and so united with it, that the idea of the one determines the mind to form the idea of the other, and the impression of one to form a more lively idea of the other. (p. 170)

Hume's reduction of 'causality' to the status of a purely psychological construct planted a seed of doubt regarding the status of scientific knowledge which, after more than a century of subterranean irritation, resurfaced in the positivist philosophies of science of Mach and Clifford in the 1890s[22]. He tries to rescue things by avowing that 'Our reason must be consider'd as a kind of cause, of which truth is the natural effect'; though he immediately adds: 'but such-a-one as by the irruption of other causes, and by the inconstancy of our mental powers, may frequently be prevented' (I. 4. i, p. 180). But the damage is done, and Hume is swept deeper into sceptical waters in considering the testimony of the senses, plaintively concluding:

> This sceptical doubt, both with respect to reason and the senses is a malady, which can never be radically cur'd, but must return upon us every moment, however we may chace it away, and sometimes seem entirely free from it. (I. 4. ii, p. 218)

Things get worse. First, it transpires that 'there is a direct and total opposition betwixt our reason and our senses' (p. 231), but it is when Hume comes to ponder 'personal identity' (in I. 4. vi) that his doubts reach a climax. Indeed, he verges on what we may anachronistically term authentic existentialist *Angst*. Whenever he tries to 'enter most intimately into what I call *myself*' (p. 252) he finds only particular perceptions. 'I can never catch *myself* at any time without a perception' (*ibid.*). Mind and Self are nothing but concatenations of ideas, perceptions, impressions, linked by the principles of association. The Self constantly threatens to dissolve. Book I ends with a famous skirling lament which contrasts dramatically with his opening hopes:

> Methinks I am like a man, who having struck on many shoals, and having narrowly escap'd ship-wreck in passing a small frith, has yet the temerity to put out to sea in the same leaky weather-beaten vessel, and even carries his ambition so far as to think of compassing the globe... The wretched condition, weakness, and disorder of the faculties, reduces me almost to despair, and makes me resolve to perish on the barren rock, on which I am at present, rather than venture myself upon that boundless ocean, which runs out into immensity. This sudden view of my danger strikes me with melancholy; and as 'tis usual for that passion, above all others, to indulge itself; I cannot forbear feeding my despair, with all those desponding reflections, which the present subject furnishes me with in such abundance. (I. 7. vii, pp. 263–4)

This strikes a tone hitherto unheard in Western philosophy. Not to put too fine a point on it, Hume's *Treatise* may arguably be considered as the point at which the truly 'psychological' emerges as a central philosophical *problem.* For Hume, the principles of Association were of the nature of natural laws; he views himself as operating, at least partially, *within,* not transcending, 'natural philosophy'. He has cast aside the consoling scaffolding of religious faith, finally abandoned any theological agenda, and found himself gazing with appalled fascination on the flimsy and insecure psychological foundations on which all human knowledge, belief, and our very sense of identity rest.

The remaining two books of the *Treatise* concern the 'passions' and morality. Again, Hume's conclusions are at odds with the prevailing sanguine confidence of the 'Age of Reason'. Reason itself cannot provide motives for action, these must originate in some 'instinctive passions'. While pleasure and pain provide the 'chief spring and actuating principle of the human mind' Hume avoids simple hedonism: there are numerous passions arising from 'natural impulse' or 'instinct', which are 'perfectly unaccountable'. 'Reason is, and ought only to be the slave of the passions, and can never pretend to any other office than to serve and obey them' (II. 3. iii, p. 415). His analysis of morality opens the doors for ethical relativism, but he fends this off to a large extent by placing the principle of 'Sympathy' in a central role. While we must here forgo any further detailed discussion of his accounts of the Passions and Morality, one important consequence of these must be highlighted: a subsequent widespread and influential acceptance, in both ethics and Psychology of the subordination of reason to non-rational motivational forces (see Midgley, 1979 for a critique of this position). It is to Hume that we owe the origin of this *topos* in its modern form, and it provides a perennial theme cutting across philosophical and psychological thought.

Hume's alleged (and probably genuine) atheism was a matter of lifelong notoriety in his native Edinburgh, but its detrimental effects were offset by a charismatic personality and the robustness of his friendships with such people as Adam Smith. He died in 1776 with a calm demeanour which Smith acclaimed, but which disturbed pious clerics,[23] who felt that atheists had no right to die in so serene a manner.

What, then, is Hume's significance for Psychology? Again we may take Leahey (1987) as a reference point. His summary of Hume's main tenets is excellent, but there is a persistent tendency to force his concerns into a modern mould. His sub-section on Hume is entitled 'Habit over Reason' (p. 110): 'In Hume's work we see the first glimmerings of the psychology of adaptation' (p. 114). He sees Hume as wishing to replace speculative metaphysics by Psychology as the foundation for all science, and is eager to downplay Hume's scepticism – it being *moderate* scepticism only that Hume advocates. This is a traditional reading, of course[24]. Behaviourism and Freud are both anticipated.

Concerning Hume's scepticism and proto-adaptationism, it is undoubtedly true that he recognized scepticism as a 'malady', and that for practical purposes one must accept the habitual and customary as providing the basis for human life. What Leahey misses, however, is the psychological dynamic of Book I of the *Treatise*; quite clearly, by Hume's own testimony, as we have just seen, he did at one point find himself driven into radical scepticism, with its attendant despair and melancholy. This may be a 'malady', but he never claims it to be an *error*. Rather, he can but return, a wiser and a sadder man, to the practical concerns of living. His acceptance (and advocacy of the acceptance) of the primacy of habit and custom (and, indeed, instinct) comes not in the nature of a happy quasi-scientific *discovery* but as a psychological prophylactic against despair. The sacrifice of the primacy of Reason is not done lightly, for this, after all, is the faculty to which he, as philosopher, is necessarily intellectually committed. It is a sacrifice achieved only by a profound personal struggle – *a struggle of which his text is itself an account*. Nor is it, in the final analysis, an entirely satisfactory outcome, precisely because it is so paradoxical – for while conceding the point at one level, modern psychologists espousing the doctrine are, by virtue of being 'scientists', denying it in practice. Abandoning the primacy of Reason is essentially a sceptical move, and – paradoxically indeed! – as impracticable to maintain as the primacy of Reason appeared, in the face of Hume's 'experimental' evidence, to be in the first place. Finally, to claim that Hume wanted to replace speculative metaphysics with Psychology is highly anachronistic – the term 'psychology' does not, so far as I am aware, occur in his work. True, he wants to create a 'Science of Man', but the *Treatise* in itself does not constitute anything which would now be called a 'science'. He actually *excludes* from it the topic of perception and, unlike Hartley, evinces no interest in physiology. Hume's despair regarding the success of his 'Psychology' is confirmed by the fact that in the subsequent *Enquiry Concerning the Human Understanding* he virtually abandoned the ambitions for a scientific Psychology which appeared to be his aim in the *Treatise*.

I am genuinely unclear how far Hume (as against Hartley) saw himself as engaged in Natural Philosophy; as often noted, his principles of Association have a Newtonian air about them, and he uses the term 'experiment' to describe his method. Yet he clearly does not identify himself with the physical sciences, and I suspect that my lack of clarity on the matter reflects his own. If there is an anticipation of modern Psychology to be found here, it is with the discipline's perennial status dilemma – the relationship between eighteenth-century 'Moral' and 'Natural' philosophies being as muddied as that between the 'Humanistic' branches of modern Psychology and its avowedly 'scientific' ones. In this respect Hume's ambiguity is an early and significant, if not unique, case.

Hume's direct influence on philosophy appears far greater than any he has had on Psychology, except as mediated by subsequent generations of rather more humdrum Associationists such as James Mill. I do not wish to deny that 'adaptationism' is present in Hume (but even Leahey discerns only 'the first glimmerings'). I would, however, deny that this is the most significant thing about him. It appears significant only if one construes one's task as primarily about identifying such glimmerings. Hume's significance is at once greater and yet more covert than Leahey indicates; his is a fully secularized philosophical consciousness (far more so than Hartley's or Reid's) trying to rely on Reason to confront and explore the psychological – and returning, wryly chastened, into a personal wisdom rather than freighted with scientific knowledge. As the first kind of such close encounter, we can recognize in it the arrival on stage of 'the psychological' as a coherent realm of enquiry. Hume's position is nodal, and we are at risk of overlooking this if we are overeager to trace only a continuity of thought from Locke to the Mills.

(e) Thomas Reid's 'Common Sense' School

The sceptical implications of a thoroughgoing Associationist empirical epistemology, as formulated by Berkeley and Hume, drew forth strong reactions. Was philosophy taking us into such absurd conclusions as that matter did not exist? That we could know nothing for certain, not even our own identity? Johnson, quite irrelevantly, famously kicked a stone, harrumphing 'Thus I refute Berkeley!' In Scotland a self-dubbed 'Common Sense' school of philosophy more successfully strove to bring things down to earth; its leading figures were Thomas Reid (1710–96), Dugald Stewart (1753–1828) and, less eminently, the polymathic and peculiar judge Henry Home, Lord Kames (1696–1782). One initially turns to Reid with a sense of mild foreboding, conscious only that virtually all British philosophical debate on psychological matters in the last third of the century was being conducted under his aegis. Between Hartley in 1749 and James Mill in 1829 British Associationism was in fact creatively moribund, its revival owing much, as we saw earlier, to Horne Tooke's linguistic theory at the turn of the century. (Thomas Brown's semi-Associationist *Lectures on the Philosophy of the Human Mind* [1820] might arguably be picked in lieu of Mill, but it hardly alters the picture.) This foreboding is not entirely justified; reading Reid's collected works is more of a difficulty typographically than stylistically, and his philosophical position turns out to be less crass than generally portrayed.

Reid opens his campaign with the *Inquiry into the Human Mind* (1764), an essentially reactionary text opposing most of those features in the works of Locke's various successors which we have identified as progressive in the sense of marking moves towards a modern Psychological orientation; he is strongly hostile to Hutcheson's sorties into mathematical analysis, recoils from the 'existentialist' issues implicit in both Berkeley's Idealism and Hume's scepticism, and has no truck with Hartleyan – or any other kind of – mechanistic physiology. His (up to a point) loyal acolyte, Dugald Stewart, can nevertheless write, in all seriousness:

> The idea of prosecuting the study of the human mind, on a plan analogous to that which had been so successfully adopted in physics by the followers of Lord Bacon, if not first conceived by Dr Reid, was, at least, first carried successfully into execution in his writings. (Reid, 1863, p. 8, all references are to this edn)

At the opening of the *Inquiry* we read, with a sense of *déjà vu*:

> I claim no other merit than that of having given great attention to the operations of my own mind, and of having expressed, with all the perspicuity I was able, what I conceive every man, who gives the same attention, will feel and perceive . . . The experiments that were to be made in this investigation suited me, as they required no other expense but that of time and attention, which I could bestow. (p. 96)

He hopes 'to justify the common sense and reason of mankind, against the sceptical subtleties which, in this age, have endeavoured to put them out of countenance . . .' (*ibid.*)[25]. One would have thought that by 1764 the fact that a whole succession of philosophers from Hutcheson onwards had claimed to be doing the same thing, yet failed to reach agreement, would have alerted Reid to the deficiencies in this methodology. Perhaps it did, for he is soon writing:

> To attend accurately to the operations of our minds, and make them an object of thought, is no easy matter even to the contemplative, and to the bulk of mankind is next to impossible. . . . it is his own mind only that he can examine with any degree of accuracy and directness . . . such a prodigious diversity of minds must make it extremely difficult to discover the common principles of the species. (p. 98)

The essence of Reid's philosophical position is that metaphysics is in a parlous state because Descartes, Malebranche, Locke, Berkeley and Hume have been led to raise serious doubts about matters which no sane man ever questioned: 'A man that disbelieves his own existence, is surely as unfit to be reasoned with as a man that believes he is made of glass' (p. 100)[26]. As for Descartes's *Cogito, ergo sum*, 'it is evident he was in his senses all the time, and never seriously doubted of his existence' (*ibid.*). ('The nature of the Cartesian Doubt and its solution is here misapprehended,' Sir William Hamilton drily notes.) These absurdities, which are bringing philosophy into such disregard, are all traceable to the doctrine of 'ideas' as entities representing the external world:

> . . . they are a mere fiction and hypothesis . . . this hypothesis of

> ideas or images of things in the mind, or in the sensorium, is the parent of those many paradoxes so shocking to common sense, and of that scepticism which disgrace our philosophy of mind, and have brought upon it the ridicule and contempt of sensible men. (p. 106)

The afore-cited philosophical succession have progressively reasoned themselves deeper into the mire; Berkeley at least attempted to render spirit secure by partitioning it off from matter, but then Hume 'wantonly sapped the foundation of this partition, and drowned all in one universal deluge' (p. 103).

It is their failure to keep themselves rooted in the empirical evidence – the 'true touchstone . . . of facts and experiments', as Home (1779) put it – that has led his illustrious predecessors astray. Reid clearly felt seriously threatened by the 'Abyss of Scepticism'; even though his tone in writing of it is one of mockery, it provokes in him periodic flights of rhetorical excess such as 'I despise Philosophy and renounce its guidance – let my soul dwell with Common Sense' (p. 101) and 'I see myself, and the whole frame of nature shrink into fleeting ideas, which, like Epicurus's atoms, dance about in emptiness' (p. 103). Intellectually intimidated by the exalted targets of his protest, he turns this into a virtue:

> It is genius, not the want of it, that adulterates philosophy, and fills it with error and false theory. A creative imagination disdains the mean offices of digging for a foundation, or removing rubbish, and carrying materials . . . (p. 99)

Seeing himself as faithfully abiding by Newton's strictures against speculation, hypothesis and theory – all of which thus become pejorative terms – Reid poses as a humble unimaginative anatomist of the mind, confining his task to a 'just induction from facts', adherent of 'the way of observation and experiment'. Philosophy severs itself from Common Sense at its peril, it is an 'unequal contest'; philosophy 'will always come off both with dishonour and loss' (p. 101).

Reid's use of the term Common Sense was a rhetorical move which has, in the long term, backfired on him. He was far from wanting to accept, unexamined, the commonplace opinions of *hoi polloi*. What he wishes to maintain is that there are a number of self-evident truths or beliefs which cannot be further analysed, reduced or explained. That I exist is one of them. That it is actually objects themselves, not ideas of them, which I experience is another. This latter rejection of a representational or causal theory of perception was unusual, especially for a mind–body dualist, and in the event Reid never succeeded in formulating a coherent alternative[27]. There are 'certain principles' in the 'constitution of our nature' which we have no alternative but to accept. In this respect Reid's critique of Hume has affinities with that subsequently mounted by Kant, his principles of common sense adumbrating Kant's Transcendental *a priori* categories (such as space and time) without which any experience at all is impossible (Drever 1966; Robinson, 1986).

The triad Sensation, Memory and Imagination are basic 'Operations of the Mind'; they do not differ simply, as Hume held, in terms of the degree of strength or vivacity of the 'Ideas' to which they apply. There is some confusion as to whether Sensation is, for Reid, an Operation of the Mind or the object of its operations; rather, he introduces the term 'simple apprehension' for the basic datum of experience. We get a somewhat better account of the underlying logic of his argument in the 'Preliminary' chapter of the *Essays on the Intellectual Powers of Man* (1787), where he discusses language. As we saw earlier, he observes that as definitions of words consist of other words, an infinite regress can be avoided only by accepting that some words cannot themselves be defined; their meanings are obvious, we all use them without any difficulty, and we have to accept them as first principles.

As Grave (1965) points out, there is a problem in giving a positive defence of Common Sense theories since, being first principles, there are no more ultimate truths from which they can be derived: 'Their positive defense thus becomes a matter of drawing attention to their authority'. They are imposed on us by the very constitution of our ultimately Divine natures.

There is surely a tension between Reid's ardent acceptance of the basic categories of folk Psychology (sensation, memory, imagination, will, etc.) as fundamental principles of Common Sense and his frustrated complaint at the opening of the *Inquiry*:

> It is hardly possible to make any innovation in our philosophy concerning the mind and its operations, without using new words and phrases, or giving a different meaning to those that are received

> – a liberty which, even when necessary, creates prejudice and misconstruction, and which must await the sanction of time to authorize it . . . (pp. 98–9; see above, pp. 116–117 for the full paragraph)

Even so, Reid's discussion of language was far from naive and raises questions not further addressed until the present century; his discussion of definition, in particular, adumbrates the problems raised by twentieth-century debates on meaning and verification, and how certain basic psychological terms (like 'pain') are used. The nature of sensations is also, for Reid, 'analogous to the work done by words' (Grave, *op. cit.*), except that whereas sensations are 'natural signs', words are 'conventional signs' which must be learned. The class of 'natural signs' – signs the meaning of which is directly known – includes also gesture, facial expression (echoes of John Bulwer) and intonation (Grave, *op. cit.*). If Grave is right, this is very similar to J. Yolton's interpretation of Descartes's own position (see above, p. 33), which would not have pleased Reid.

The task of Reid's 'anatomy' of the mind, therefore, is to delineate its powers and operations. In adopting this approach he is, it should be stressed, doing no more than conforming to the general Scottish Enlightenment concept of Natural Philosophical enquiry, summed up by Bryson (1945):

> Attention was not so much directed to finding out how things actually work as it was to classifying observations under some already accepted principle of explanation[28]. (p. 17)

The body of the *Inquiry* is limited to discussing the five senses in the light of Reid's critique of the doctrine of 'Ideas'. Unlike Berkeley's work on vision, its impact on perceptual theory has effectively been zero. In the *Essays on the Intellectual Powers of Man*, a fuller scheme unfolds. As Sir William Hamilton conveniently summarizes it in a footnote (p. 221), Reid's system has the following structure: The Powers of the Mind can be classified as Active or Passive and as Natural or Acquired. This yields four possibilities: Natural Active powers are what we call Faculties (these were, in effect, affective in character, or 'conative' powers of the will; see Spoerl [1936], p. 223); Natural Passive ones are Capacities or 'Receptivities' (in effect cognitive 'Intellectual Powers'; Spoerl [*ibid.*]), Acquired Active Powers are Habits and Acquired Passive ones are Dispositions. Spoerl's Table (see Table

3.1) comparing the natural faculties proposed by Reid, Stewart and Gall (reproduced in Allport [1937], p. 84) identifies 25 'Active Powers', and under 'Intellectual Powers' includes the five senses plus six others. 'Imitation' and 'Language' are – somewhat arbitrarily perhaps – allocated to the former. Brooks (1976) manages to tease out no fewer than 43 'faculties' from Reid's works. Although his catalogue is very different from the traditional rationalist quartet of Sensation, Thinking, Feeling, and Will, Dugald Stewart went some way towards integrating the two approaches by grouping the various mental phenomena into Feeling, Thinking and Willing (with Sensation included under Thinking or 'Intellectual Powers', as just noted). Down to Bain (1855) Reid's successors continued to juggle with – and argue about the details of – his classification, though they did not challenge its basic rationale.

Reid's thought is more than a simple *lumpen* backlash against scepticism. He is, however, his own worst enemy in many respects – patronization, sarcasm, false modesty, long-windedness and mockery figure far too prominently in his stylistic repertoire. There is also, I feel, a genuine failure on his part fully to appreciate what his philosophical predecessors were all about – his arguments against them too often seem at cross-purposes. That Hume replied so kindly and civilly to Reid in response to an advance look at the manuscript of the *Inquiry* only enhances our esteem for Hume's equanimity – but by then Hume had little concern to defend the masterpiece of his youth. As far as the history of Psychology is concerned, we must now reconsider the roles respectively ascribed to the Associationist and Scottish Common Sense traditions.

Seekers after anticipations of modern Psychology might, as noted above, see Reid's account of perception as foreshadowing J.J. Gibson's 'ecological' theory; psychometricians could find, in his analysis of the various powers and faculties, far clearer auguries of their work than anything in Locke, Hume or James Mill; he even yearns for 'a full history of all that hath past in the mind of a child', which 'would probably give more light into the human faculties, than all the systems of philosophy about them since the beginning of the world' (p. 99) – Reid as aspiring genetic epistemologist? This last may have inspired at least one contemporary empirical investigation of child development (see below, p. 225). Or again, his account of language in some respects anticipates C.S. Peirce's Pragmatism. It is commonplace to refer to

Table 3.1. Comparative table of Faculties

THOMAS REID, 1780	DUGALD STEWART, 1827	FRANZ JOSEPH GALL, 1810
Active Powers	*Active Powers*	*Determinate Faculties*
Self-Preservation		
Maintenance of Habits	Propensity to Action and Repose	
Hunger and Thirst	Hunger and Thirst	
Lust	Sex	Instinct of Generation (1)
	Acquired Appetite for Drugs	
	Desire of Society	
Instinct of Imitation	Instinct of Imitation	Mimicry, Imitation (25)
Language		Verbal Memory (14)
Desire for Power	Ambition	Vanity, Ambition (9)
Self-Esteem	Self-Love Self-Confidence	Pride, Self-Esteem (8)
Desire of Knowledge	Desire of Knowledge	Educability (11)
Confiliate Affection	Parental Affection Filial Affection	Love of Offspring (2)
Gratitude	Gratitude	
Pity and Compassion	Pity Sympathy	
	Universal Benevolence	Good Nature (24)
Esteem of the Wise and Good	Desire of Esteem	
	Veracity	
Friendship	Friendship	Friendship, Attachment (3)
Sexual Affection	Sexual Affection	
Public Spirit	Patriotism	
Emulation	Desire of Superiority	
Animal Resentment Rational Resentment	Resentment	Courage, Self-Defence (4)
Transcendent Good	Interest	
Duty	Sense of Duty	
Veneration	Veneration	Theosophy, Religion (26)
	Hope	
	Decency, Regard to Character	Firmness of Character (27)
Imagination (–invention)	Imagination	Poetry (23)
	Instinct for Construction	Mechanical Aptitude (19)
	Sense of Similarity and Contrast Sense of the Ridiculous	Wit (22)
Beauty	Memory for Colors	Sense of Colors (16)
	Time	
	Music	Music (17)
		Wish to Destroy (5)
		Cunning (6)
		Sentiment of Property (7)
		Cautiousness (10)
		Mathematics (18)
Intellectual Powers	*Intellectual Powers*	
The Five Senses and Their Faculty of Perception	The Five Senses and Their Faculty of Perception	
	From	Memory for Persons (13)
Size and Novelty	Size Novelty	
	Locality	Local Memory (12)
	Language	Memory for Languages (15)
Memory	Memory	
Judgment and Reason	Judgment and Reasoning	Comparative Sagacity (20)
Abstraction	Abstraction	Metaphysical Depth (21)
Conception	Conception	
	Attention	
Moral Taste	Moral Taste	
	Association of Ideas	

Sources: Thomas Reid, *The Works of Thomas Reid*, ed. Sir William Hamilton (2 vols., 8th ed.; London, 1895); Dugald Stewart, *Elements of the Philosophy of the Human Mind*, ed. Sir William Hamilton (3 vols., 2nd ed.; Edinburgh, 1877); and F.J. Gall, *On the Functions of the Brain and of Each of Its Parts, etc.*, trans. Winslow Lewis, Jr., ed. Nahum Capen (6 vols.; Boston, 1835).

Gall's numbering of the faculties is in parentheses; he alone used numbers.

From H.D. SPOERL (1936), p. 222

Associationism as the dominant indigenous British tradition. What, then, are we to make of the fact that Reid's fellow Aberdonian, Alexander Bain, widely accepted as the transitional figure from 'the older intellectualism and associationism to the activist and hormic psychologies which supplanted it' (Hearnshaw [1964], p. 9), begins his 1855 *Senses and the Intellect* with a critique of the relative virtues of the various faculty classifications of Reid, Stewart and Hamilton then on offer? According to Hearnshaw (*ibid.*) Bain 'disagreed with the Scottish school on fundamentals' but 'borrowed from it in details'. This understates the matter – the very titles of Bain's two key texts (*The Senses and the Intellect*, *The Emotions and the Will*), as well as his later work on character, suggest an underlying acceptance of the Scottish Faculty framework. If his Psychology marks a highly significant move towards an 'active' concept of mind, this too is a Reidian orthodoxy, while his whole vocabulary is pervaded with such characteristic expressions as 'Active Powers', 'Intellectual faculties', 'Volitional signs', 'Retentiveness' and 'Moral sentiments'.

It is at least arguable that the discursive, descriptive, less analytical Scottish school had a greater impact on the British psychological vocabulary than did ascetic Associationism, and that its 'anticipations' were no less numerous. It almost certainly provided the intellectual soil in which phrenology was later to flourish (see Chapter 6). In general histories of Psychology only Murray (1983) moves towards exploring Bain's Scottish Enlightenment connections in a more balanced way. One confusing factor, perhaps, is that while not Associationist, Scottish Common Sense philosophy was Empiricist; thus the expression 'British Empiricism', often used as synonymous with 'British Associationism', should really include the Scottish school. Indeed, in Reid and Home one constant charge against Associationists is their failure to be good Empiricists. (See the comments at the opening of this chapter.) Associationism *and* Reid's faculty account are, equally, psychological faces of British Empiricism.

In fact such writers as Samuel Taylor Coleridge, Thomas Brown, George Combe, Sir William Hamilton, James Mill and Bain were *au fait* with the thought of all parties. They incorporated the various viewpoints in a more piecemeal fashion than the simple historical formula of a binary opposition of 'schools' allows. To their contemporaries Hume and Reid could appear on occasion to differ only in emphasis, as Thomas Brown's comment to Sir James Mackintosh indicates: '"Yes", Reid bawled out, "We must believe in an external world"; but added in a whisper, "We can give no reason for our belief". Hume cries out, "We can give no reason for such a notion"; but whispers, "I own we cannot get rid of it"' (Graham [1908], p. 253). For all his distant affinities with some of the concerns of modern Psychology, Reid, like most of his contemporaries, is motivated by religious and moral considerations and his devotion to 'experiment', like Hume's, means no more than a broad affirmation of Empiricism. This is equally true – to cite one instance – of Home, Lord Kames, whose major psychological work, *Essays on the Principles of Morality and Natural Religion* (1751, 3rd edn 1779), while fairly comprehensive in its survey of psychological matters, is basically an attempt to reconcile the Calvinist, anti-Arminian doctrine that everything is determined by God with the notion of liberty (i.e. the determinism versus free will issue) – a reconciliation he claims to find in the doctrine of 'moral necessity'. As long ago as 1966 Drever argued that the 'British Associationist' tradition was largely nonexistent. The picture emerging in papers such as Robinson (1986) supports the present argument that for Psychology the 'Common Sense' school is as significant as Associationism, while even Associationists such as the Mills in fact accepted some of Reid's criticisms of extreme Humean Associationism.

How far, then, were the eighteenth-century British philosophers doing Psychology? There is no disputing that whatever they were doing, they frequently touch on issues currently considered to be the province of Psychology. Even if outright neologisms were rare, the vocabularies they evolved in analysing such issues also provided much of the technical conceptual repertoire which nineteenth-century founders of the discipline took as their point of departure. Even so, as we have seen, the agendas in pursuance of which these psychological analyses and conceptual developments were generated differed fundamentally from any we would now recognize as governing Psychology. Their worries were metaphysical and moral; even when they were claiming to create a 'Science of Human Nature' (or some such phrase) they could not conceive of this as serving purposes other than those of Moral Philosophy or epistemology. Nor could they conceive, apparently, of any appropriate methods of enquiry other than those of analytical reasoning on the one hand and appeals to common experience on the other. Since Natural Philosophers were breaking new ground methodologically throughout the century, this methodological conservatism, even among those adopting a rhetoric of 'experiment' and 'science', demands an explanation, and this surely lies in our earlier observation that they were simply not asking the kinds of question to which the new methods could obviously offer answers.

In particular they remained preoccupied with the following themes: (a) a core set of basic psychological terms such as *idea, sensation, faculty, impression, reason* and, later in the century, *sentiment*, are continually being reshuffled, redefined and re-evaluated in order to discover a way of structuring their interrelationships which matches the 'self-evident' criterion of an introspectively known psychological reality; (b) they are seeking a rational basis for morality consistent with – but not derived from – religious doctrines, this being essential for the maintenance of society; (c) they are concerned with mapping the emotions, 'affections' and 'passions', generally in the context of moral philosophical issues; (d) in tackling all these themes due obeisance must be made to Natural Philosophy. In regard to the last however, this amounts, first, to constraining oneself within current Natural Philosophical knowledge and 'experience' and, secondly, to accepting Newton's authority as a guiding spirit forbidding 'speculation', and accepting 'Natural Law'. Their treatments of these themes are framed within the context of a deeper preoccupation with the relationship between Soul and Body, Thought and Matter.

In the light of Danziger (1983) it can surely be argued that as long as the mind–body problem underpinned the theoretical agenda, there was no way in which a properly experimental Psychology could emerge. The problem simply could not be formulated in terms amenable to empirical evaluation. Nor has Psychology at any time since succeeded in doing so. Fechner is the rule-proving exception, for while his *Elemente der Psychophysik* (1860) was conceived as facilitating an assault on this very issue, it was his methodology, not his views on the mind–body problem, which earned him an honoured place in the discipline's historical annals. It is an intractably philosophical conceptual riddle. The changes in neurological theory initiated by Whytt involved, as we will see later, a shift in attention from the mind–body problem to the nature of the organism's relationship to its environment. This created the conditions in which empirical experimental studies of behaviour could indeed be envisaged. While Whytt's physiological successors pursued this new paradigm, it seems that eighteenth-century philosophers remained unaffected. If Danziger's argument and the linguistic argument proposed in Chapter 2 are both sound, then the absence of an Enlightenment Psychology was considerably overdetermined.

In short, in pursuing an agenda of the kind just outlined, there was indeed no apparent role for the sort of systematic data-gathering, experimentation and measurement which we take to be the hallmark of empirical science. In K.O. Apel's terms, their 'goals of knowledge' were communicative understanding and self-emancipation, not prediction and control. Their methodological conservatism is itself prime evidence that we are dealing here with *mentalités* fundamentally different from those which, a century later, could conceive of Psychology as a branch of natural science. Nevertheless, the psychological transformations required were, by the century's end, of no major proportions; indeed, had arguably already occurred in some areas other than philosophy, as we shall see.

2 Political and Social Philosophy

In so far as British and French philosophy extended beyond the agenda just discussed, it was outwards into considerations of the nature of society and social life, rather than inwards into the depths of the psyche. The emergence of new general images of human nature is more apparent in this work than in that of the post-Lockean philosophers discussed so far, wherein ultimately we see only the intensification of the battle between the materialist tendency and defenders of the soul. The more holistic images of human nature expounded in Political and Social Philosophy were of varied kinds. One of the earliest and most scandalous of these was Bernard Mandeville's cynical *The Fable of the Bees* (1723). Subsequently Jean-Jacques Rousseau's *The Social Contract* (1762) had a Europe-wide impact and, with his other works, introduced the concept of the 'Noble Savage' (the antithesis of Hobbes's image), a notion bolstered by new anthropological reports[29]. It also elaborated a (not unproblematic) notion of the 'general will' as a basis for the legitimacy of governments.[30] In Britain the Scottish social philosophers Lord Kames, Adam Ferguson, Adam Smith, Lord Monboddo and John Millar provided less Romantic images of human nature, although Smith's *Wealth of Nations* was unusual in offering a fundamentally 'selfish' version. They were nevertheless influenced by Rousseau and Montesquieu, and also by Natural History of the kind being developed by Buffon; indeed, in so far as there was a 'scientific' model for the sociological and 'Psychological' enquiries of the Scottish Enlightenment thinkers, it was Natural History rather than Newtonian physics (Wood, 1990). In English, as opposed to Scottish, thought, social philosophy became dominated by Jeremy Bentham's 'Utilitarianism', which remained influential until the 1840s. Speculative histories of human society and the rise of civilization begin to appear both in Britain and on the European mainland (especially in France and Germany)[31]. The British work was essentially aimed at justifying and reforming the existing order, the German simply at its justification and the French, as often as not, at subverting it. One difficulty in relating continental and British 'Psychological' writing at this time is that both in France and in Germany there arose traditions of enquiry calling themselves '*anthropologie*'. Georges Buffon's (1707–88) *L'Histoire naturelle de l'homme* (1749) (a major influence on the Scots) was adopted as their founding text by French anthropologists, while in Germany Kant, for example, used the term (while believing it could not be a true science), both writing on and teaching the subject, from the 1770s. Throughout the century *anthropologie* included psychological matters among its topics of enquiry, but in practice the continental work concentrated on the marshalling of cross-cultural evidence concerning variation in physique, social customs and institutions (such as marriage). In England the term is rarely used (though known) and such researches are largely absent. Only among the Scots do the psychological *and* the social levels seem to be genuinely integrated in people like Monboddo and Kames (who feuded interminably with one another). Again, need I say, continental '*anthropologie*' texts do not figure in the standard histories of Psychology, even though other texts by their authors may.

In the background lay an important difficulty. Natural Philosophy still saw the natural world as somehow immutable and perfectly governed by Natural Laws; on the Continent the Leibnizian argument that this was the best of all possible worlds remained widely influential. The contents of this perfect universe comprised a *scala naturae*, a 'Great Chain of Being' from the highest to the lowest in which, many believed, there could be no gaps[32]. It was thus still an essentially static picture. But the emphasis was beginning to shift from the descending to the ascending character of the scale, raising the possibility, addressed by Charles Bonnet (1720–93), that the universe was perfectible over time: that Nature displayed a perfect unfolding, rather than resting in a static state of perfection. In attempting to bring the Natural Philosophical spirit to bear on human society, social philosophers naturally strove to identify both Laws and a 'natural scale'. Yet if anything was obvious about human society, it was its imperfection. If the rich man in his castle and the poor man at his gate is the natural hierarchy, and if social morality rests, at the psychological level, on a mechanistic 'moral instinct' or moral perception, then both the great chain of social being and the fundamental laws of society inevitably shift in status. They can no longer be conceived of simply as describing a natural reality, but become normative. They become prescriptions for how society should be organized, not accounts of how it actually is. However debatable the question of whether Nature was static or dynamic, human society also clearly had a history and – it seemed self-evident – a *progressive* one at that. The lesson inevitably drawn was that human society was perfectible and, indeed, in the process of becoming perfect: an end conditional on the recognition of – and adherence to – these 'natural' laws and principles of society and social structure. The implicit contradiction. of course, is how a 'natural' law can ever be infringed in the first place[33].

We can now consider five of the major eighteenth-century social philosophy texts: four British and Rousseau's *Social Contract*, the influence of which permeated throughout Europe and, indeed, North America.

(a) *Bernard Mandeville's The Fable of the Bees: or, Private Vices, Publick Benefits* (1723)

This work was at once scandalous and enormously influential. In particular, it prepared the ground for the later emergence of Economics as a distinct discipline in Adam Smith's *Wealth of Nations*. Its scandalous character is encapsulated in the subtitle;

Mandeville sought to demonstrate how social order, justice and prosperity arose as the net effect of individuals pursuing their own pleasures and gratification. Ethical concepts, on this account, become, in Hundert's words, 'rhetorical artifacts, terminological devices deployed as weapons by social actors in their pursuit of recognition' (Hundert, 1986, p. 316). Whether an individual 'really' believes in moral principles or merely simulates such belief for opportunistic purposes is in practice irrelevant. That out of the apparently selfish behaviour of individuals (Mandeville uses the terms 'vanity' and 'pride') a higher level of law-like, seemingly rational, principles of social organization emerges, regardless of the actors' individual intentions, was an argument of a radically novel kind. Adam Smith's notion of 'the Invisible Hand' was its direct successor. In a way it was a distant anticipation of modern 'Chaos Theory'. Mandeville's work was satirical and ironic in tone, but the argument was nevertheless clear and cogent[34]. While Natural Philosophy had by then established itself as the appropriate mode of investigating Nature, investigation of Society had remained firmly in the province of prescriptive moral and theological philosophizing. The works of writers such as Hobbes and Bossuet[35] were explicit moves in contemporary political and ideological debates and struggles, providing blueprints of reform or defences for insecure establishments. Mandeville's sceptical, mocking orientation ostensibly treated society as it was: as a quasi-natural phenomenon. Of course the ideological dimension is there; after all, it provides a fair rationale for competitive capitalist economic individualism, but this rationale is presented as an account of how society operated, as a matter of fact. Again, one can see adumbrations of events a century later.

This 'naturalization' of society, of humans at the collective level, as an object of Natural Philosophical enquiry anticipated the battles of those, from William Lawrence (1819) to Charles Darwin, who would argue the same for humans at the individual level (and in the event, with a similar ideological message). Winning this latter point was a necessary, if insufficient, condition for Psychology's appearance as a discipline studying 'Man' as a natural object of enquiry rather than a privileged spiritual being half outside of Nature. We might, then, discern in Mandeville's *Fable* a significant conceptual shift towards the possibility of a Psychology. He would also, we can assume, have enjoyed Richard Dawkins's *The Selfish*

Gene (1976).

Another aspect of Mandeville's *Fable* which is of interest is his view, virtually unique for his century, of language as a social product. It is not basically a medium for communicating thoughts and ideas, let alone a representation of the world, but an instrument – a weapon, even – deployed by individuals in the social arena to further their egoistic ends in pursuit of status, pleasure and wealth. Indeed, rhetoric has a central mediating role in the social process as a whole[36].

Unfortunately for those wishing to see a direct lineage from Mandeville to modern economic theory and sociobiology, appreciation of the nature of his achievement was long delayed. His eighteenth-century reputation was as a sceptical Augustan satirist, and his book was condemned as corrupting by the righteous. It was for subsequent centuries to provide the intellectual contexts in which *The Fable* could receive the kinds of reading which would discern within it the insight and profundity with which it is now credited[37]. Adam Smith might be seen as an immediate successor, but one who condemned Mandeville's moral scepticism, terming his system one

> of which the tendency is . . . wholly pernicious . . . Though the notions of this author are in almost every respect erroneous, there are, however, some appearances in human nature, which, when viewed in a certain manner, seem at first sight to favour them. These, described and exaggerated by the lively and humorous, though coarse and rustic eloquence of Dr. Mandeville, have thrown upon his doctrines an air of truth and probability which is very apt to impose upon the unskilful. (Adam Smith, *The Theory of Moral Sentiments*, 1759, Part VII, Sect. II)

He then, not unskilfully, proceeds to deconstruct Mandeville's central concept of 'vanity' to unveil the linguistic sleights of hand by which the argument was so plausibly managed. None the less, Smith's economic theory clearly derives much from Mandeville (see below, pp. 187–188).

(b) *Jean Jacques Rousseau's The Social Contract* (1762)

In *The Social Contract* and *Emile* (see below, pp. 216–219), Rousseau is credited with providing a very different image of human nature. While Rosenow's (1980) critique of *Emile*, discussed below, may apply here also, the received version holds that for Rousseau humans were naturally good, disinclined to strife and altruistic, the very opposite of Hobbes's brutal savage tameable only by submission to an absolute monarch, to whom his subjects delegated the exercise of force. The problem is that *The Social Contract* is – at least in late-twentieth-century retrospect – a very ambiguous text. Take, for example, the statement of the 'social compact' itself:

> Each of us places in common his person and all his power under the supreme direction of the general will; and as one body we all receive each member as an indivisible part of the whole. (1947 edn p. 15)

What to his contemporaries sounded like an ideal egalitarian creed, a recipe for social harmony and justice, with everyone freely labouring in the common interest, carries rather darker resonances to us. 'General will' sounds an ominously specious concept, an excuse for crushing rather than liberating the individual. It is now impossible to read this except in the light of the modern excesses of regimes which claimed to find in it their ideological roots. The famous opening line 'Man is born free, and yet we see him everywhere in chains' (p. 5) is fine rhetoric, but what kind of liberation was Rousseau actually offering? In the event he largely baulks at offering one at all, even holding that 'Liberty not being a fruit that every climate will produce, it is not within the abilities of all peoples' (p. 69) and that the question 'Which is absolutely the best government?' 'is as insoluble as it is indeterminate' (p. 74). The nearest he approaches to identifying the hallmarks of good government is:

> That government is infallibly the best, all other things being equal, under which, without employment of any external means, without the naturalization of strangers, without receiving any new colonists, the citizens increase and multiply. (1947 edn p. 75)

Even allowing for the fact that the eighteenth century had not heard of population explosions, this is surely pretty feeble stuff, hardly more sophisticated than Old Testament injunctions to 'go forth and multiply'. But what of the 'Noble Savage'? This is more properly an image derived from *Emile* than from the *Social Contract*, where the character of the 'first societies' receives a bare page's attention. We are told that 'The earliest and the only natural societies are families' (*ibid.*, p. 6), these apparently being of a patriarchal nuclear kind.

Children break away on reaching maturity, and the 'bond of nature is dissolved' (*ibid.*), though 'a voluntary union' may persist (*ibid.*).

True, Rousseau mounts powerful attacks on the notion of a 'right of force', on slavery, and on arbitrary despotisms and tyrannies of all kinds, which earned him the acclaim of later political radicals. It must be confessed, though, that his own analysis of the foundations for a just society gets irremediably bogged down in seeking felicitous formulations of the relationship between the individual as subject and the individual as a component of the 'Sovereign', agent of the 'general will'. Every form of smaller scale 'association' interposing between the atomic citizens and the totality of the State represents a threat to the ideally all-powerful 'general will'. In discussing the principle of decision by majority voting, he says:

> When . . . the motion which I opposed carries, it only proves to me that I was mistaken, and that what I believed to be the general will was not so . . . This is indeed supposing that all the characteristics which mark the general will still reside in the most votes: when that ceases to be the case, whatever measures may be adopted, it means the end of liberty. (*ibid.*, p. 96)

Again, this seems to us to have a darker side: it is one thing to agree to abide by majority decisions, another to accept them as infallible guides. One can accept being in disagreement with the 'general will', but the tenor of Rousseau's writing in discussing this continually seems be suggesting that this 'general will' is the final and absolute arbiter of what is morally right, if not of Truth itself.

Reading Rousseau with justice at the end of the twentieth century is difficult. In *The Social Contract* he was confronting for the first time many genuine problems in Political Philosophy, problems central for formulating a social ideology appropriate for post-monarchic, secular democracies. In doing so it was perhaps inevitable that Rousseau would underestimate the complexities of such issues, blithely straying in directions which, if pursued, lead not to liberty and freedom but, ironically, back to tyranny of an even worse order than anything that had gone before. This ambiguity – particularly his recurrent flirting with collective absolutism and submersion of individuality, as well as his happiness with such concepts as 'general will' and 'The State', of which we have learned to be so suspicious – renders Rousseau's own position particularly elusive. For nigh on two centuries its underlying message seemed basically clear, even though commentators like G.D.H. Cole recognized shortcomings and contradictions in some of Rousseau's formulations[38], but by 1947 the editor of the Hafner Library edition, Charles Frankel, is writing:

> Practically all sides agree as to its truth or at least partial truth, or feel it best to pretend to do so; they disagree only as to its proper interpretation. (1947 edn, p. ix)

This work – revolutionary in its contemporary impact, banned in France and Switzerland – undeniably had a catalytic role in changing the basic terms in which political philosophy was conducted. It led directly to the ideas which justified the French Revolution, and to Tom Paine's *The Rights of Man* (1791–2). At this remove, by contrast, it has become more of a thematic apperception test into which political ideologists of any persuasion can read a confirmation of their own credo. The immediate messages – that government was the servant, not the master of the people, that 'men' were equal, had natural rights, were not naturally sinful or savage, and were entitled to overthrow rulers who affronted the 'general will' – were, by contrast, clear-cut.

Of further psychological interest is Rousseau's *Confessions* (1782), although the work contains little in the way of new Psychological doctrines, it represents a landmark in self-disclosing autobiography, the title deliberately echoing St. Augustine's *Confessions*. While space prevents us from discussing the work here, it might be added that by this point in his life Rousseau has come to believe himself the target of a Europe-wide conspiracy.

(c) *Adam Ferguson's An Essay on the History of Civil Society* (1767)
The notion of a natural sociality existing between people formed the psychological basis of Ferguson's study of the nature of society, although he himself argued against the distinction between 'natural' and 'unnatural', these terms being 'the least determinate in their meaning' (1768 edn, p. 15). In spite of its title, the work does not take a historical approach to human nature itself – on the contrary this, for Ferguson, is always and everywhere the same:

> If we are asked . . . Where is the state of nature to be found? we may answer, It is here; and it matters not whether we are understood to speak in the island of Great Britain, at the Cape of Good Hope, or the Straits of Magellan. (*ibid.*, p. 12).

Speculative histories of our rise from a 'state of nature' are thus rejected outright, in any case:

> . . . whatever may have been the original state of our species, it is of more importance to know the condition to which we ourselves should aspire, than that which our ancestors may be supposed to have left. (*ibid.*, p. 16)

While we may trace the rise of 'Civil Society' through various stages, this represents, in modern terms, a 'sociological' development, not a psychological one. Human nature itself, including its 'desire for perfection', and the 'principle of progress' are universal, regardless of material conditions.

Affection is the basic 'principle of Union among Mankind', but ironically, far from having grown, it is at its weakest in 'commercial society':

> It is here indeed, if ever, that man is sometimes found a detached and a solitary being: he has found an object which sets him in competition with his fellow-creatures, and he deals with them as he does with his cattle and his soil, for the profits they bring. (*ibid.*, p. 31)

While this might be cited as evidence for the appearance of the new self-contained, autonomous mode of individuality, now widely ascribed to this period, it can hardly be said to be constituting or endorsing it. Far from saying that competition is natural, Ferguson – with Mandeville no doubt, in his sights – reserves severe condemnation for the doctrine that 'self love' or 'selfishness' is the engine of society. His critique of this remains sound:

> In the case before us, they [i.e. advocates of selfishness as the basic human motive] have actually found that benevolence is no more than a species of self-love; and would oblige us, if possible, to look out for a new set of names, by which we may distinguish the selfishness of the parent when he takes care of his child, from his selfishness when he only takes care of himself. For according to this philosophy, as in both cases he only means to gratify a desire of his own, he is in both cases equally selfish. . . . The fact is, that we should need only a fresh supply of language, instead of that which

> by this seeming discovery we should have lost, in order to make our reasonings proceed as they formerly did. (*ibid.*, p. 23)

In another dig at Mandeville, he jeers at those who

> with acrimony pretend to detect the fraud by which moral restraints have been imposed, as if to censure fraud were not already to take part on the side of morality. (*ibid.*, p. 55)

On the contrary, we have an 'amicable disposition' which serves as a foundation of

> a moral apprehension . . . and the sense of a right which we maintain for ourselves, is by a movement of humanity and candour extended to our fellow creatures. (*ibid.*, p. 57)

The 'Psychological' content of the book is confined to Part I of six, the rest being sociological and economic. While the passages cited here are, by and large, optimistic, Ferguson does not dispute that 'War and Dissension' are part of the human lot too. But he does not derive them from some innate brutishness:

> They are sentiments of generosity and self-denial that animate the warrior in defence of his country; and they are dispositions most favourable to mankind, that become the principles of apparent hostility to men. (*ibid.*, p. 38)

Man, he argues, is disposed

> to employ the forces of his nature against an equal antagonist; he loves to bring his reason, his eloquence, his courage, even his bodily strength, to the proof. (*ibid.*)

And

> Without the rivalship of nations, and the practice of war, civil society could scarcely have found an object or a form. . . . [h]e who has never struggled with his fellow creatures, is a stranger to half the sentiments of mankind. (*ibid.*, p. 39)

Even War and Dissension are thus assimilable to his benign vision.

Curiously, while the doctrine of human nature as 'naturally good' is so often associated with Rousseau, Ferguson's far less ambiguous – if also less Romantic – version is generally overlooked. For Ferguson, after all, there is no polarity between an innocent state of nature and corrupt civilization; we are good now, and always have been.

Ferguson's influence was not confined to the *Essay on the History of Civil Society*; as Professor of Pneumatics and Moral Philosophy at Edinburgh he was a central figure in Scottish Enlightenment thought and in his other works (*Institutes of Moral Philosophy* [1769; an outline of his lecture course] and *Principles of Moral and Political Science* [1792]) he expounded on psychological issues in somewhat more detail. His account of the mind in the *Principles* differs somewhat from Reid's in identifying 12 traits as opposed to about 28, but his approach and rationale are fundamentally similar[39].

(d) *Adam Smith's The Theory of Moral Sentiments* (1759), *The Wealth of Nations* (1776)

The Theory of Moral Sentiments culminates that genre of treatises on moral philosophy which began with Ashley Cooper and Hutcheson, and continued with Lord Kames's *Essays on the Principles of Morality and Natural Religion* (1751). It marks a significant move away from the analytical, philosophical mode of treating the issue towards a more 'Psychological', or at least 'phenomenological', approach. A second difference is that while his predecessors aimed at discovering rational grounds for morality as a basis for social life, their focus had been primarily on the individual, in whom they sought some innate moral instinct or moral perception. Adam Smith's discussion, by contrast, focuses on social relations from the outset. His central psychological concept is 'sympathy', the natural 'fellow-feeling' which we have for one another's 'passions' (joyous as well as suffering). In surveying the operation of this principle he is able, in Part One, to build up a complex picture of the dynamics of social relationships, ranging from our differing reactions to physical and emotional distress in others to our 'disposition to admire the rich and the great' (and its morally corrupting effects). On the former the following joke still works:[40]

> The loss of a leg may generally be regarded as a more real calamity than the loss of a mistress. It would be a ridiculous tragedy, however, of which the catastrophe was to turn upon a loss of that kind. A

> misfortune of the other kind, how frivolous soever it may appear to be, has given occasion to many a fine one. (1853 edn, p. 36)

While a full synopsis of the work cannot be attempted here, it is of interest to note some of the topics to which Smith turns his attention. Having dealt extensively with the notions of Justice and Beneficence in Part Two, he addresses the apparent disparity between the rational basis for moral evaluation as lying in the actor's intentions, and the reality, in which moral evaluation is greatly affected by the actual outcome of an action (e.g. its success or failure), regardless of intention:

> That the world judges by the event, and not by the design, has been in all ages the complaint, and is the great discouragement of virtue. Every body agrees to the general maxim, that as the event does not depend on the agent, it ought to have no influence upon our sentiments, with regard to the merit or propriety of his conduct. But when we come to particulars, we find that our sentiments are scarce in any one instance exactly conformable to what this equitable maxim would direct. (*ibid.*, p. 152)

Irrational though this may appear, it nevertheless transpires that nature in 'implant[ing] the seeds of this irregularity in the human breast, seems, as upon all other occasions, to have intended the happiness and perfection of the species' (*ibid.*). If 'baseness of the thought' elicited as much outrage as 'baseness of the action', social life would clearly become impossible. Thus:

> [T]hat necessary rule of justice . . . that men in this life are liable to punishment for their actions only, not for their designs and intentions, is founded upon this salutary and useful irregularity in human sentiments concerning merit or demerit, which at first sight appears so absurd and unaccountable. (*ibid.*, p. 153)

In Part Six he expatiates on 'Of the Order in which Individuals are recommended by Nature to our care and Attention', exploring what would nowadays be called 'social distance' in relation to the power of sympathy. Its most intense level, within the family, we term 'affection', but 'what is called affection is in reality nothing but habitual sympathy' (*ibid.*, p. 323). Unlike modern sociobiologists when discussing altruism, Adam Smith rejects any notion that biological kinship *per se* is involved: 'This force of blood, however,

I am afraid, exists nowhere but in tragedies and romances' (*ibid.*, p. 326). There are tensions, though – for instance, between 'the strongest of all natural affections' and 'a regard for the safety of those superiors upon whose safety often depends that of the whole society' (*ibid.*, p. 333) – where personal conscience alone can decide priorities.

Finally, we might mention some interesting observations in Part One illustrating the greater power of 'immediate' than 'remote' effects of objects over our imagination.

> A prison is certainly more useful to the public than a palace; and the person who founds the one is generally directed by a much juster spirit of patriotism, than he who builds the other. But the immediate effects of a prison . . . are disagreeable; and the imagination . . . does not take time to trace out the remote ones . . . A prison, therefore, will always be a disagreeable object; and the fitter it is for the purpose for which it was intended, it will be the more so. (*ibid.*, p. 46)

> Trophies of the instruments of music or of agriculture, imitated in painting or in stucco, make a common and an agreeable ornament of our halls and dining-rooms. A trophy of the same kind, composed of the instruments of surgery . . . would be absurd and shocking. Instruments of surgery, however, are always more finely polished, and generally more nicely adapted to the purposes for which they are intended, than instruments of agriculture . . . Instruments of war are agreeable, though their immediate effect may seem to be in the same manner [i.e. as surgical instruments] pain and suffering. But then it is the pain and suffering of our enemies, with whom we have no sympathy. With regard to us, they are immediately connected with the agreeable ideas of courage, victory, and honour. (*ibid.*, pp. 46–7)

In identifying the motivational basis of social behaviour as a universal natural capacity for 'sympathy', immediate and beyond conscious control, Adam Smith is most directly rejecting the egoistic utilitarian analyses of many of his contemporaries (*ibid.*, p. 448). He is also offering a less clearly rational 'Psychology' than that of either these utilitarians or his own later *Wealth of Nations*. The apparent irrationalities of what we might term his 'sympathetic calculus' nevertheless turn out to be strategies by which a wiser and more cunning Nature ensures the maintenance of society. Yet *The Theory of Moral Sentiments* remains typical in being prescriptive as well as descriptive, in diagnosing rectifiable pathologies of 'sympathy' in addition to treating it as a natural law-like phenomenon. The acceptance of many of the manners and *mores* of his own Scottish society as representing universal ethical standards also often prevents Adam Smith from clearly differentiating morality from 'Propriety' (one of his favourite words). This is especially evident in the high esteem given to the suppression of emotional display (e.g. an aristocrat who wept on the scaffold being considered as having disgraced himself).

The Theory of Moral Sentiments is none the less at least halfway to being Social Psychology. Purely philosophical analysis and *a priori* classification of passions, and so on, take a clear second place to discursive descriptions of typical social behaviour. The image of 'Man' here is less that of a calculating egoist or aggregate of component ideas than a rather too easily misled but essentially unmalicious social creature whose concern for others usually – *in extremis*, at least – outweighs self-interest. The similarity with Adam Ferguson here is obvious, Ferguson's 'principle of Affection' and Smith's 'sympathy' serve almost identical functions.

The Wealth of Nations, on which Adam Smith's historical reputation as the founder of modern Economics rests, need detain us only briefly, since it is indeed mostly concerned with such topics as the division of labour, rent, accumulation of stock and the 'Natural Progress of Opulence'. The work's main point of interest for us is that the underlying image of human nature on which the economic theory rests differs considerably from that provided in *The Theory of Moral Sentiments*. Sympathy now plays a very faint second fiddle to egoistic self-interest. Unlike animals:

> . . . man has almost constant occasion for the help of his brethren, and it is in vain for him to expect it from their benevolence only. He will be more likely to prevail if he can interest their self-love in his favour, and show them that it is for their own advantage to do for him what he requires of them. (1974 edn, p. 118)

> We address ourselves, not to their humanity but to their self-love, and never talk to them of our own necessities but of their advantages. (*ibid.*, p. 119)

We uniquely possess, it seems, a 'certain propensity in human nature' to 'truck, barter, and exchange one thing for another' (*ibid.*, p. 117). It is from the exercise of this propensity in the service of 'self-love' that division of labour (the key to economic progress) gradually develops. This in turn facilitates the variety of talents and dispositions so characteristic of humans, a variation ascribed to the effects of upbringing after the age of six to eight rather than to innate differences in 'natural talents' (*ibid.*, p. 120). Although some species (Smith cites dogs) do vary enormously, this avails them nothing, since they lack the bartering propensity which endows individual talents with value. This 'Psychological' content, however, is confined to a bare four pages (Book One, Chapter 2). The image of economic man as rationally calculating his own best interests (women figure little in all this) nevertheless underpins Smith's entire model of economic behaviour.

Adam Smith's own labours thus appear to be divided regarding human nature. The earlier work seems to herald the rise in humanitarian concern associated with Romanticism and the semi-deification of 'Humanity' in *fin-de-siècle* political radicalism and German *Naturphilosophie. The Wealth of Nations*, by contrast, provides an economic ideology for the Industrial Revolution, a rationale for *laissez-faire* capitalism, a 'naturalization' of the economic system as a law-governed, self-adjusting phenomenon. The laws of supply and demand govern the operations of a free marketplace inhabited by rational self-interested egos, and from this the optimum solutions to all economic problems emerge. There is, in the famous phrase, an 'Invisible Hand' guiding the whole business of business[41].

(e) *Jeremy Bentham (1748–1832) and Utilitarianism*

Among the numerous significant points in the history of modernity, one which was beloved of Foucault (though he was hardly the first to see its significance), is Samuel Bentham's idea of the 'Panopticon': a prison designed like the spokes of a wheel, from the hub of which the inmates could be kept under constant surveillance. Jeremy Bentham promoted and developed his brother's brainchild enthusiastically for years, although finally to no avail (other than eventual government reimbursement of the £23,000 he had spent on the project). The Panopticon is taken to epitomize the appearance of a new, 'modern' concept of the nature of social power and its management. For Bentham and his contemporaries this Panopticon was an instrument not of oppression but of humanitarian reform, and he drew up analogous schemes for dealing with the impoverished and the unemployed. It is easy to see in Bentham the forefather of the bureaucratic State, the prophet of techniques of mass control and a philistine whose principle of 'The Greatest Happiness of the Greatest Number' was simply too crass to bear the weight of ethical, moral and legal theory placed upon it. Figures as varied as Nietszche and Keynes have poured vituperation on him (Mack, 1962).

The main source of difficulty is that Bentham was unusual among British writers in centring his life-work on law and legislation[42]. The law, he believed, constituted the overarching, superordinate factor determining the quality of our lives as social beings. It could not, of itself, make us happy, but it could both punish and provide frameworks for the pursuit of happiness. It is therefore upon the legislator that the task of justly ordering society ultimately falls. Nevertheless, although the law is the hub of Bentham's work, this is underpinned by a comprehensive grasp of, and interest in, contemporary philosophy. His 'Utilitarian' creed is rooted in British and continental Enlightenment philosophy, notably Locke, Hume and the French philosopher Claude-Adrien Helvétius (1715–71), in whose controversial *De l'Esprit* (1758), which he read at the age of twenty one, he found the inspirational key to his vocation. Bentham's driving motive was always to devise practical methods of reducing the amount of human misery, with which he felt a lifelong empathy. While we cannot discuss here his whole politico-legal philosophical system, which was far more complex than the caricatures suggest, his central psychological doctrines of human motivation are of interest on several accounts. Unlike the writers just discussed, Bentham provides no single text in which these doctrines can found; they permeate his work from *The Principles of Morals and Legislation* (1789) onwards[43].

First, we have to consider his 'Felicific' (or 'Hedonistic') Calculus. Hedonistic theories of human motivation were, of course, nothing new, but in Bentham this ceases to be a simple philosophical or psychological thesis, becoming an *applicable* scientific foundation for legislation and social policy. As we have seen, several of his predecessors, such as Hutcheson and Hartley, had provided fairly sophisticated analyses of the varieties of human pleasure, but Bentham systematizes them to an unprecedented degree. Following Everett (1966, pp. 48–50) these can be divided into four 'privative' pleasures, eleven 'expansive' ones and a final sixteenth religious one ('piety'). In the case of the 'privative' ones my own enjoyment of them is generally at someone else's expense; they are sense (I am unclear about this; presumably it refers to sensual pleasures), wealth, power and malevolence. Such pleasures are of the lowest type. Expansive pleasures include the three social pleasures of amity, good name and benevolence, and those of art and science: skill, memory, imagination, association, expectation and relief. In addition, Bentham identified seven dimensions along which these pleasures might vary, rendering quantification potentially possible: certainty, 'propinquity' (proximity to goal), purity, intensity, duration, fecundity (i.e. generation of further pleasures) and extent. The inclusion of such items as 'benevolence' in this scheme indicates that Bentham's 'hedonism' was not simply reductionist. Indeed, Mack (1962, p. 220) argues that Bentham's concept of 'pleasure' was an extremely broad one, ultimately 'synonymous with all pro-words, "pain" with all anti-words'. On Mack's reading, the role of the pleasure/pain distinction is as fundamental terms in a formal 'logic of the will', and it is incorrect to understand Bentham as proposing a conventional 'hedonistic ethical theory'. None the less, his intentions notwithstanding, it is as the most systematic form of hedonistic theory that Bentham's Utilitarianism has been historically understood.

A second feature of Bentham's thought, especially germane to us, is his explicit espousal of a linguistic position similar to Horne Tooke's; he, like Tooke, read Locke's *Essay* – indeed metaphysics in general – as essentially about how words are to be used. He accepts that to be meaningful a word must eventually be translatable into concrete (usually visual) terms. Thus a great many psychological and political concepts are in fact fictions, and, typically, he identified numerous levels of fictionality. To uncover the meanings – if any – of such terms, he developed a technique he called 'Paraphrasis', 'whereby words were arranged in sentences and defined by simpler equivalent sentences suggesting material images' (Mack, 1962, p. 49). This is significantly different from Tooke's etymological method and more akin to the twentieth-century logical positivist strategy. Late in life he drafted a short 'Conjectural History of Language' (1826), which appears to differ from others we have encountered in taking not the word but the entire utterance as the basic unit (*ibid.*, pp. 157–8)[44]. Like Coleridge and Whewell he was an inveterate – indeed, notorious – neologizer, and over time his yearning for linguistic clarity led him into syntactic innovation also, as well as a dislike of verbs ('Substantives', he wrote, 'are the only real entities: situations, motions are imaginary entities' – quoted by Mack, p. 196). The outcome was that Bentham, a lifelong seeker for and advocate of simplicity and clarity, ended up writing some of the densest, least comprehensible prose ever penned. His accounts of language are in some respects protean musings in which anticipations of almost all later doctrines – positivist, Wittgensteinian and even deconstructionist – may be discovered. His success in getting his neologisms accepted, and bringing about PL innovation, was in the event, unlike Coleridge's, minimal. Apart from aesthetic reasons, this is primarily because they arise in the context of an attempt to devise a science of legislation, of managing and structuring social power. Eventually he abandoned motivational questions as irrelevant to legislation, which can deal only with actions, and wryly recognized that people are frequently unaware even of their own motivations.

Bentham is often depicted as representing the political face of British Associationism. This is understandable in view of his close connections with the Mills and the fact that he and the Associationists tended to share their political agendas. His ostensibly scientific approach was also congenial to their own. Nevertheless, his doctrines themselves are only partly captured by such a label, and his Psychological thought is influenced by other schools as well. The fundamental distinction he espoused was between Will and Understanding, although he recognized these as 'fictions'. Bentham's final achievement, as far as Psychology is concerned, is in creating a framework in which the discipline would eventually discover a role in managing and guiding social reform and legislation. He well understood that power was central to social life, and his system sought to ensure that its exercise was in the interests of 'The Greatest Happiness of the Greatest Number'. At the same time he recognized, as a philosopher, the ultimately 'fictional' and 'socially constructed' (even 'linguistically constructed') nature of the law, and the central concepts on which we necessarily depend such as 'right', 'liberty' and 'obligation'. The irony, perhaps, is that while, since Foucault, Bentham's work has been seen as *symptomatic* of the advent of a modern bourgeois *mentalité*, his work itself contains anticipations of this very analysis.

Bentham's influence was incalculable, and extended worldwide. Initially it was greater abroad than at home, owing to the labours of his French disciple Etienne Dumont. A Panopticon was eventually built according to the original blueprint at Joliet Penitentiary in Illinois, and the term became a common Central American word for any jail. In Britain, numerous pieces of nineteenth-century legislation governing public health, penal reform, even the 1832 Reform Bill itself (given Royal Assent the day after he died), were to a large degree implementations of schemes Bentham himself had drafted, realized by followers such as Owen Chadwick. Whether Benthamite Utilitarianism strictly *caused* these social reforms may be disputed, but it played a major role in determining the manner in which they were mediated.

Conclusion

The varieties of Social Philosophy propounded during the eighteenth century exercised a great effect both on Psychology as a potential discipline and even more, perhaps, on European psychology. They served variously to promote, construe, criticize and analyse the deep changes in social and economic structure which European culture as a whole was undergoing, particularly in Britain, France, Germany and North America. These changed and changing circumstances demanded new formulations of 'Human Nature' in several respects. The place of 'Man' in Nature could no longer be answered by traditional Christian doctrines in the light of accumulating scientific and anthropological knowledge; the place of 'Man' in Society could similarly no longer be stated in terms of traditional rhetorics of loyal subjectivity and a Divinely ordered status quo; and the management of newly emergent forms of social and economic life itself required different kinds of analysis of human motivation and social behaviour to those which drama and literature offered. Social Philosophers responded, as we have seen, in a variety of ways, but all of them, from Rousseau to Bentham, pushed proto-Psychological thought in new directions. They share, in various degrees, in the process of what A.O. Lovejoy called the 'temporalizing' of the Great Chain of Being while for the most part continuing to accept this traditional doctrine. Even so, tangible evidence of conceptual novelty regarding the psychological before the last decades of the century is as elusive in Social Philosophy as in metaphysics. Certain ideological and political notions, such as 'humanity' and 'democracy', move centre-stage, but apart from terms directly derived from these ('humanitarian', 'democratic') the PL vocabulary itself is not immediately affected, rather the existing one is co-opted and occasionally systematized (for example by the Scots and Bentham) to accord with the new philosophical systems.

The underlying axis of debate among Social Philosophers was between those who sought to ground their account of human society in the existence of universal Natural Laws or principles, particularly moral laws, and those adopting a more relativistic position. The former included Montesquieu, the Scots and, in an idiosyncratic fashion, Mandeville; while among the latter were Lockeans such as Condillac and other French *philosophes*, as well as Rousseau, Bentham, and German Romantics such as Herder. The extension of the concept of Natural Law to morality, initiated by Shaftesbury and pursued by Hutcheson, Ferguson, Kames and Adam Smith, was central in determining the character of their 'Psychological' thought. While the Associationists sought to bring Human Nature under the aegis of Natural Philosophy via a reductionist, sensationalist epistemology, their Scottish opponents, motivated by more practical social concerns, sought the same end by developing the notion of these natural moral laws. Eventually, nineteenth-century positivist science would reject this extension of the concept of Natural Laws as confounding the distinction between the world of objective natural phenomena properly amenable to scientific enquiry and the subjective realm of human values and culture. Evolutionary theory eventually returned morality to the scientific realm, but at the price of reductively explaining it in terms of morally neutral principles of adaptation – and these principles would leave the cosmos itself essentially amoral. In terms of the development of psychological ideas, however, the 'Moral Law' project stimulated wide-ranging empirical studies of human social behaviour, attributes and 'powers' of no less significance than the more respectably 'scientific' Associationist and sensationalist investigations of perception and epistemology.

4
Practical Pressures: Nerves, Madness, Sex and Education

Introduction

We now turn from philosophy, however broadly construed, to other kinds of discourse which anticipated, in some degree, the concerns of Psychology. In doing this we find ourselves increasingly embroiled in contextual issues, in 'psychology' rather than 'Psychology'. Although the net could easily be cast more widely, I have concentrated on three main areas: first, physiology and medicine, the most relevant aspects being neurophysiological theory and madness. Second, we will look at eighteenth-century sexuality, which has received considerable academic attention in recent years. Lastly, some educational works will be discussed, since these occupy a nodal point in the mediation of proto-Psychological thought into practice, and the meeting of psychology and Psychology. It is argued that these commonly neglected writings prove quite central to the creation of the climate in which Psychology could eventually emerge, and that in some cases at least they were clearly more fruitful than philosophy in generating new psychological ideas.

1 Physiology and Medicine

Two principal topics relevant to Psychology concerned eighteenth-century doctors and physiologists, of which neurophysiology ultimately proved the most significant. In reconceptualizing this, the Edinburgh-born doctor Robert Whytt perhaps played the major role. The later part of the century also saw growing interest in the brain itself. The second, which had more contemporary impact, was the nature of insanity and mental disorder. Although there was sometimes considerable interaction between doctors and philosophers (crucially in relation to insanity) the physiological and medical research traditions had a quite distinct input into the repertoire of psychological ideas. None the less, physiologists tend to share certain underlying philosophical assumptions with Empiricist philosophers – not least, of course, a mechanistic orientation and a belief in the physical basis of psychological phenomena – indeed, as in the cases of Hartley and La Mettrie, physiology and philosophy were mutually reinforcing in this respect. Regarding the brain, notwithstanding Thomas Willis's earlier groundbreaking efforts (see Chapter 1), British physiologists played a minor role during the eighteenth century; the major work was undertaken by continental physiologists such as G.B. Morgagni, Bichat, Rolando, and Gall (who went on to create 'phrenology'). This topic will be discussed in Chapter 6, since historically its interest here is as an integral part of the background to phrenology.

A 'physicalization', if not a simple mechanization, is one of the most salient features of normal Enlightenment psychological discourse. It is no longer in terms of the soul's destiny but in terms of the vicissitudes of the body that self-experience is encoded. It is from the spleen, the vapours, nervous distempers, or 'blunt and obtuse intellectual Organs' (Cheyne, 1742)[1], that people suffer, not the ravages of Puritan guilt; a medicalized 'melancholia', not a spiritually resonant Burtonian melancholy. This is a direct consequence of that victory of reason over the theological which accompanied the Williamite settlement and the advent of a new proto-capitalist, proto-bourgeois economic order. It is particularly evident in the language of madness:

> This disqualification of spiritual authority, the possessors dispossessing the possessed, the provident annexing Providence, took many forms, but one lay in a reductionist psychiatry curing the voices of enthusiasm. (Porter, 1988, p. 15)

The number of treatises on insanity was legion, but the broad dimensions of debate for the first half of the century continued along the lines of a battle beween an old guard maintaining a pessimistic view and seeing madness as a mysterious, if no longer spiritually significant, condition of the Soul[2], and an ultimately victorious new guard of optimists influenced by Locke for whom it all boiled down to a physiologically caused misassociation of ideas.

A key episode in this is the controversy between Alexander Munro (old guard) and William Battie (new guard) in the 1750s, Arnold (1782, 1786) representing the new orthodoxy which emerged. This naturally entailed changes in the language used to classify and describe. Although the century saw the rise of specialist 'mad-doctors', it did not see psychiatry established as an organized sub-branch of medicine; mad-doctors were highly individualistic (and unregulated) in their practices. The new guard's victory was short-lived, for their physiological theories of madness yielded few therapeutic rewards, and as optimism waned, more psychological approaches began to flourish at the end of the century, involving atheoretical 'moral treatments' exercised by charismatic physicians or asylum owners. The picture of eighteenth-century British psychiatry (although the term is anachronistic) emerging from works such as Andrew Scull's *Museums of Madness* (1979) and Roy Porter's *Mind Forg'd Manacles* (1988) (themselves at odds on certain points) diverges considerably from that famously provided by Foucault (1967) for France. The latter clearly cannot be generalized in an unqualified way to the British situation. Common to both the pre-'moral treatment' schools of thought was an attitude to madness which dehumanized and bestialized the insane as having, as it were, lost either their souls or their reason, the Enlightenment hallmark of humanity. 'Moral treatment' will be discussed in Chapter 8, since its impact fell primarily in the following century.

(i) Neurophysiology

While Jaynes (1973), in his usual rumbustious fashion, casts Descartes as heroic initiator of the 'stimulus–response paradigm', for Descartes and his early-eighteenth-century successors the two central neurological questions were (a) how to formulate an account of the way nerves worked which would enable 'animated motion' to be assimilated to the mechanistic laws of motion (hence the plethora of hydraulic, spring, pulley-and-string and similar models); and (b) how to characterize the relationship between the soul, or mind, and this fleshy apparatus (i.e. the mind–body problem). Any adequate theory would have to solve both these riddles. One solution was to take La Mettrie's route – simply deny the second problem altogether and opt wholeheartedly for materialist mechanism. As we have seen, neither question favours the development of Psychology: the first converts psychological questions into physiological ones (see Chapter 1); the second confines them within philosophy. Furthermore, the second question also hinders physiology in separating itself from philosophy.

A way out of this impasse gradually consolidates during the latter half of the eighteenth century.[3] The solution, in simple terms, was to introduce a new kind of 'mechanism' for explaining organic processes – namely, that nerves, muscles and perhaps other organs (much controversy surrounded the details) possessed the properties of 'irritability' and/or 'sensibility' which enabled the organism to react to stimulation in a 'wise', self-preserving manner. It ceased to matter, in effect, whether stimulation originated externally (in the form of sensations) or internally (from the conscious mind). The 'soul' in a way pervades organic matter, but its operations need not be conscious and are governed by mechanical laws (albeit of a new kind). Neither 'sensibility' (an organism's ability to react to stimuli) nor a nervous tissue's 'irritability' (its localized ability so to respond) necessarily entails consciousness. The organism as a whole is a *self-regulating* machine; there is an 'animal oeconomy' analogous to the self-regulating political economy portrayed by proto-economists. As Danziger (1983) (on whom I am drawing heavily here) notes, the invention of self-regulating machines was a major feature of contemporary technology from around 1745 (Watt's centrifugal governor or 'planetary valve', which ensured the smooth operation of the Boulton-Watt steam engines, being a famous, but far from unique, case). In this 'animal oeconomy' the mind or soul no longer rules from above like an absolute monarch but becomes integrated more and more into the day-to-day running of affairs, as one component in the complex set of self-regulatory feedback loops (to put it anachronistically). Very few physiologists were prepared to deny the existence of an independant rational soul altogether, but it ceased to be directly relevant to their enquiries.

Even after 1781, when the idea was seriously challenged by Felice Fontana (1730–1805), the tubular nature of nerves remained widely, if not universally, accepted; indeed, according to Liddell (1960) Fontana held nerves to be cylinders filled with gelatinous fluid. Emancipation from the 'nerves as tubes' model was a protracted business, having to await Jan E. Purkinje's (1787–1869) work in the 1830s, using new achromatic microscopes, for its final resolution. The term 'animal spirits' remained in common use, along with more modern-sounding expressions like 'nervous fluid'; but such terms were increasingly understood as metaphorical and hypothetical in character. The consequence of the new kind of organic 'mechanism' in this respect was rather to promote – in some quarters, anyway[4] – notions of a vitalistic life-force mediated by a *vis nervosa*, which underlay the pervasive capacity for sensibility. Electrical fluids were also frequently invoked as either analogous to, or identical with, this mediating factor[5]. (How many of us now, by the way, think of 'current' in 'electric current' as a fluid metaphor?)

The principal figures in the story of this transformation were G.E. Stahl (sometimes spelled Staahl) (1660–1743), Albrecht von Haller (1708–77), Robert Whytt (1714–66), J.A. Unzer (1727–99), Georg Prochaska (1749–1820) and P.J.G. Cabanis (1757–1808). While Stahl himself eventually repudiated physiological research, his German successors did not, and Prochaska's 1784 *A Dissertation on the Functions of the Nervous System* (transl. Laycock, 1851) develops the notion of a division between the 'soul-sensorium' and the 'body-sensorium', each operating according to a law of self-conservation. Prochaska also addresses the question of localization of function in the brain, considering it 'by no means improbable, that each division of the intellect has its allotted organ in the brain' (1851 edn, p. 447). By 1800 the stage was set for Bell and Magendie (who differentiated the afferent and efferent nerves) and Marshall Hall (who coined the noun 'reflex' in 1833), as well as Flourens's work on the brain and E.H. Weber's proto-psychophysical studies of the senses. The most significant shift which had occurred was that attention could now be paid to the nature of the organism's responses to environmental events or stimuli, and the structure, properties and sensitivities of the sensory organs. True enough, Descartes had seen behaviour as triggered by external events, but the issue had remained grounded in a quest for the machinery by which this was transmitted via the senses to mind or muscle. There was no space here for studying 'sensitivity' to stimuli, no concept of the organism as a holistic entity whose behaviour had to be understood in self-regulatory terms. For Descartes and his followers there was 'no fundamental distinction between the way in which animate and inanimate bodies responded to external influences that impinged upon them' (Danziger, 1983). By 1800 this had ceased to be the case.

Of the figures listed, Robert Whytt is perhaps the most 'advanced', although in broader terms than neurophysiological theory von Haller is more historically eminent[6], and Prochaska more directly influential in Europe. But it is Whytt who, in his *On the Vital and Other Involuntary Motions of Animals* (1751), raises the term 'stimulus' to the status of a technical concept and sees the need to distinguish animate from inanimate motion[7]. While Stahl had invoked an almost mystical pervasive 'soul', and von Haller (with whom Whytt engaged in a protracted controversy) remained ultimately entangled with the older dualistic mechanistic model of mental versus physical causes, Whytt was able to steer a middle path by clearly distinguishing the 'sentient soul' from the 'rational soul', thus countenancing a third level mechanism, governed by neither reason nor Cartesian mechanics[8]. Unzer and Prochaska develop this further, progressively attenuating the role of the soul and, in Prochaska's case, articulating the self-regulatory nature of organic processes[9]. Cabanis, in the last year of the century, hints at a hierarchical notion of the nervous system (a view later to dominate nineteenth-century neurophysiology), differentiating between behaviours governed centrally and those governed peripherally.

In the transformation of neurophysiological thought in the eighteenth century we discern several interweaving themes: the weakening hold of theological considerations over physiological research; the impact, as Danziger suggests, of novel technology in providing new theoretical schemata; a widening gulf between philosophy and physiology in how the psychological was being approached (though this, as we will see, was bridged in part by contemporary accounts of madness) and the input of new technical concepts (often by giving existing terms more specialized meanings) which feed into contemporary PL – irritability, sensibility, stimulation, sympathy, nervous, and the like. Finally in all this, we should perhaps spare a thought for the multitudes of decapitated frogs upon whom much of this edifice of new knowledge was erected.

(ii) Insanity

Throughout the 1970s and 1980s the history of psychiatry was a flourishing area, to some degree unleashed by Foucault's seminal *Madness and Civilization* (1967, partial English translation 1971[10]). The literature, even on the eighteenth century, is now of a scale which precludes any brief synthesis of its findings. We have already indicated the broad lines of the mid-century debate between Battie and Munro. Since Battie's *A Treatise on Madness* (1758, actually December 1757) is most likely to be encountered (along with Munro's reply) in the Hunter and Macalpine reprint of 1962, a slight digression will be perhaps in order to draw attention to what appears to be a seriously misleading claim in their introductory essay. They argue (p. 15) that Battie's distinction between what he called 'Original' and 'Consequential' forms of madness anticipates that between 'non-organic' mental illness (mental illness proper) and organic conditions which are the mental manifestations of cerebral disease. It must be stressed that Battie is quite explicit that all madness is ultimately due to 'some disorder of that substance which is medullary and strictly nervous' (Battie, 1758, p. 41). He has no notion of 'non-organic' madness, simply acknowledging that some forms are 'original'. These do not appear to 'follow or accompany any accident' (*ibid.*, p. 59), may be hereditary and are extremely difficult to treat, requiring management more than medicine (*ibid.*, p. 68). Nowhere does he suggest that they are less physiologically based in the 'medullary substance' than any other forms of madness. Rather, since they are somehow endemic, there is no way of rendering the physical pathology accessible to the physician's attentions – unlike fractures of the skull or gluttony and idleness which he lists as causes of Consequential madness. This is an important point, because the Hunter and Macalpine reading would ascribe to Battie a more psychological view of 'Original' madness than he in fact possessed.

Numerous works by Andrew Scull, Klaus Doerner, Roy Porter, W. Bynum, and Vieda Skultans are now available which provide detailed accounts of eighteenth-century psychiatric practice and institutional organization, while Denis Leigh (1961) remains an important source of basic information, albeit historiographically unsophisticated[11]. Mark S. Micale has recently published two most important critical reviews of the history of hysteria (Micale, 1989, 1990). Stanley Jackson's survey (1986) of changing theories of melancholy and depression also contains much on this period. Little would be gained by systematically reviewing their readily available findings here, although reference will be made to them on occasion. Instead I will look more closely at the language used in Thomas Arnold's *Observations on the Nature, Kinds, Causes, and Prevention, of Insanity* (1806, 2 vols; originally published in 1782 and 1786) as the most detailed exposition of the approach initiated by Battie.

Arnold offers a fully elaborated attempt at utilizing Hartley's version of Lockean epistemology as a basis for analysing the nature of madness and classifying its varieties. This he strives to integrate with the theories of Whytt and Haller. The result is a classification radically different from that traditionally adopted. Instead of a primary division between Melancholy and Mania/Phrensy/Fury, a distinction going back to the Ancients, he offers one between 'Ideal Insanity' and 'Notional Insanity'. The former was a distinction between symptoms; Melancholy being 'a permanent delirium, without fury, or fever, in which the mind is dejected, and timorous, and usually employed about one object' (vol. I, pp. 26–7), the latter 'a permanent delirium, with fury and audacity' and, in the case of 'phrensy', fever also. Arnold finds this unsatisfactory on numerous counts, and attempts to get beyond the symptoms to the underlying source of the madness. His new division rests on whether this lies (a) in a disturbance of Sensations or 'Ideas' used to refer to strictly mental representations of objects of sensation; or (b) in a disturbance of the processes of 'Reflection' – that is, whether we are dealing with an 'Ideal delirium' in which a person's ideas about the external world are at fault (and this may happen as a result of fever as well as of madness) or a 'Notional delirium' in which their 'notions' (i.e. Locke's 'Ideas of Reflection') are affected, which, he is inclined to believe, is unique to madness (vol. I, pp. 55–7). Ideal insanity is due to erroneous images, Notional insanity to erroneous associations (vol. I, p. 66). The latter may relate to notions of good and bad, in which case we have the 'Fool', who suffers from Moral but not Medical insanity wherein it is notions of cause and effect which are at fault. James Cowles Prichard's later introduction of the concept of 'Moral Insanity' is partly foreshadowed here, but Arnold's meaning is more restricted and ancillary to his main nosology.

Table 4.1 Thomas Arnold's Classification of Insanity (1782)

Ideal Insanity	*Notional Insanity*	
Phrenetic	Delusive	Vain, or self-important
Incoherent	Whimsical	Hypochondriacal
Maniacal	Fanciful	Pathetic*
Sensitive	Impulsive	Appetitive
	Scheming	

* *Varieties of 'Pathetic'*

amorous	jealous	avaricious
misanthropic	arrogant	irrascible
abhorrent	suspicious	bashful
timid	sorrowful	distressful
nostalgic	superstitious	fanatical
desponding		

adapted from Thomas Arnold (1806), p.93

Sir Alexander Crichton's Classification of Insanity (1798)

Genera 1.	Delirium	
species 1.	Mania furibunda	raving-fury
" *2.*	Mania mitis	raving-gaiety
" *3.*	Mania melancholia	dejection
Genera 2.	Hallucination or Illusion	
species 1.	Hypochondriasis	re-health
" *2.*	Daemonomania	communion with spirits
" *3.*	Vertigo	rotating notion of objects
" *4.*	Somnambulensis	?
Genera 3.		
species 1.	Fatuitas	imbecility
" *2.*	Memoria imminuta	memory problems
" *3.*	Perceptia imminuta	perceptual problems
" *4.*	vis idearum associandi	confused thoughts
" *5.*	vis fingendi "	'total want of genius . .'
" *6.*	vis judiciandi	want of judgment

adapted from D. Leigh (1961), p.45

With this binary distinction in place, he ventures a full classification of the varieties of insanity (see Table 4.1). What is immediately striking is that with a few exceptions, this remains couched in folk-psychology terms. Like Reid, Arnold cannot move beyond a systematization of existing categories, except in the initial differentiation of the Ideal from the Notional. The only other technical terms are 'Phrenetic', 'Hypochondriacal', 'Pathetic', 'Appetitive' and, possibly, 'Nostalgic'. Even these are mostly long-established expressions in the medical argot of the early modern period. 'Appetitive' is perhaps a euphemism, since it seems to refer only to nymphomania and satyriasis. He has abandoned the term 'Melancholy' as a basic category, although he uses it in the text – basically as synonymous with Hypochondriacal, nor does he make much use of 'Hysteria', although it does occur. The difference from modern psychiatric diagnostic categories is striking: psychotic, paranoia, catatonia, schizophrenia, hebephrenic schizophrenia, amentia, anorexia, even neurosis and the like all *sounding*, at any rate, as if they are scientific medical terms, and all originating within psychiatry.

Although the framework provides a structure for methodically reviewing all the varieties of madness he has encountered, it is painfully obvious that the Lockean distinction between the two levels of epistemological processing – sensation and reflection – is actually inadequate for medical purposes. The weakest point of the system, however, is reached when he comes to the Pathetic subvariety of the Notional insanities, which 'exhibits a striking and melancholy picture, of the empire of the passions' (vol. I, p. 185), where one passion completely controls the mind. The sixteen varieties he names as most common are hardly more than a list of the passions themselves. When he is elaborating on the features of each type of madness the clarity of the Ideal/Notional distinction can also become blurred – for example 'Sensitive insanity' (which is an 'Ideal type') refers to such identity delusions as people believing they are:

> . . . wolves, dogs, lions, cats, cows, oxen, game-cocks, sparrows, cuckoos, nightingales, earthen vessels, pipkins, jars, tea-pots, bricks, candles . . . wax, butter, glass, leather, or straw (vol. I, p. 122–3)

while Delusive insanity (a Notional type) includes imagining that one possesses such powers as being able to fly, etc., and 'Vain or Self-Important' would include believing one was a king or a pope. The difference in logical type between the delusions of believing yourself an earthbound cuckoo, and believing yourself a flying human, is surely rather fine, however polarized their symbolic tenors. ('Tis p'raps clearer 'twixt pope and pipkin.)

Arnold nevertheless provides us with a rich seam of case histories and observations. His image of the mind is not, despite his Associationist theory, an entirely passive one, for reflection proper is an essentially active process:

> . . . the mind must have a perpetual motive, of some kind or other, for the exertion of its active powers [a Reidian phrase], and must ever be engaged in the pursuit or avoidance of what it likes or dislikes, relative to knowledge, virtue, or pleasure. (vol. I, p. 52)

Elsewhere the possibility of unconscious motivation briefly surfaces:

> But as we cannot easily conceive of conduct without motives, or motives without notions; and must therefore suppose notions of some kind or other, to be the immediately antecedent causes of every voluntary action; we may safely, I think, rest satisfied that the conduct of these sorts of patients [i.e. Impulsive variety of Notional insanity] is regulated by notions, however they may conceal themselves from our observation. (vol. I, p. 169)

The view of 'notions' as 'causes' is also prophetic of one of the most problematic Freudian formulations. Arnold actually uses the term 'unconscious' in discussing our unawareness of the sensations of breathing and habitual actions (vol. II, pp. 42, 52).

Turning, in the second volume, to causes of insanity, Arnold distinguishes far more unambiguously than Battie between Bodily and Mental. While he rages at the outset against 'the more early modern writers' who 'have been as uselessly, as they have been indefatigably, minute' in enumerating 'causes with the most insignificant and disgusting refinement, and have multiplied distinctions without end' (vol. II, p. 2), his own list of causes fares little better, extending (among the physical) to 'worms in the nostrils' – a cause as minute and disgusting as any one could wish for.

The mental causes are also really a hotchpotch, although they are ordered under three headings as due to study (plus business, schemes and other 'prolonged employments of the mind'), passions (with too great activity of the imagination) and imbecility. This is followed by an excursion into neurology, from which he derives six categories of stimuli: following Whytt, he accepts that stimuli can be corporeal or mental, the former can be accidental or natural (e.g. light, motions of air on eardrum), the latter necessary (producing involuntary changes in the body, such as appetites and passions) or voluntary (acts of will). Accidental corporeal stimuli are further broken down into mechanical, 'acrimonious' (arising from 'peculiar sensible properties' of objects such as 'bitter, salt, caustic, ignited', etc.) and 'specific' (such as some 'vegetable poisons' which 'do not possess any very conspicuous sensible properties') (vol. II, pp. 36–7). How these analyses actually relate to the Lockean model introduced in Volume I is unclear, although presumably they allow for the possibility of diagnosing with more specificity the points at which faults may develop in either sensory input (erroneous images) or notions (erroneous associations).

Arnold ends with various wise words of counsel on how to stay sane – temperance, exercise, regulating one's passions and developing rational views of religion being among the best strategies. What he does not do in this work – and its absence from the title may have been noted – is to say anything about treatment and cure. This he appears to have intended for a future work, but he is conscious from the outset that improvements 'in the Healing Art' have made little progress compared to other fields, and particularly so in the treatment of madness. Leigh (1961) rightly admires Arnold's appreciation of the psychological, as well as physiological, nature of madness.

The terms of Arnold's nosology were in marked contrast to those offered shortly afterwards by Sir Alexander Crichton in his *An Inquiry into the Nature and Origin of Mental Derangement* (1798) (see Table 4.1). Here folk language is replaced by a Latinate medical terminology organized in terms of genera and species; thus we find the Genera 'Amentias' including 'Fatuitas' (imbecility) and '*vis idearum associandi*' (confused thoughts – Arnold's 'Incoherence'), for example. Leigh (*op. cit.*) praises Crichton's classification as an advance on Arnold, but it is surely an advance for which a considerable price has been paid.

The appearance of Arnold's compendious but fatalistic survey of the varieties of madness coincided with a major shift in attitudes towards treatment throughout Europe. Interpretation of this has been controversial ever since Foucault challenged the optimistic, heroic received account of Pinel's casting off of the chains of the inmates of the Bicêtre Asylum in Paris in 1789. This supposedly enlightened giant step from darkness and fear towards humane medical wisdom was recast as a giant step forward in the bureaucratic management of social deviancy, providing incarceration with new, more powerful medical rationales. In Britain, the Quaker William Tuke's famous 'Retreat' at York, founded in 1792, was the first and most famous institution to employ Moral Therapy. The subsequent rise of 'moral treatment' in Britain coincided not only with needs for bureaucratic management and pressures for professionalization among 'mad doctors', but also with rising humanitarianism and Romanticism's revaluation of the irrational. Not that these are clearly demarcated; humanitarianism in particular was the mode in which management pressures were most powerfully expressed and advocated (and I am implying no hypocrisy here). The appearance of this new approach was, as we shall see in Chapter 8, far from welcomed by the medical profession, revealing as it did the almost total ineffectiveness of the medical treatments of madness.

2 Sex and Education

Eighteenth-century sexuality has been the target of a considerable body of recent historical research, stimulated principally from two directions. The first is the rise of feminist (and also to some extent gay) scholarship since the late 1960s, which has striven to uncover the history of gender relations. Since these are implicated at every level of social life, this has naturally led researchers to examine issues ranging from the economic to the psychological. Secondly, much of Michel Foucault's work, and especially *The History of Sexuality* (1979), opened up new theoretical perspectives towards – and raised new kinds of questions about – the very nature of 'sex' as a category in Western culture, adding further weight to feminist critiques of conventional wisdom. These developments took place against a background of increasing interest in social history – including family history, historical demography and the like – which had been under way since the late 1950s, culminating perhaps in Lawrence Stone's monumental *The Family, Sex and Marriage in England 1500–1800* (1977). The crucial role of the 'Enlightenment', the 'Age of Reason', in the emergence of Western culture (as well as the approbatory nature of these traditional labels themselves) placed it high on the agenda for historical scrutiny and reappraisal. The present discussion, like that of psychiatry, must necessarily be somewhat restricted with regard to how much of this contemporary scholarship can be taken on board.[12] Of the many issues raised we are in any case concerned here with a fairly limited subset: how, and why, did ideas regarding the nature and meaning of sex and sexuality change in Britain during this period? How *psychological* (as opposed to biological or moral, for example) was the eighteenth-century understanding of sexuality?

The interest in education which developed at this time is particularly significant for the history of Psychology, since in focusing attention on the child and on learning processes it was one of the first areas in which a genuinely exploratory empirical investigation of psychological issues manifested itself. Only the study of perception clearly preceded it. While it was late in the century before any significant educational reforms actually took place, the cultural climate enabling these changes had been building up ever since Locke's *Some Thoughts Concerning Education*, which first appeared in 1693.

(i) Sex

The popular image of attitudes to sex in Hanoverian England is that they were 'rollicking, naughty, fun-loving, liberal, permissive, advanced and enlightened, frank and frolicsome' to borrow Roy Porter's (1982) list (or, if you prefer, 'disgusting, decadent and debauched'). Promiscuity reigned from London to Bath and Tunbridge Wells, uninhibited by the ever-present threat of the 'clap' or 'pox' – treatments for which were an unabating topic of coffee-house speculation by Boswells and beaux; Tom Jones and Fanny Hill forever tumble in laughing, vigorous, guilt-free copulation. Nor is this caricature entirely fictitious, although the reality was considerably more complex.

As a schematic outline, the trajectory of attitudes towards sex seems to run somewhat as follows. First, a Court reaction after the Restoration against Puritan and traditional Christian views of sex as inherently sinful for purposes other than procreation and a temporary suspension of the double standard which condoned, or paid only lip-service to condemning, male adultery and promiscuity while strongly reprehending such behaviour in women. Participants in the relatively short-lived period of outrageous Court profligacy self-consciously aimed to shock and scandalize. Beyond Court circles the emergence, in the middle class, of a more companionate – as opposed to arranged, economically based – concept of marriage was also accompanied by a corresponding acceptance of the non-procreative value of sex in sustaining conjugal relations, though the double standard persisted. Secondly, in the early eighteenth century what we might term the 'secularization' of sex continued, and a more 'laid back' (pardon the expression), permissive acceptance of sexuality gained sway, although not all sectors of society were equally affected. The difference in attitudes between this phase and that of the Restoration Court may be seen by comparing John Cleland's best-selling pornographic novel *Fanny Hill* (1749) with Rochester's poems. Cleland strives to present sexuality elegantly as a happy, harmless, healthy activity (using no four-letter words, incidentally; see Brooks-Davies, 1982), while Rochester's verse is calculated to outrage, full of expletives, and gratuitously prurient. After 1750 the momentum of permissiveness appears to accelerate, accompanied by a well developed sex industry of pornographic books and prints, sex aids and brothels catering for special tastes (particularly flagellation). Mistresses (and their offspring) again become publicly acknowledged by the aristocracy. By the 1780s, however, a reaction was beginning to set in which Porter (1982) sees as taking two forms: first, the anti-hedonism of the Evangelical revival (which gained increasing force after 1800 and evolved into full-blown Victorian repression); second, the Romantic spiritualization of sexuality found in Blake and Shelley. Both equally rejected the 'mundane sexuality of the Enlightenment' (Porter, *ibid.*, pp. 20–21).

As Stone stresses, this picture must be seen against a darker background of horrendously unhygienic living conditions, medical ignorance, appalling gynaecological risks for women in child-bearing, lack of effective contraception (*coitus interruptus* or *coitus reservatus* being the most common, condoms being used primarily for prophylactic reasons in extra-marital relations and then available only in London in the latter half of the century), and widespread venereal disease. According to Stone, single-parenthood apparently increased dramatically as the century progressed for complex demographic reasons such as the rise in bachelor younger-sons unable to support families and greater levels of unchaperoned social contact between young people. The data are problematical, however, because in 1753 the Clandestine Marriage Act greatly narrowed the definition of marriage with the result that offspring of unions (e.g. 'common-law' marriages) hitherto legally recognized were subsequently classified as 'illegitimate'[13]. Masturbation became a topic of anxiety early in the century, but did not attract the intensity of obsessional loathing and fascination characteristic of the mid nineteenth century.

Turning to our first question, then, how did ideas regarding the nature and meaning of sexuality change during this period? Sex, it has been said, involves a triad of concerns: love, lust and procreation. Its meaning at any time can be considered as the interrelationship which is seen as holding between these. Within the faithful companionate marriage lust is admissible only as sanctioned by love, with procreation as an occasionally desired, but not necessary, outcome. In practice the double standard ensured that for males lust was acknowledged to possess its own imperatives independent of love, and a satyr like Boswell was continually racked with guilt about his inability to reconcile the two needs within the bounds of a monogamous loving marriage. It can be argued that it is during this century that the view of women as 'sex objects' really establishes itself in Western, and particularly British, culture. Whilst female sexuality had always been acknowledged, in the previous century it had remained integrated (in Donne and Marvell, for instance) with romantic love, while the image of woman as 'procreator' had dominated her role as wife. With the decline in the power of religion in defining the meaning of sexuality, lust becomes 'decoupled' (pardon this expression too) from both love and procreation. As the middle-class *ménage* becomes more child-centred and infant mortality rates fall after mid century, the procreative role *per se* becomes de-emphasized in favour of the nurturing-mother role[14]. When, towards the end of the century, her traditional domestic roles become delegated to nurses, maids and governesses, while professional work remains unavailable, the middle- and upper-class wife suffers an increasingly restricted scope for personal fulfilment. The burden, in consequence, falls progressively more heavily on her being sexually satisying to her husband and embodying a more idealized, quasi-spiritualized, image of 'motherhood' for her children. This latter involves her own infantilization as playmate and consoler, as well as rendering her an authority on matters of morality.

By the end of the century the moral authority of this idealized, pious, self-sacrificing 'mother' (embodied in women, often not actually mothers, like Hannah More, Sarah Trimmer, Maria and Honora Edgeworth and Elizabeth Hamilton) was beginning to exert itself as a lust-taming force. Hedonism was a value from which the mother had herself become increasingly excluded, her consolations, such as they were, deriving from sublimation and self-abnegation in the service of her children, or charity works. The number of unmarried women had also increased (see below, p. 228); this meant that such women were frequently led into governess type roles where their 'moral authority' and anti-hedonistic attitudes were heightened. As these voices become more widely heard – especially, as we will see, through the dominance of women writers on education at the turn of the century – would-be hedonistic males have no option but to appear, at least, to come guiltily to heel. Within marriage itself lust is again subordinated to love, but in a different form, for female lust itself is now being inhibited by the anti-hedonistic value system which woman has had to evolve for psychological survival. She submits out of love, but her lust remains in check. The male Romantic response to this (e.g. in Blake, Shelley, and *Naturphilosophie*) is to concede the rejection of materialistic hedonism but to reconstrue lust as an integral part of a more transcendental kind of love in which both flesh and spirit are fused as aspects of a single cosmic process. In the event, as the nineteenth century progressed, the initial sensuality of Romanticism rapidly attenuated, while its ideal of spiritual love and fusion determined the overt (if not covert) hedonistic tone of Victorian heterosexual relations.

From the late eighteenth century onwards, sexuality was doomed to be an area of profound psychological conflict (though it had never been totally otherwise). No single sexual ideology could hope to gratify all sections of society. The anti-hedonistic values instilled in the respectable bourgeois home could not, for men, be reconciled with those of the male-dominated world of work and urban street life. There were conflicts, too, for single women (in an era of excess of women over men) competing for husbands, since the qualities which males found alluring were frequently at odds with the values they had internalized at their mothers' knees. While male involvement in parenting had at times increased during the eighteenth century, and father–child relationships had become far less formal, by the end of the century the tide had reversed again. For both sexes procreative fecundity was an ambiguous virtue: for males it exacerbated their economic burden; for females it was downright dangerous. In the middle classes, however, it at least served to consolidate women's domestic power-base and provide a focus for lives denied other sources of satisfaction, simultaneously boosting the male's self-image as an important patriarch.

In Britain, the net psychological effect of eighteenth-century shifts in the construal of sexuality was to render it problematical in a way unprecedented in European culture. Disinhibition of lust as an accepted component of sexuality created tensions of several kinds: conflicts between emotional life (the ethical arena of love) and sexual life (the biological arena of the 'animal oeconomy'), anxiety about performance, anxiety about the ethics and effects of masturbation, problems of social control in balancing one sector of society's permissiveness against the other's demands for decency. While both male homosexuality and lesbianism remained largely underground, here too (particularly in the former case) the century's close sees an increase in concern. Sexual preferences were not seen as defining psychological identity until later in the nineteenth century – a man may be a bugger or a sodomite but 'the homosexual' as distinct personality type or psychopathological syndrome is a Victorian achievement[15]. It is worth noting that early-eighteenth-century homosexual 'sodomites' tended towards misogyny, their effeminacy becoming the target of proto-feminist satire[16]. In sum, the eighteenth century sees the gradual emergence of sexuality as a psychological *topos*: (a) in the growing focus on – and conflictedness of – female sexual identity between 'sex object', 'spiritualized mother' and 'procreator' at the expense of other roles; (b) in male inabilities to integrate lust and love; (c) anxiety about masturbation; and (d) in the Romantic effort to purify or spiritualize sexuality. While the earlier part of the century still construed sexuality in a mixture of religious and biological terms, focusing on either its immorality or its effects on health, by 1800 the weight of concern is shifting towards its role in the individual psyche.

(ii) Education

While relatively little practical reform in education was achieved during the eighteenth century, projects and proposals were numerous and discontent accelerated in its closing decades. These had been anticipated in the previous century by the educational reform schemes – never implemented – of Hartlib and Comenius. In the eighteenth century a number of experimental schools did briefly flourish, the best-known being William Gilpin's at Cheam, David Manson's in Belfast (both founded in 1752) and the Rousseau-influenced David Williams's Laurence Street Academy in Chelsea, London (1773)[17]. While they paved the way for nineteenth-century projects like Robert Owen's in New Lanark, they had little effect on the normal running of education in Hanoverian Britain. Elementary schooling was served by generally dismal 'dame schools' ('little more than baby-minding establishments': Barnard, 1961); private day schools – typically, if not always, equally grim; and a variety of religiously orientated charity and work schools or 'schools of industry', which trained labouring class children in practical skills. In the 1780s Sunday Schools also came on to the scene. Secondary education for boys took the form of grammar and public schools dominated by an increasingly irrelevant classics curriculum and characterized, especially in top public boarding schools like Eton, by harsh and brutalizing regimes. There were occasional pupil rebellions at these as late as 1851 (at Marlborough)[18]. For girls, numerous private boarding schools provided tuition in genteel skills like lacquering and domestic arts, but in some cases also a rather broader general-knowledge curriculum which could, ironically, result in their emerging better educated than their Latin-bound brothers. Even so, the quality of middle-class female education was usually poor (and for poorer sisters nonexistent).

English university education was, if anything, in even worse shape. Oxford and Cambridge, effectively intellectually moribund until the 1790s (especially the former), served as little more than playgrounds for idly rich youth and lacked any form of written examination. In any case, attendance was confined to Anglicans.

A few Nonconformist academies briefly flourished in the 1750s and 1760s (notably Warrington Academy, where Joseph Priestley taught), offering far superior courses to Oxbridge. In Scotland the situation was rather different, with four universities (Aberdeen, Edinburgh, Glasgow and St Andrews) to England's two, all non-sectarian and offering a wide range of courses seriously taught and assessed. There was, in short, no state education as such, no official monitoring of standards, and no official educational policy throughout the eighteenth century. For the wealthy there was always, of course, the option of private tutors and governesses. Teaching at all levels thus came under increasing criticism as the century progressed, on grounds ranging from the crudity of teaching methods, via the corrupting moral climate, to the irrelevance of the curriculum.

Two texts dominate any consideration of eighteenth-century educational thought (if not practice): Locke's *Some Thoughts Concerning Education* and Rousseau's *Emile*. The former, first appearing anonymously in 1693, was based on correspondence between Locke and Edward Clarke concerning Clarke's elder son's education. The final version (the 1705 fifth edition) remained in print throughout the century[19]. Works on education had, of course, appeared before this, the Catholic Obadiah Walker's *Of Education. Especially of Young Gentlemen* (1683) being perhaps closest in its agenda to Locke's work, although it retained features in common with the traditional 'courtesy book' genre[20]. Rousseau's work became available in English in the 1760s and again stayed in print thereafter. Subsequent works by Richard Lovell and Maria Edgeworth and Elizabeth Hamilton are characterized by efforts to integrate the rather different insights of these two authorities in a religiously orthodox form. Hannah More, by contrast, is fighting a rearguard action against Rousseauism, while at the opposite pole Mary Wollstonecraft adopts a radical feminist stance regarding the education of women. Thomas Sheridan's *British Education* (1756) offers a quite separate analysis of how the woes of the nation stem from its educational deficiencies. Although it had little direct impact on educational thought, Sheridan's book is nevertheless of considerable historical interest, as we shall see. The number of works on education increases considerably after the 1760s[21]. One outcome of this discovery of the child via education was, it will be suggested, a historically crucial psychological development.

(a) Locke

Apart from a passing recommendation of the extension of work schools for the labouring classes, Locke offers few ideas regarding the reform of the education system – for which, unlike Comenius, Hartlib and Milton, he has little time, preferring education by private tutor. The essence of his message is that since 'The little, or almost insensible Impressions on our tender Infancies, have very important or lasting consequences' (para. 1)[22], great care must be taken throughout childhood in ensuring that the mind is 'made obedient to Discipline, and pliant to Reason' (see para. 34). One must begin early:

> A Compliance and Suppleness of their Wills, being by a steady Hand introduced by Parents, before Children have Memories to retain the Beginnings of it, will seem natural to them, and work afterwards in them, as if it were so, preventing all Occasions of struggling or repining. (para. 44)

Invoking the principles of Awe, Respect and Reverence as the instruments for attaining this happy outcome, he observes:

> . . . he that has found a Way how to keep up a Child's Spirit easy, active, and free, and yet, at the same time, to restrain him from many Things he has a Mind to, and to draw him to Things that are uneasy to him, he, I say, that knows how to reconcile these seeming Contradictions, has, in my Opinion, got the Secret of Education. (para. 46)

Locke is not, however, a strict disciplinarian, and attacks the 'dangerous Disease' of 'breaking the Mind' (para. 51). It is not physical rewards and punishments but psychological ones which he holds paramount:

> *Esteem* and *Disgrace* are, of all others, the most powerful Incentives to the Mind, when once it is brought to relish them. (para. 56)

Beating (preferably delegated to a servant) should be reserved for '*Obstinacy* and *Rebellion*' and even then 'it should be Shame which is the greatest part'. Children's minds should not be clogged with numerous 'Rules and Precepts', 'which they often do not understand, and constantly as soon forget as given' (para. 64). As in the work of his successors, the problem of servants subverting parental schemes (para. 69) or frightening children with tales of 'goblins', etc. (para. 138) is a recurrent leitmotiv. There is much advice on tutor selection and taming the child's love of '*Dominion*', which exceeds even its love of liberty (see para. 103). Locke appreciates that children cannot constantly exhibit high levels of motivation, and 'Seasons of Aptitude and Inclination' should be 'heedfully laid hold of' (para. 74). Children should be taught 'an Abhorrence of *killing*, or tormenting any living Creature' (para. 116).

Turning to specific subjects, he suggests various techniques for teaching reading (e.g. using dice with letters on their various faces [para. 149]), recommending a separation between learning by heart and learning to read, and goes so far as to propose a systematic sequence for introducing subjects – each facilitating the understanding of its successor. Thus, beginning with Geography we move to Arithmetic, thence to Astronomy and use of Globes, which in turn provide a basis for Geometry. At this point 'chronology' and History can be introduced, so leading on to Ethics, Law, Rhetoric and Logic, and Natural Philosophy. On the latter he has a passage which is hardly what we expect from one supposedly imbued with the spirit of the Scientific Revolution:

> The works of Nature are contriv'd by a Wisdom, and operate by Ways too far surpassing our Faculties to discover, or Capacities to conceive, for us ever to be able to reduce them into a Science. (para. 190)

The history of the Bible and the study of 'spirit' should precede the 'Study of Bodies' (paras 191–2). Among the works recommended for Natural Philosophy is – again somewhat surprisingly – the Neo-Platonist Cudworth's *Intellectual System*. Dancing 'cannot be learned too early' (para. 196), but he does not think much of Music. Latin and language are, however, 'the least part of Education'. He ends by stressing the individual uniqueness of children and the need to tailor education accordingly.

While he views education as aimed at instilling Reason as the ruling guide, Locke is humane, eminently sensible and relaxed in his recommendations. Of course obedience and discipline figure prominently, but their value depends on their subordination to this higher goal. He counsels against spoiling and overindulging young children, since the earlier they are taught to control their desires the better, and the easier it will be for them later. Locke rarely uses the technical language of his *Essay*, but his philosophy is implicit throughout, especially in his discussions of early infancy.

The child depicted in *Some Thoughts Concerning Education* is a being with natural desires for liberty and 'dominion', but capable, with enlightened guidance, of achieving rational control over these without too much difficulty. There is no privileging of religion and little overt concern with morality, sin, or the fate of the soul. It is taken as read that Reason encompasses morality – the processes of socialization and subordination to Reason are, we may assume, identical. Under Locke's scheme the privately educated gentlemen of the Enlightenment would honestly and rationally manage society – a role that is both their birthright and their duty. Though it is not a textbook of 'Developmental Psychology', *Some Thoughts Concerning Education* marks an important step towards rendering childhood an object of rational enquiry. But not until the end of the eighteenth century were further significant moves made in this direction.

(b) Jean Jacques Rousseau

The image of childhood conveyed by Rousseau's educational classic *Emile* (1762) was, unlike Locke's, a radical assault on conventional wisdom. The format used is fictionalized narrative rather than philosophical treatise, depicting an idealized account of the form education should take. The traditional reading of Rousseau, more or less since the first publication of Emile, has been that he was concerned with enabling the child to grow 'naturally', uncorrupted by civilization. The fictional tutor, devoted to rearing Emile in idyllic isolation for the first twenty-five years of his life, operates covertly, negatively but humanely, like a gardener removing impediments and subtly directing the natural unfolding of the child's potential. The result is that Emile finally enters society and marriage (to Sophie, his equally ideally reared mate) feeling himself to be a free and unconflicted individual. It has usually been held that Rousseau heralded modern child-centred progressive education, respecting the special character of childhood and the organic nature of its development. Culturally, *Emile* firmly established in European educational thought, later developmental Psychology and even personality theory an image of the child as a unique spiritual being full of potential which it was the pedagogue's vocation to nurture to fruition. In the context of the history of psychological ideas, this is a major move towards the concept of the fully individualized psychological subject. Education is to be about shaping the child's mind – not in the sense of arbitrarily moulding it, but rather in the sense of cultivating its own 'natural' or innate potential to the full. It thus facilitates the growth and maturation of the child's own desires and inclinations, enabling it to be 'free'. The teacher stands behind the child, nudging, suggesting, hinting, distracting, but all in the child's 'best interests'. For W.A.C. Stewart (1972):

> The key idea of the book was the possibility of preserving the original perfect nature of the child by means of the careful control of his education and environment, based upon an analysis of the different physical and psychological stages through which he passed from birth to maturity. (p. 15)

Following its appearance in English in 1762 there was what Stewart (*ibid.*) terms an 'outbreak of Rousseaumania' lasting into the 1790s. Imitative novels appeared, the most successful being *Sandford and Merton* (1783–89) by Thomas Day. *Emile*'s influence on European education has been greater than that of any other single work. So it is that European developmental Psychology's greatest centre this century has been Piaget's long-time academic home, the Institut Rousseau in Geneva.

It is, as observed above, what writers are understood to be saying, rather than what they actually said, which is historically most important. None the less, in the case of Rousseau, Rosenow's reappraisal of *Emile* (1980) is instructive – indeed, rather unsettling. If he is right, the totalitarian aspect of the novel's programme has possibly remained influential in spite of being overlooked, for it is an essential component of Rousseau's vision. Rosenow argues very plausibly that Rousseau's aim is the rearing not of a 'natural', 'free' child, but of one who will uncritically conform to the demands of the 'general will', whose individuality is utterly dissolved, desiring no more than to fulfil their duties as a citizen, acknowledging all egoistic desires as contrary to 'necessity'. The apparently 'progressive' educational techniques involved in achieving this, far from being natural, amount to complete manipulation of the child at every stage, the tutor achieving his (definitely!) ends by cunning and dissembling, ruthlessly controlling the child's mind at every turn under the guise of being a detached friend. How else are we to construe such a passage as this?

> . . . let him [the pupil] always think he is master while you are really master. There is no subjection so complete as that which preserves the form of freedom; it is thus that the will is taken captive . . . No doubt he ought only to do what he wants, but he ought to want to do nothing but what you want him to do. He should never take a step you have not foreseen, nor utter a word you could not foretell. (Rousseau, 1966 edn, pp. 84–5; quoted in Rosenow, 1980, pp. 217–18)

It is not the 'natural man' but the 'perfect citizen' whom Rousseau aims to create – a citizen entirely, unrebelliously subservient to the collective:

> . . . Emile gains one basic advantage, which Rousseau considers worth any price: he is at one with himself and has no conflicts whatsoever. He has no desires. He desires no property, since he has learned that property subjugates and that ownership implies dependence. He does not desire to be honoured and respected, since he knows this implies his subjugation to public opinion. He does not desire power, since he knows that it means dependence on his subjects. Emile has no ambitions whatsoever, he does not want to reform the social order, and he has no wish to improve or educate men: he accepts reality as it is. 'I only desire what is and I should never fight against fate,' concludes Emile in his summarising speech. (Rosenow, *ibid.*, pp. 219–20)

Far from being 'individuated', Emile has become a mere cipher, and instead of *Emile* being a radical plea for 'freedom', 'freedom' has been become synonymous with total self-alienation. For Rosenow, *Emile* is the first and most thoroughgoing distopia, distant ancestor of Aldous Huxley's *Brave New World* and George Orwell's *Nineteen Eighty-Four*. But even more closely, he observes, it anticipates – albeit from a very different theoretical direction – B.F. Skinner's *Walden Two*. Not only is the status of *Emile* as a manifesto for child-centred learning and free education ironic: 'The question is, whether we have not adopted, unaware, together with Rousseau's principles, both the interpretation he has given them and the use he has made of them. If this is indeed the case, then the irony is a twofold one and Rousseau's cunning triumphs over us too' (Rosenow, *ibid.*, p. 223).

In the event, sunnier readings of *Emile* prevailed, and English educational writers such as the Edgeworths and Elizabeth Hamilton, as well as continental reformers like Rousseau's fellow countryman Pestalozzi, are usually lavish with their praise, taking issue only with details. But given that some of them, especially after the French Revolution, were actually engaged in trying, via education, to control and manage a potentially rebellious labouring class, Rousseau's – to us – totalitarian tendencies would have been a recommendation, especially since they were packageable as humanitarian. Opinions of Rousseau, however, were divided, with Hannah More[23] ('From Liberty, Equality and the Rights of Man, Good Lord deliver us!') and John Wesley among anti-Rousseau crusaders, believing in the child's original wickedness and the need to break its will (Stewart, 1972). Such evangelical opponents aside, a wide range of writers found Rousseau's thought congenial, and this should at least give us pause for thought before we assume that his educational message was universally read as radically libertarian. At any rate, given such passages as that quoted above, which are hardly ambiguous in their message, we are left with the condundrum of why Rousseau's historical image has been socially constructed as it has – as benign advocate of the rights of childhood and pioneer of enlightened pedagogy.

(c) Thomas Sheridan

I now – somewhat quirkily – devote a few pages to a man (alluded to in Chapter 2) who was of relatively little historical importance (in terms of influence) but, I suggest, of underestimated significance. Irish-born actor, theatre manager, lecturer, teacher of elocution and dictionary compiler, Thomas Sheridan (1719–88) was a familiar figure in mid-century London and Dublin society, though less well known to posterity than his playwright son Richard Brinsley Sheridan. Samuel Johnson, having fallen out with him, told Boswell: 'Why, sir, Sherry is dull, naturally dull, but it must have taken him a great deal of pains to become what we now see him. Such an excess of stupidity is not in nature.' His life, though, certainly wasn't dull, but we cannot go into that here. His thespian background none the less provides the key to his diagnosis of Britain's ills, expounded in *British Education: or the Source of the Disorders of Great Britain* (1756, repr. 1769).

He opens with polemics against the 'irreligion, immorality, and corruption' of the times, and the neglect of education to which this is due:

> Important as it is to the state, education hath never once claimed the attention of the legislature since its first institution. . . . [N]o one topic has less employed the pens of our writers. . . . We have in our whole language but two treatises [i.e. an essay by Milton and Locke's *Some Thoughts* . . .] of any note expressly written on that subject. (1769 edn, p. 11)

The aim of gentlemanly education is 'to make them good men' who can serve their society, 'to shape their talents, in such a way, as will render them most serviceable to the support of that government, under which they were born' (p. 13). To this end, the present education system is useless. His paean of praise to the role of gentleman is worth quoting here; it is:

> . . . to animate and give motion to the whole body of the people; to be an example and model to all; the fountain of manners and source of principles . . . (p. 25)

Sheridan is soon into a lengthy critique of the applicability to Britain of Montesquieu's analysis of the principles of the different known forms of government. Montesquieu had identified these as follows: Republicanism is based on Virtue, Monarchism on Honour and Despotism on Fear. But in applying this to Britain, 'he has not' says Sheridan, 'made use of that clearness and precision which appear so evidently in the rest of his work' (p. 37). Britain, it transpires, is a happy blend of all three types, and a superordinate principle must be found to integrate and control the interplay of Montesquieu's triad without letting any one of them dominate. This 'can be no other than Religion' (p. 41) – a conclusion Sheridan feels Montesquieu suppressed for fear of being seen to support reformed religion.

So far so good, but here the second-best tragedian to Garrick (according to the *DNB* entry) unveils the real reason for the decline in religion, education and British culture as a whole – the neglect of Oratory. Oratory is 'the basis of our constitution, and pillar of our state' (p. 52) as well as the primary instrument of religion. What ensues is a 450-odd-page-long sermon on the character and condition of the English language, comparisons with Latin being made constantly. Sheridan's aspiration is to render English the third and finest classical language, and without Oratory this cannot be achieved.

Written English had, in the seventeenth century, gone from being a transcription of oral speech into an essentially separate medium, adapted to philosophical and Natural Philosophical discourse. Hobbes's and Wilkins's antipathy to figurative language was in part a rejection precisely of the kind of rhetoric which rendered spoken oratory powerful. Sheridan sees this clearly; the clergy have abandoned the weapon of rhetoric for logic and come off – not surprisingly – the worse:

> By this method, our divines have not only changed their celestial armour made by God himself, of proof against all human force, for such as was made by the weak hands of imperfect man; their weapons tempered in pure aetherial fire, for those of brittle steel; they have also swerved from the example, and deserted the method pointed out by their great founder. It was by preaching, not writing, that our blessed Saviour propagated his doctrines. . . . It was the gift of the tongues, not of the pen, which was miraculously bestowed on the apostles.. (pp. 87–8)

Only Oratory is an instrument of sufficient force and 'sufficient dignity' to support religion (p. 89). The perfection of both Greek and Latin was founded on Oratory, and their slow degeneration began with its decline. Education must turn from being centred on the classics and focus instead on the cultivation and study of English. In particular, our priority must be to systematize and order a national tongue:

> which like our commons is suffered to lie desolate, uncultivated and waste, to the great prejudice, in point of wealth, as well as ornament, of this fair island. (p. 205)

Potentially English is better than all other languages put together. The metaphor shifts slightly and soon Sheridan is saying:

> . . . the soil is now so luxuriant that it requires more than ordinary

> cultivation and tillage, in order to produce useful and profitable crops, instead of being over-run with gawdy flowers and noxious weeds. (p. 209)

Instead of attending to this:

> How many excellent scholars, now pining in want, make no other use of their Latin, but to lament in Virgilian strains, that ever they were acquainted with Virgil, or knew any other but their mother tongue? (pp. 210–11)

Sheridan's vision is of English as a language out of control – a tongue running riot, and in so doing sapping clarity of thought and burying his contemporaries under a rising heap of literary trash. If 'correct style' became necessary for the success of books, an 'army' of writers would be released to 'become useful members of society by carrying muskets against the enemies of their country' (p. 216). English must be pruned and brought into order, like French. The written must again be rendered subject to the spoken word, stabilized by the standards of Oratory and rhetoric, in terms of both pronunciation (he despairs of the variety of dialects) and grammar. The 'Disorders of Great Britain' boil down, it seems, to logorrhoea, and the cure is to make Oratory and English the gentleman's core curriculum. The maze of philosophical systems will disperse, scepticism will evaporate, suicide rates will fall (he believes them to be higher in England than anywhere else: p. 500), poets will, he hopes, abandon the barbaric Teutonic device of rhyme[24], and Great Britain will bequeath to the world a tongue finer than Latin, not least because, unlike Latin, its oratorical roots will lie in the holier soils of Christian faith – future English rhetoric will, we infer, be divinely inspired. Curiously Sheridan's other shorter work on education, *A Plan of Education for the Young Nobility and Gentry of Great Britain* (1769), while reiterating the need to 'methodize' English, proposes a more down-to-earth scheme of vocational training with six streams (for those 'born to be' legislators, in Holy Orders or Doctors of Physic, lawyers, military, in 'civil employments or the mercantile profession' and those of 'independent fortunes'). Like Locke, to whom he generally defers, he is against both corporal punishment and music.

Why spend so much time on Sheridan's forgotten manifesto? First because, although he so often gets the wrong end of the stick, his diagnosis of the linguistic situation is in many respects quite acute – for example, he penetratingly sees certain kinds of recent linguistic change as a major culprit in the declining fortunes of religion. Ironically, his complaints echo those of Hobbes and Wilkins, who also see in unruly language a curable source of controversy, slipshod thinking and public confusion. But their cure is Sheridan's disease. The Sheridan position is a mirror-image of the Hobbes/Wilkins one, and he is not – to be fair – their inferior in his expertise on the nature and significance of language as a social institution. He has a quite complex model of the interaction between the spoken and the written, of the sources of linguistic stability, and of the powerfully pervasive, diverse roles of language in social life. He torpedoes himself principally on two main counts: first, a narrowness of vision which cannot get beyond seeing Latin as an ideal – thus the highest destiny he can envisage for English is to surpass Latin; secondly, a temperamental antipathy (characteristic of the age) to seeming disorder and disharmony. He sees language as floundering in a distressing state of anarchy, and can discern in this nothing creative. He wants to stop the language, to tame it, to 'methodize' it and thereby, he thinks, bring concord where discord reigns, especially in matters of philosophy and religion.

Secondly, Sheridan's return to rhetoric and oratory marks a clear, if ill-fated, move back towards a creative literary view of language consistent with active PL generation, though of course I am not claiming that he was actually concerned with this issue. As part of the 'Literary school' identified in Chapter 2, his inhibitions on this would be the same as theirs. It is no coincidence that his intellectual heroes include his father's friend Swift[25], a great mocker of Natural Philosophy and the Wilkins account of language, and Milton, most Latinate of English poets.

Finally, at the more mundane level, Sheridan is indeed very concerned with education, and clamouring for State involvement. Although he rests for the most part on Locke as far as 'Educational Psychology' goes, he clearly envisages a professional role for the educational expert beyond anything Locke proposed. Education should be vocational, it should be officially managed, it should be humanely operated. Since this aspect of his thinking is outweighed by his forgotten linguistic obsessions, his reputation as an educational reformer is now marginal. Nevertheless, it is at least a hypothesis worth raising that he was among the first since Comenius and Hartlib fully to grasp the centrality of education for modern society in practical, as opposed to Romantic Rousseauesque, terms. And this need provided of course, in time, a major base for Psychology's disciplinary emergence. Nobody could pretend that Sheridan's impact approached that of Rousseau. Rousseau's legacy, whatever ambiguities may now come to light, was a radically revised image of childhood as a psychological phase, an image which spread across Europe and played a major part in determining Educational Psychology's agenda. Accounts of this are legion however, while Thomas Sheridan has long been in eclipse.

(d) Richard Lovell and Maria Edgeworth

The Edgeworths' compendious *Practical Education* (1798) comprises an exhaustive treatment of all aspects of the education of young children, though it is little concerned with formal schooling. While it is in many respects an expansive gloss on Locke, there is a major difference in tone: the Edgeworths have become preoccupied not only with the child's moral and intellectual maturation but with respectability and genteel decorum, with socializing the child into a set of bourgeois values and behaviours (which for them are hardly distinguishable from moral virtue as such). The child is, for example, to be kept entirely away from servants: 'If children pass one hour in a day with servants, it will be in vain to attempt their education' (p. 126). This is far stronger than anything in Locke, an attempt at rigidly consolidating class divisions:

> Children who are at ease with their parents, and happy in their company, will not seek inferior society; this will be attributed to pride by servants, who will not like them for this reserve. So much the better. (pp. 131–2)

There is also a peculiar humourlessness, a priggish disapproval of levity: 'We should not *even* in jest talk nonsense to children, or suffer them *even* to hear inaccurate language' (p. 140). Parental passion is to be kept firmly under control, on grounds partly of 'propriety' (p. 245). On the other hand, the Edgeworths share Locke's distaste for severe punishment, and their view of the learning process is essentially his:

> The general principle that we should associate pleasure with

> whatever we wish that our pupils should pursue, and pain with whatever we wish they should avoid, forms . . . the basis of our plan of education. (p. 713)

For those seeking anticipations of Child Psychology themes, *Practical Education* is a rich seam. There is an analysis of moral development (pp. 242 ff.), an anecdote about how a small child's irritating singing was stopped by his sister putting him on an 'unsteady board' – 'his attention was occupied, and he forgot his song' (p. 183), and an appendix of observational notes by Honora Edgeworth of the kind which became common later in the following century. She was:

> resolved to write notes from day to day of all the trifling things which mark the progress of the mind in childhood. She was of opinion, that the art of education should be considered as an experimental science, and that many authors of great abilities had mistaken their road by following theory instead of practice. (pp. 733-4)

The passage by Reid on the potential value of studying the development of children quoted above (p. 169) is invoked in support of this enterprise.

As far as Rousseau is concerned, while they believe that he was misled by 'a false idea of the pleasures of liberty' (p. 177), 'whenever Rousseau is in the right, his eloquence is irresistible' (p. 178). Moreover, their goal is not that far from Rousseau's, if we accept Rosenow's reading, for it is the 'enlightened obedience of rational beings' (p. 716).

If the product of Locke's scheme is a sturdily independent-minded, rational yet dutiful gentleman, the Edgeworths' product will be a refined class-conscious conformist, displaying exquisite taste, decorum and an aversion to overt exhibitions of emotion. They could well be obnoxiously pious into the bargain. Maria Edgeworth, like Hannah More, wrote vast numbers of children's books and poems which suffused her value system throughout middle-class Britain. They were a major medium via which the new anti-hedonistic (often Evangelical) voice of domestically based female moral authority was propagated. Those confusing combinations of genuine child-centredness and moral stuffiness, sensitive caring insight and emotional blackmail, worthy moral earnestness and status-consciousness which have characterized the

British middle classes ever since are all there in embryo in the Edgeworths. They are also axes of tension which have underwritten the agendas of Child Psychology on a far wider scale.

(e) Elizabeth Hamilton (1758–1816)

Elizabeth Hamilton's *Letters on the Elementary Principles of Education* (1801) is similar in its message to that of the Edgeworths: again an explicit belief in 'association' as the key to learning and, like Locke, a stress on the importance of early infancy. She is typically opposed to harsh discipline, and 'child-centred' in her approach. For Hamilton, however, the goal of education is more explicitly dominated by religious considerations; in the end it is the fate of the child's soul which takes precedence, and this must not be lost sight of. It is important, therefore, that the associations formed in relation to religion are positive, the Bible must be seen as 'the constant companion of your serious hours, the subject of your daily and delightful meditation', ensuring that:

> they will associate the idea of superior excellence with the bible, before they are able to read. But on the contrary, if they see it only brought out upon a tedious and gloomy Sunday, and then read as a duty and a task, the prepossession that will take place in disfavour of its contents will probably never be eradicated. (vol. I, p. 151)

Class-consciousness is relatively downplayed; she disagrees strongly with the Edgeworths about servants, believing that there is no problem if they are selected carefully, and if the parents themselves live according to genuine Christian principles. 'Miss Edgeworth's' advice, even if practicable (which she doubts), would be 'dangerous to enforce by precept':

> . . . to suffer them to consider servants in the light of noxious animals, whom they must carefully shun, I should apprehend to be injurious. (vol. I, p. 95)

The second volume of the work surveys the cultivation of the 'Intellectual Faculties': perception, attention, conception, judgement, imagination and taste, abstraction and reflection. In structuring the work under these headings, Hamilton is making a further move towards integrating the study of the child with the putative, but as yet primarily philosophical, 'Science of Man' being advocated by the Scots.

The differences in nuance between Hamilton and the Edgeworths are interesting. Hamilton (herself unmarried and childless) is at once more relaxed – less obsessed with censoring everything the child reads, for example – and clearer in her moral goals. Though she is occasionally prone to blur the boundaries between matters of taste and of morality, she does not, like the Edgeworths, treat them as virtually synonymous. She is far more philosophically astute and aware than they are, and her application of Lockean principles is explicit and carefully elaborated. It is revealing that she feels so diffident and apologetic about writing as a woman, with constant references to her 'feeble pen' and extending 'beyond my sphere' – which come across as more honestly felt in her case than similar passages in Hannah More, who milks them for all she is worth.

What Hamilton has done, in effect, is harness Locke and Scottish Enlightenment philosophy alike to the service of a religion-centred education. The philosophers' role has become to provide techniques, or conceptual bases for developing them, rather than acting as metaphysical authorities. While not exactly a Romantic, she is in tune with the contemporary revival in religion, and motivated by the imperatives of faith.

As a woman, Hamilton, like Maria and Honora Edgeworth, Sarah Trimmer, Hannah More and Mary Wollstonecraft, is in a position to evaluate the practical value and accuracy of existing male wisdom regarding childhood and education. In their roles as mothers, governesses and live-in aunts on regular babysitting duty, such women could bring the philosophy of mind to earth in a practical context. Though Locke and Rousseau are the canonical authorities of the period, we must ask how great their practical impact would have been if their views had not been subjected to the more realistically informed evaluation and scrutiny of this group of late-eighteenth-century women writers. Hamilton subsequently became an advocate of Pestalozzi, Rousseau's direct intellectual heir with regard to education but, unlike him, a dedicated working teacher (Hamilton, 1815).

Not least among these writers' concerns, of course, was the education of women, which they had, after all, directly experienced. Their complaints may, perhaps, be summed up in Hannah More's remark that 'moral and intellectual degradation increases in direct proportion to the adoration which is paid to mere external charms' (More, 1799, p. 3); female education was seen as aimed primarily at enhancing marriage chances in an era when the proportion of women remaining single was rising rapidly – as high as 25 percent in the upper classes[26]. To this end, critics felt, their studies concentrated on superficial and frivolous skills at the expense of cultivating their moral and intellectual faculties; thus vanity took precedence too often over virtue: 'false associations . . . annexe ideas of importance to what is trifling and insignificant, and . . . connect ideas of glory with silly admiration of fools and coxcombs' (Hamilton, *Letters*, vol. II, p. 266). Naturally, the voices of these critics vary from the out-and-out feminism of Mary Wollstonecraft and the pious Christianity of Elizabeth Hamilton to Hannah More's insufferable Evangelical fascism. There is a broad consensus among them regarding the nature of the system's shortcomings; it is the place and character of woman herself that is in dispute.

At the heart of education is the child, and it is through concern with education that a new cultural interest in the nature of childhood is aroused. Behind this lie such complex demographic and economic changes as the decline in infant mortality, industrialization requiring a more skilled workforce, the management of the modern bureaucratic State, and the rise of 'companionate' marriage based on affection. Philosophers, too, were coming to see in the study of childhood a potential route to answering some of their own epistemelogical questions. Others (like Rousseau and Sheridan) were viewing education as a key factor in social reform. By 1800 the study of childhood, at least in an educational context, was firmly on the agenda in Britain and across Europe, where Itard's study of Victor, the 'Wild Boy of Aveyron'[27] and the publication of Teten's pioneering treatise on human development (1777) were important proto-Psychological texts. Out of this comes a very important psychological idea: the idea of childhood itself as a distinct phase of life qualitatively different from adulthood, a phase with a dynamic of its own which may be empirically investigated. This child has peculiar needs and interests which the pedagogue and 'preceptor' must understand if education is to succeed.

Rousseau's image of the child as somehow nearer Nature received a more down-to-earth expression in the first section of the Scots doctor John Gregory's popular *A Comparative View of the State and Faculties of Man with those of the Animal World* (1765, 'new edition' 1798). In childhood, instincts are still 'the immediately impelling principles of action' (p. 16). And instincts are not savage: 'Where the voice of Nature and Instinct is clear and explicit, it will be found the surest guide' (p. 20). Gregory's musings lead him to speculate, a century early, on the eugenic possibilities of improving the species by applying animal-breeding principles: '. . . it is amazing that this Observation was never transferred to the Human Species where it would be equally applicable' (p. 21). He vehemently opposes swaddling, assails the 'preposterous management' of ignorant midwives, and praises breastfeeding (which, he appreciates, also inhibits pregnancy). In fact the whole section is a remarkably sensible and tolerant plea on behalf of childhood. He observes: 'The faculties of the mind disclose themselves in a certain regular succession' (p. 73). Childhood is 'that period of life where Instinct is the only active principle of our Nature, and consequently where the analogy between us and other Animals will be found most compleat' (p. 79). Gregory, Reid's cousin, Professor of Medicine at Edinburgh, friend of Hume, Monboddo *et al.*, can reasonably be taken as voicing here the mainstream Scottish Enlightenment concept of childhood. As the century drew to a close, this view of 'childhood as natural' could easily be infused with Romantic or Blakeian images of childhood innocence.

From this, a new, intense adult awareness of the presence of the child, this vehicle of Nature, creates a new social relationship – the adult–child relationship – which the adult may explore and cultivate. In so doing the adult is drawn back to his or her own childhood; in the adult's 'entering into the child's mind', the child's mind, conversely, enters the adult's. There is now an arena of respite from the demands of adult society, a legitimate field for the adult's own play and fancy in which childhood becomes a lost Arcadia, the innocent opposite of the 'real', vicious, adult world. Expressions of this can be as sublime as Blake's or as trite as the flood of sententious moralizing children's books which begins to lap around every middle-class nursery. Adults begin to articulate, under the guise of education, their own idealizations of virtue, heroism, fate, loyalty and parenthood, representing these to children as depictions of the 'real' world. This is a complex and unresearched psychohistorical development, all I wish to stress here is the importance, both psychologically and Psychologically, of the unprecedented reconnection of adult to child within the adult psyche – a reconnection which has only continued to strengthen. The issue of how far the adult is subjectively projecting on to the child, and how far he or she is indeed recovering childhood subjectivity, is a knot I will refrain from striving to untie here.

5
Rethinking Eighteenth-Century Psychology

It would be premature to claim that a clear picture is yet possible of the dynamic interrelationships of the various strands of psychological and proto-Psychological thought we have been examining. What is clear is that the schematic account of this period presented, with only minor variations, in traditional history of Psychology texts is not only far too simple – it is actually wrong, even in its own terms, on several counts. The task of this chapter is to suggest a number of questions and hypotheses which could form the basis for a new research agenda. These may, for convenience, be said to fall into three groups.

First, there are those pertaining to my initial analysis of the linguistic conditions underlying (and, I argued, actually constraining) PL innovation within disciplinary contexts. Secondly, there is the more specific question of the relative roles of Associationist (Anglo-French) and Scottish Enlightenment thinkers as sources of Anglo-American Psychology. Associationists have traditionally been given the honours here, with – until very recently, at least – little notice being given to the Scots. This urgently needs rectifying. (The German situation will be addressed in Chapter 7.) The roles of physiology, educational writings, Social Philosophy, physiognomy and phrenology, and texts on madness, are also in need of evaluation. Thirdly, there is the knotty problem of relating this proto-Psychological work to ongoing psychological change in the culture at large: changing attitudes towards – and concepts of – sex, children, madness, marriage. Ideally this would incorporate the mediating role of literature as a new mass medium articulating and embodying such kinds of psychological change.

This leads directly to the elusive question of the 'Self'; the emergence of the notion of the individual psyche, self, mind, or 'moral domain' (in Nikolas Rose's terms [1987]) as an object of enquiry. There is, as already noted, a current consensus that Western individuality underwent some deep change during the eighteenth century (though it began in the previous one). If so, then how does its alleged 'self-contained', 'possessive' character square with the end-of-the-century upsurge of humanitarianism, and post-French Revolutionary moral backlash on which the Victorian mentality was ultimately founded (*and* the complex interrelationships between these two)? These three will be discussed in turn, but we must begin on a more negative note by pulling together the case for the absence of a clear precursor to Psychology in the eighteenth century.

1 The Eighteenth Century without Psychology

That Psychology had more than one source of origin before the mid nineteenth century is obvious. Even so, articulations of this generally take the form of an identification of one or two major 'taproots' which account, so to speak, for most of the variance. Philosophy, or philosophy plus physiology, are the usual candidates. It is this which, in Britain's case at least, is at issue here. The first and most patent difficulty is that the category 'Philosophy' does not possess the unitary character ascribed to it. The Scottish Enlightenment tradition is not only distinct, philosophically, from the English one, but itself comprises a variety of types of enquiry, including proto-anthropological and proto-sociological researches inspired by the Natural History paradigm and drawing, too, on continental writers such as Montesquieu, Buffon and Rousseau. (This will be discussed further in Section 3.) Secondly, it ignores the possibly crucial roles of such diverse writers as the turn-of-the-century female educationists and the linguist Horne Tooke in changing and refocusing philosophical debates in a more 'Psychological' direction. As far as the physiology side of the equation is concerned the situation was similarly lacking in overall coherence; Hartley (who usually stars) and Whytt have little in common and the latter, not (as is usually implied) the former, was the more influential in advancing the cause of psychophysiology (while neither relates clearly to Gall's physiological input via phrenology). The most immediately 'Psychological' inferences from physiology are found in proto-psychiatric texts, phrenology and Mesmerism. Far from being monopolized by one or two 'taproot' disciplines, the kinds of issue with which Psychology is now concerned prove, if they are present at all, to be scattered across a whole range of textual genres – some, indeed, concerned with philosophy (from several different perspectives) and physiology, but others with anthropology, sociology, economics, linguistics, education, madness, sexual medicine, physiognomy, ethics, literary criticism and aesthetics, theology and politics. Nor are such genres always distinct among themselves. Even so, there are absences; where in eighteenth-century Britain are the disciplinary forebears of comparative Psychology and ethology (apart from a few pages in John Gregory, though French natural historians had more to say), or of counselling, psychophysics, psychometrics of any kind (Hutcheson?), and modern research on memory? Perchance anticipatory works on such topics will turn up – absence of evidence is not evidence of absence – but if they do, they will not be found in the well surveyed mainstreams of Associationist Philosophy or physiology. The interesting question now becomes: If there was no Psychology, then why not? The aspiration to create a Science of Mind or of Man was constantly being voiced. It is on this that the linguistic situation promises to shed some light.

2 The Language Question

In Chapter 2 I argued that none of the quite numerous accounts of the nature of language offered during the century was compatible with the generation of new psychological ideas within a disciplinary framework. This is not to say that the century was devoid of new PL – quite the contrary – but this rarely, if ever, came as the result of a 'Psychological' enquiry. One exception might be Hartley's 'vibratiuncles', but it is doubtful if anyone has ever used the term outside discussions of Hartley. It certainly never caught on, and not solely for aesthetic reasons; it simply failed to come to signify anything anyone was actually experiencing because Hartley provided no route for enabling it to do so[1]. Only in 1810 did Dugald Stewart finally appreciate the situation, and even then he was unable to follow his insights through.

The upshot was that aspirants towards a Science of the Mind tended, putting it simply, to adopt one of two strategies: they took either a materialist reductionist tack, seeking to dissolve the psychological into the physical, or a Natural History tack, which sought to systematize the existing folk-psychological vocabulary. Not that the process by which PL was generated was unrecognized

– everyone from Locke onwards sees that 'concrete' terms are the basis for 'abstract' and 'moral' ones. What eludes them is the ontological problem thereby raised for the status of the latter's referents; they cannot escape the notion that the vast received folk-psychological vocabulary refers to some pre-existing, fixed, and probably universal categories of psychological phenomena. They are not uncritical of this conceptual repertoire, of course – hence the urge to systematize and clarify it – but they cannot significantly add to it. They can see that it is often muddled and misleading, and different schools of thought frequently accuse their opponents of falling into just such errors, but they remain essentially content with the language itself.

Before leaving this, a qualifying digression is called for. Although I have argued that it was via physiology that the new natural sciences affected psychological ideas, there is a partial exception to which attention should be drawn. Approaching the issue from what might be termed a rather 'orthogonal' position, the Australian historian Jamie Kassler published a paper in 1984 with the enticing title 'Man a Musical Instrument: Models of the Brain and Mental Functioning before the Computer'. Although it is only partially concerned with events falling within our current period of concern this elicits the presence of a powerful leitmotiv in physiological and philosophical thought from the seventeenth century onwards in which analogies with musical instruments are deployed as models of psychological and psychoneurological processes (e.g. Diderot's '*clavecin sensible*'). Instruments so chosen vary from organs to violins and flutes. In some ways this is a subvariety of Cartesian mechanical models, but it has its own distinctive features. While such phenomena as vibrating strings and air columns may be used in a fairly orthodox way to represent mechanical principles, the situation is made more complex by drawing attention to such things as fingering and the player–instrument relationship itself. If the body is a machine like a musical instrument, who or what is playing it?

Diderot affected a circumvention of this question by making the '*clavecin sensible*' a self-playing instrument, but as Moriarty (1987) shows this negates the very coherence of the metaphor. Such mechanistic models thus point beyond pure La Mettrie-type mechanism to the need for a superordinate level of agency and control. While musical instrument imagery rarely dominates a text, and thus appears relatively unremarkable in any specific instance – a conventional literary device – the ubiquity, persistence and variety of such analogies disclose the covert power and richness of the metaphor. While musical instruments are not exactly products of science, they were certainly, by this time, in a more technically complex category than the fountain or even the windmill; their production increasingly required mathematical knowledge of harmonic principles and a specialist grasp of some basic physics. Nevertheless, although the musical instrument provided a valuable body of metaphors and schemata for physiologists and philosophers alike, it never served as a basis for an explicit Psychological theory as opposed to being a ready source of apt analogies. Nor – apart, perhaps, from reinforcing the constant invocations (hardly new) of 'harmony' in every sphere from politics to physiognomy – is there an immediately obvious linguistic impact on PL vocabulary[2].

To return to the main issue: the irony is that when Psychology eventually emerged, it was not because this linguistic problem was solved but because the original insights into the nature of PL generation were simply forgotten or ignored. The assumption that PL categories referred to something 'real' and pre-existing the PL used to refer to them was retained. None the less, PL generation itself was disinhibited and proceeded within a 'scientific' disciplinary framework by reflexively applying new concepts from the physical sciences as schemata for construing the new psychological phenomena which its active experimental (or at least empirical) researches created. If the preceding analysis is correct, then, it also illuminates why previous historians of Psychology have overlooked it, for to admit it would be to raise deep problems about the scientific status of the discipline – the very thing they are generally motivated to celebrate.

This argument is surely one issue which should inform the future research agenda. Its fuller evaluation would involve, among other things, a deeper investigation of the differences between the Materialist Sensationalist view of language derived from Locke and the view of it held, in particular, by Scottish Enlightenment thinkers. The development of the latter from Reid to Stewart appears to mark a significant move towards a more modern pragmatic understanding, while the former heads ever more deeply into a reductionist materalist mode. This has further implications for events in the decades from around 1820 to 1860. Further elucidation of the nature and impact of Romantic linguistics (not least Coleridge's) and its relationships with the other approaches is also needed. Finally, the issues raised at the end of Chapter 2 concerning the role of linguistic thought and discourse in the rise of the new individuality identified by many current writers should be explored.

3 Associationism, Common Sense and Neurophysiology

Of the many questionable features of the received account, a most striking one is, as we have seen, the relative neglect of both Scottish Enlightenment thinkers and – albeit to a lesser degree – neurophysiology. Besides the 'taproot' discipline of philosophy the Scottish Enlightenment contribution extends to several other genres which warrant consideration: the various histories of human, or 'Civil', society which (along with the equally neglected continental '*anthropologie*' tradition) constitute founding texts for anthropology and sociology, Monboddo's work on language, the neurology of Robert Whytt, and numerous works on aesthetics, education and ethics. As long ago as 1945 Gladys Bryson observed, regarding the Scottish school:

> We shall not be guilty, then, of a false perspective in looking to them for knowledge of the eighteenth century's best efforts toward a science of man.. (1968 edn, p. 2)

The extent of this downplaying is apparent if we consider the relative coverage given to English and Irish Associationists (Locke, Hutcheson, Berkeley, Hartley, Priestley, James Mill, John Stuart Mill) and Scottish Enlightenment thinkers (Hume, Reid, Stewart, Kames, Monboddo, Ferguson, John Gregory, Adam Smith, Whytt) in general History of Psychology texts (see Table 6.1). David Hume is the rule-proving exception; if anyone is a Scottish Enlightenment thinker it is he, and he ranks second only to Locke in terms of coverage. The reason is, of course, that Hume is the arch-associationist, the only one in the Scottish camp.

It may be protested that – Hume aside – the Scots simply do not compare in eminence or philosophical calibre with those on the other side. But eminence and philosophical calibre as such are not the only criteria relevant to assessing the nature and importance of a thinker's role in the historical development of a corpus of ideas, a mode of discourse or a disciplinary tradition. (There is also the question-begging nature of the protest – how do we know that they are not of the same eminence and calibre? Because, in part anyway, they are not covered in the texts.) Nor is it only the Scots who are excluded, but early anti-Lockeans too, such as Broughton and Peter Browne.

The omission becomes more curious when we examine what these respective camps were actually writing about, and how far it resembled contemporary Psychological concerns. It would indeed be possible to make out a case for the weightings being the very reverse. Such an argument could claim that regardless of their philosophical greatness, from Psychology's point of view the Associationists remained sidetracked in the rather futile quest of trying to figure out how atomistic sensations can be cobbled together into what we actually experience, running round in circles juggling with a handful of basic concepts such as Idea, Sensation, Impression, and the like. With these, plus a Pleasure and Pain principle to serve the motivational side, they seek to account for the entire range of psychological phenomena. Isn't it all a bit like trying to whistle the Ring Cycle? Berkeley, the critic might claim, drifts off into mystic reverie, Hume terrifies the life out of himself and switches to writing history, and Hartley is, to be honest, a historical curiosity with no direct legacy. By contrast, in the Scottish school we find writers sensibly refusing to be drawn into metaphysical abstractions but diligently surveying the whole spectrum of the human mind's powers, passions and faculties, both active and passive: this invariably entails attempts to review the realms of social behaviour and the basis of morality, and often extends even more widely into the very nature of human society and humans as social animals. In the process they are continually throwing off ideas about such things as the desirability of studying child development (Reid, Gregory), the pragmatic character of language (Reid and Stewart), education (Kames), social psychology (Smith)[3] or the significance of individual differences (Smith again), which sometimes directly stimulated further empirical research, but in any case really did anticipate modern Psychological concerns. The Associationist tradition, however, played a rather minor part in founding Psychology (though this is masked by casting Bain erroneously as exclusively Associationist). The origins of modern Psychology in Britain are surely, such an argument would run, to be

Table 6.1 Coverage of British Associationist and Scottish Enlightenment Writers in Sixteen General Histories of Psychology

	R	MK	EGB	Lhy	Shlz	Blwn	Ba	Bb	Brn	GM	RIW	Wert	Kln	LH	DNR	MS	*Total*
a. English Associationists																	
Locke	12	18	43	14	7	9	15	59	23	13	23	7	85	21	66	10	425
Berkeley	6	5	23	13	6	4	7	13	10	7	16	6	76	4	30	8	234
Hartley	1	23	18	6	3	1	9	22	9	23	9	3	39	6	14	8	194
Bentham	0	6	3	5	1	1	0	0	2	5	1	1	3	1	16	0	45
Mill, J.	3	11	25	5	3	1	3	16	20	7	8	3	33	3	8	10	160
																	1058
b. Scottish Associationists																	
Hume	10	6	18	25	5	11	7	44	15	3	13	8	85	11	63	6	330
Brown T.	7	16	3	3	0	1	2	7	9	15	7	1	38	1	4	6	120
Hutcheson	0	0	0	1	0	1	2	1	0	0	0	0	6	0	3	0	14
																	464
c. Other Scottish Enlightenment writers																	
Reid	3	7	11	16	0	1	4	11	8	6	2	1	40	5	15	5	135
Stewart	1	0	9	6	0	1	2	5	0	0	2	1	22	2	5	2	59
Hamilton W.	3	8	1	0	0	2	4	12	0	5	0	1	14	2	1	1	54
Fergusson	0	0	0	0	0	0	1	0	0	0	0	0	0	0	0	0	1
Whytt	0	0	6	0	1	0	1	1	0	0	0	2	0	1	0	0	12
Smith, A.	0	4	1	1	0	1	1	1	0	1	0	0	5	2	3	0	20
Kames (Home)	0	0	0	0	0	1	0	0	0	0	0	0	0	0	0	0	1
Monboddo	0	0	0	0	0	0	0	0	0	0	0	0	0	1	0	0	1
Gregory	0	0	0	0	0	0	0	0	0	0	1	0	0	0	0	0	1
																	284

Summary	[no]	[%]
English Associationists	1058	58.6%
Scottish Associationists	464	25.7%
Total Associationist	**1522**	**84.3%**
Other Scot. Enlightenment	284	15.7%
Total	**1806**	**100.0%**

Figures refer to number of pages entered in index. Where an index differentiates passing, footnote and/or bibliographic mentions from principal textual discussions these have been omitted.

Sources abbreviated as follows:

MK	Murphy & Kovach (1972)	EGB	Boring, E.G. (1950)
Lhy	Leahey, T.H. (1987)	Blwn	Baldwin, J.M. (n.d.)
Ba	Brett, G.S. Vols 2.&3. (1921)	Bb	Brett's History of Psychology ed. R.S. Peters (1953)
Brn	Brennan, J.F. (1982)	R.	Roback, A.A. (1964)
Kln	Klein, D.B. (1970)	LH	Hearnshaw, L. (1987)
GM	Murphy, G. (1932)	Wert	Wertheimer, M. 1979)
RIW	Watson, R.I. (1968)	Shlz	Schultz, D. (1975)
DNR	Robinson, D.N. (1981)	MS	Misiak & Sexton (1966)

found mainly in works such as Smith's *Theory of Moral Sentiments*, John Gregory's *A Comparative View of the State and Faculties of Man with those of the Animal World*, Lord Kames's *Sketches of the History of Man*, and the philosophical writings of Reid and Stewart. While conceding that Hume and Berkeley were great philosophers, their Psychological legacy was, the argument would conclude, far less significant.

Though plausible, this simple reversal of the pecking order is not a particularly fruitful move. Locke's role, from whatever perspective, was absolutely crucial, and both Berkeley and Hume remain indisputably central in shifting the terms of reflexive discourse. The more important question is how serious the effects of the omission of the Scots have been on the historiography of Psychology, and why this omission occurred.

Addressing this, we see that the picture has been distorted in the direction of portraying Psychology's origins as resting far more firmly within the 'positivist', reductionist, 'materialist' tradition of thought than they in fact did. Even in evaluating Hume, it is his supposed 'adaptationism' and discernible positivist tendencies which are focused on, not the phenomenological 'confession' which comprises the first Book of the *Treatise*. Due recognition to the Scottish thinkers would involve an admission of the centrality to the story of their more humanistic and phenomenological concerns. A particular stumbling block is that the Scottish writers were fundamentally concerned with morality – they are, after all, usually labelled *Moral* Philosophers[4] – and this concern underpins most of their wide-ranging agenda. Their goal, from Hutcheson onwards, was to provide a natural foundation for morality in an era when religious diktat alone no longer sufficed. But since positivist science classically aimed at a value-free objectivity, such moral goals were tackled more peripherally. It would be rhetorically *inconvenient* at best, therefore, to locate the origins of a would-be positivist Psychology in eighteenth-century Scottish Moral Philosophy[5]. The Moral Philosophical dimension to Scottish proto-psychological thought continues, as we will see later, down to George Combe's *Constitution of Man* (1828), which remains similarly marginalized by disciplinary historians, and for much the same reasons.

In the event, the founding of Psychology involved the fusion of both approaches (plus some others), not the simple metamorphosis of Associationism. The late-nineteenth-century and early-twentieth-century positivist shift in Psychology was, it could be argued, a result (at least in internalist terms) of three new and major factors: the massive increase in physiological knowledge, the influence of Wundtian experimental psychophysics erroneously construed as a German version of Associationism, and the Darwinian evolutionary perspective – although the last was more ambiguous in its effect. If this is true, then the hiatus between Psychology's eighteenth-century prehistory and its history looks far greater than the orthodox story concedes, and the direct influence of *any* of the philosophers discussed so far appears fairly minimal. In order to salvage a role for the eighteenth century we would have to examine far more closely how eighteenth-century philosophical thought was mediated via transitional forms of discourse which did genuinely feed directly into mid-nineteenth-century Psychology. Three candidates immediately offer themselves: (a) educational writings which drew eclectically on philosophical thought of all kinds; (b) physiognomy and phrenology, the latter of which came to incorporate the Faculty Psychologies of Reid and Stewart and via Combe's *Constitution of Man* also contributed to the advance of evolutionary thought; and (c) proto-psychiatry. There may well be others.

Turning to neurophysiology: Danziger's thesis suggests a key role for the Scottish physiologist Whytt in creating a conceptual framework for a 'neuropsychology' freed from metaphysical issues, while phrenology also played a major role in determining the nature of subsequent 'functionalist' neuropsychological research on the brain, as even Gall's opponent Flourens readily acknowledged[6]. The importance of physiological thought for British Psychology is fully recognized by Hearnshaw (1964) and Danziger (1982)[7], but the eighteenth-century background was outside Hearnshaw's agenda (which began at 1840). Whytt and Sir Charles Bell, whose researches revolutionized neurophysiology and whose work on emotional expression influenced Darwin, also happen to be representatives of the Scottish school. The orthodox approach is to leapfrog over the eighteenth century to Descartes and Hobbes, blind to the fact that it was a *rejection* of Cartesian mechanism, not its acceptance, which liberated neurophysiological thought – again, then, distorting the story in favour of a particular reductionist theoretical position. (These errors may be understood as resulting from those factors identified in the critique of orthodox histories of Psychology given in the Introduction, which need not be rehearsed again.) Further investigation by historians of Psychology of the period from around 1770 to the 1840s is now required if the process by which Psychological discourse emerged is to be clarified.

4 Contextual Issues and the Self

The eighteenth century saw major changes at the psychological level, affecting virtually all educated people. Such changes were associated with a variety of economic, political and demographic shifts in British and French social life. The articulation and expression of this new psychological climate required new kinds of psychological discourse. Rose (1987) has described the creation of the 'moral subject' and identifies, in the management crisis affecting such problem areas as madness, subnormality and education, the immediate context for Psychology's disciplinary debut. The broader notion of a new mode of individuality arising in the eighteenth century is shared by other contemporary writers, particularly aficionados of Foucault (see above, p. 132), but dates back to the classic sociological work of Weber, the political theorist C.B. Macpherson (on whom John Shotter draws for his concept of 'possessive individualism'), Norbert Elias (1978, [1939]) and Zevedei Barbu's (1960) psychological history.

There were also, however, a number of other factors present which we have touched on in the preceding pages. First, and most abstract, among these appears to be the issue of the individual 'Self', already adumbrated in the genre of 'private' writings discussed in Chapter 1, and continued by diarists such as Boswell. This takes a variety of forms: Hume's metaphysical anxiety about personal identity, the Scottish Social Philosophers' frequent analyses of social relationships (e.g. in Adam Smith's *Theory of Moral Sentiments*), which sometimes verge on Goffman-like concerns with the 'presentation of self in everyday life', and the kinds of spiritual striving and anxiety found in Romantic writers like Lavater and Blake as well as in educational concerns with the child as a 'moral subject'. This self-conscious individualism has complex roots: the demise of comfortable elaborated religious frameworks for construing the self, new urban social roles associated with the Industrial Revolution and rapidly developing capitalist modes of socioeconomic organization, an enlarged, relatively prosperous bourgeois class with time on their hands and brains, a new cosmological picture in which the position of 'Man' had become genuinely problematic[8], and, at a different level, a kind of continuous snowball effect exerted by texts articulating these concerns on successive cohorts of reader/writers. Not least among these texts were novels. This problem of the 'Self' is, as we will see, a factor in the successes of (a) physiognomy and phrenology, which concern the subject's 'character' rather than the traditional concern with 'fortune'; and (b) the 'Moral Therapy' approach to madness (as well as the appeal of popular psychotherapeutic cults like Mesmerism and James Graham's sex therapy). The characterizations of the new individuality given by Edward E. Sampson (1990) and John Shotter (1990) tend to be very negative – a vital dimension of social connectedness has been severed, people become fragmented, 'disembodied nomads', defined by their separateness from others (Sampson, p. 120); the 'possessive individual' 'owes nothing to society', 'owns himself', is not a 'moral whole'[9]. Rose is generally more ambivalent, as am I.

The reverse of the Self, its 'counter-term', is the Other, and a heightened humanitarianism, foreshadowed by the central notion of a natural principle of 'sympathy' in Scottish Enlightenment social thought, is a marked feature of British life at the turn of the century, providing a rationale for the kind of exercises in the 'management of individuality' which Rose discusses. Again, cultural factors ranging from the novel to the recrudescence of Evangelical Christianity and a growing number of affluent middle-class women seeking a meaningful outlet for their energies in charitable works can be invoked as fuelling this. Educational thought and Moral Therapy are the most obvious fields of proto-Psychology to benefit. Changed concepts of both Self and Other are obviously implicated in the new political rhetorics of equality and liberty, which, while wholeheartedly espoused by relatively few, nevertheless pervaded political thought much as Green ideas have done in the late 1980s and early 1990s. The psychologically autonomous citizen replaces the loyal subject defined by their place in a 'natural' social hierarchy. Criminals, the insane, the idiot, oppressed paupers, impoverished labourers, the child, now become objects of more general concern as being both fellow humans, brothers and sisters, and potential threats (children excepted) to a social order comprised of honest, free and equal citizens. But this can be only a partial explanation, and in Britain, as we have seen, a multitude of pressures were working in the same general direction – more so, perhaps, than in France.

While it is always possible to be cynical about humanitarianism, especially when retrospective sociological analysis reveals its covert roles in managing power relations, this is a posture of which we must be very wary – it slides too easily into a social version of the 'everybody is selfish' argument. If the new individualism had negative features, or could take negative forms, there were positive features and forms as well. This period sees the appearance not only of the anomic, socially alienated, egoistic, psychologically fragmented 'nomad', but of the humanitarian utopian, the lover of mankind, the social reformer and campaigner. This latter, I would suggest, is equally a product of the new individualism. And how far did this development extend to women? Or were they only additional victims?

The cultural atmosphere changed dramatically in the 1790s as erstwhile radicals recoiled from the post-Revolutionary Reign of Terror and for the first time in a century the British establishment felt itself genuinely threatened. As grim seriousness of purpose replaces permissive urbanity, a new English middle-class mentality emerges from a fusion of Nonconformist religiosity and self-conscious realization of the immense economic power diligently earned over previous decades while their betters caroused. While this is presumably one form which the 'new individualism' took, it presents a constellation of features rather more complex than the traits enumerated by Sampson (1990). It involves, for example, the creation of a new style of psychological expression in which preoccupations with morality and social status merge; there is a seemingly unquestionable belief in the objective moral rectitude of respectable bourgeois life and in the natural (if no longer Divinely ordained) character of existing social structure. This puts some obvious constraints on the actual exercise of humanitarian sentiments (susceptibility to which itself constituted one of the identifying stigmata of membership of this class). Charity is carefully directed at identifiable subgroups of deserving poor and, slavery excepted, no structural reforms of the system itself are sought. The recipient of charity is also to feel a suitable humility and gratitude. This new style of discourse appears to be almost *structurally* hypocritical, deploying an intrinsically complacent vocabulary of terms and expressions which simultaneously celebrate the user's superiority (moral *and* social) and inculcate a deliciously gratifying sense of worthy self-martyrdom.

Armoured with such a set of constructs, one could sustain a heightened sense of self-consciousness whilst remaining impervious to the risks of genuine critical self-scrutiny. The resultant rhetoric of hectoring conservative self-righteousness could be ruthlessly employed to check social unrest – for example Hannah More's attempted brainwashing of the labouring classes through cut-price moral tracts and poems on the spiritual rewards of poverty. Some, of course, saw through this genre of patronizing Evangelicism: William Cobbett claimed that its aim was 'To teach people to starve without making a noise!'. If Psychology begins in a context of human management, a first move is psychologically to justify one's right to manage. Such a discourse certainly does that. It is also a discourse which continues to evolve in sophistication throughout the ensuing century, if not beyond. But does it really reflect quite the mentality which Sampson's and others' epithets describe?

There is a close link, it was suggested, between this nascent anti-hedonism and changes in middle-class domestic life, for life in the new middle-class family served to problematize sexuality in a radical way, rendering it an area of conflict both for males (striving to reconcile lust with loving, companionate, respectable marriage) and females (torn between being infantilized vessels of spiritual ideals and fecund, sexually attractive partners). This particular nexus of psychological stress received little immediate explicit attention beyond the literature of moral exhortation, which only exacerbated the problem. It would be nearly a century before Freud could start trying to address the issue directly. Even so, sexuality does become an increasingly important Psychological and psychiatric topic thereafter, albeit in displaced forms such as medical texts on female diseases and gynaecology, quasi-medical diatribes against masturbation, popular 'advice' manuals on marriage and hygiene, fascination with 'deviance' and a preoccupation in psychiatric and anthropological works with the sexual behaviour of idiots, the insane, and 'primitive people'. Much of this literature circulated covertly, primarily among males, often under the Victorian equivalents of the plain brown wrapper, with red herring titles like *Esoteric Anthropology* (T.L. Nichols, 1873). Even *Aristotle's Masterpiece*[10] continued its closet career (cropping up in Bloom's hands in *Ulysses*). Again, much more research is required to evaluate the persistent presence of sexuality as a Psychological topic from the late eighteenth century to its surfacing a century later in Krafft-Ebing and Freud.

Summary

What we are concerned with here is really the broad question of how Psychology emerged from psychology; how the psychological climate was created in which Psychology itself became a *necessary* mode of reflexive discourse, and how this was mediated. This dimension is rarely even acknowledged at present. What I have tried to indicate at this point is (a) that while Psychology did not exist in the eighteenth century, the evolution of this psychological climate was well under way, certainly by the 1770s; and (b) that proto-Psychological texts were as much expressions and reflections of this as they were its prime movers.

The central psychological idea of 'the psychological' itself still has not really made an entrance on stage (credit for achieving general circulation of the term 'psychology' in Britain largely resting with Coleridge at the beginning of the next century), but by contrast with 1700, in 1800 there are proto-texts aplenty, and these are not confined to Associationist philosophers; *au contraire*, they are scattered across genres as varied as education and physiognomy, neurology and economics, linguistics and psychiatry. If, although in the background for most of these genres, philosophers are still present as sources of concepts and authorities to be invoked, the fact remains that their influence is as much indirect as direct, and in these indirect mediations much is added and altered. It is to these genres that historians of Psychology should now be turning their attention.

As far as identifiable, discrete Psychological ideas are concerned, the main achievement of the century was a systematization and elaboration of what remained essentially an unchanged folk-psychological vocabulary. Neologisms actually originating in 'scientific' discussions of psychological issues remain rare (though plentiful in everyday language). There are certainly some terms which are characteristically Georgian in tone: *sentimentality*, *sensibility, irritability, nervousness, 'powers', faculty, hypochondria, spleen, humane, civilized, condescension, feeling, taste, sublimity, reflection, impression,* while others, such as *conscious(ness), sympathy, feeling* and *abstract(ion),* while not in any way novel, acquire connotations during this period which need to be understood. From the 1790s onwards, many of these figure prominently in the moral rhetoric discussed above. In Reid and Stewart, and even more in phrenology a little later, we do find that in the course of cataloguing there are attempts to create technical sounding synonyms for everyday terms, even reifying them into substantive principles (such as Alimentiveness [love of food], Amativeness [sexual drive] and Philoprogenitiveness [love of children]; see Table 3.1). In retrospect, it is often possible to find writers adopting positions which appear to correspond to those now labelled as, for example, adaptationist, cognitive, evolutionary, hereditarian, top–down or bottom–up, even computational. The truth is, though, that such terms themselves were either nonexistent or differed considerably in sense from their later meanings[11], and that there is invariably little evidence that the current schools of thought so labelled directly owe anything to these apparent precursors. Such anticipations were often, for their authors, quite incidental, their main concerns being quite alien to those of modern Psychologists. There is strong evidence to support the view that over the course of the century a psychological sea change occurred across Europe (well, Britain, France, Germany and the Low Countries at least) regarding the nature of individuality, but how precisely we are to construe this remains debatable. Further consideration will be given to the nature of the emergence and origins of the new individualized mode of consciousness in the final chapter.

Thus ends an unavoidably rather rambling review of the eighteenth century – a review which has, even so, left out much of importance, particularly the role of literature. Sterne's *Tristram Shandy* is an especially regrettable gap. Other British individuals seriously missed (mostly pretty self-contained and autonomous but not all disembodiedly nomadic and none, perhaps, too damagingly fragmented) include Erasmus Darwin, Joseph Priestley, Tom Paine, Mary Wollestonecraft, Edmund Burke, William Godwin and Daniel Defoe. Gaps notwithstanding, I hope I have indicated both the complexity and the scale of the task of satisfactorily unravelling the eighteenth century's role in the history of

Psychology, as well as starting a few hares which others might find it profitable to pursue. While the nature of the task has involved concentrating on the British situation, I have attempted to indicate the major French connections (Germany is reserved for Chapter 7).

6

Reading the Body and Ruling the Mind: The First 'Scientific' Psychologies

In this Chapter I consider three movements of late-eighteenth-century origin which, I believe, have the best claim to being directly ancestral to Psychology as a would-be scientific discipline, distinct in some measure at least, from philosophy or physiology, as it emerged in the mid nineteenth century. Of these the most significant is phrenology, for in the light of Robert M. Young's *Mind, Brain and Adaptation in the Nineteenth Century* (1970) and Roger Cooter's more recent work *The Cultural Meaning of Popular Science: Phrenology and the Organization of Consent in Nineteenth-century Britain* (1984) it is now clear that phrenology played a crucial and direct role in the theoretical thought of Herbert Spencer and Alexander Bain, and that the image of human nature it advocated (highly successfully) met deep-rooted psychological needs in contemporary society.[1] Although the phrenological vision of human nature is long superseded in detail, some of its essential features have arguably underpinned the majority of Psychological theorizing ever since. Physiognomy, often confused with phrenology, was in some senses its polar opposite for reasons which we will be examining. Again, only fairly recent scholarship (e.g. Graeme Tytler's *Physiognomy in the European Novel: Faces and Fortunes* [1982]) enables us to bring it into focus. Mesmerism, the third movement to be discussed, has long been a popular topic for historians, and its place in the discipline's history is perhaps less in need of reappraisal than the places of phrenology and physiognomy. Even so, in the present context a re-examination of certain facets of Mesmerism proves illuminating.

1 Physiognomy and Phrenology

At first glance, Lavater's physiognomy and Gall's phrenology anticipate modern Psychology to a remarkable degree. First, both involved fairly intense empirical research (even eventually, in phrenology's case, quantitative research) on a specific psychological issue – namely, what is now termed 'personality' or 'individual differences'. Secondly, both were practically applied in ways directly comparable to modern Psychology – as bases for individual 'counselling' and evaluation of others in contexts such as suitability for employment. Thirdly, neither was completely assimilable to either philosophy or medicine, thereby signifying the presence of a genuine third realm of the psychological appropriate for 'scientific' enquiry. In the case of phrenology there was also a clearly articulated physiological rationale underpinning the theory, enabling it to present itself as scientific in character. Their cultural roles thus anticipated those later taken by Psychology – to the extent of the emergence in the early nineteenth century of the professional phrenologist/physiognomist, and even an occasional institutional presence[2]. Their evaluation necessarily takes us deep into the nineteenth century, when their cultural presence peaked. Their roots, it is true, are still in philosophy, but in the Romantic German idealism of Herder and Goethe, not in the supposedly dominant British Associationist tradition. Although they were European in origin (Lavater was Swiss and Gall German) their impact in Britain and the USA (especially, in the latter, phrenology) was considerable. Lavater's *Essays on Physiognomy* were Europe-wide best-sellers, and the finest British edition included engravings by William Blake. Phrenology, as expounded by Gall's apostle Spurzheim, was first adopted with particular enthusiasm in Edinburgh (where the philosophical climate was highly congenial), most successfully by George Combe (1788–1858).

One might, then, describe them, especially phrenology, as 'dry runs' for Psychology, for by the time of phrenology's effective demise as a serious enterprise in the 1860s it had become applied in such diverse areas as Education, Insanity and Ethnology[3], had developed a methodology including rating-scales and statistics (albeit crude) and had a professional organization (The Phrenological Society, founded 1820, later the British Phrenological Society), as well as serving both to determine and to articulate prevailing cultural modes of construing psychology 'character' and personality. In addition to Bain and Spencer, phrenology was taken seriously by persons as various as George Eliot, Queen Victoria and Dostoievsky, and in popular culture, phrenological books (of an increasingly ritualized and crude type) continued to be published into the present century[4]. Although in principle distinct from (and, as will seen, at heart theoretically opposed to) physiognomy, phrenological writings often in practice absorbed some of its doctrines, as well as those of the much older humoral personality typologies (e.g. George Combe, 1836). The European cultural impact of Lavater's physiognomy was no less considerable. Tytler mounts a powerful argument for giving Lavater a pivotal role in the development of the nineteenth-century novel, since many major as well as minor English, German and French novelists alike referred to him and utilized his physiognomic principles in the literary depiction of character. His impact on painting and aesthetic theory was no less considerable (see Mary Cowling, 1989).

Notwithstanding the magnitude of their cultural presence, these doctrines have received short shrift from general historians of Psychology, Flugel calling phrenology Psychology's 'great *faux pas*' (Flugel, rev. West, 1964, p. 38), and even proceeding to claim, quite erroneously, that 'we can at least console ourselves that no psychologist of note was party to the indiscretion' (*ibid.*). In retrospect they are both seen as naive, crude and fallacious. Their 'failure', coupled with the fact that their philosophical rationales lay outside the canonical mainstream lineage, has resulted in a misleading marginalization of their roles. Lavater is systematically ignored and does not even figure in R.I. Watson's bibliography of the discipline (1968). Since the questions they asked, and the methods they used to answer them, more clearly anticipate those of modern Psychology than do those of their contemporaries in philosophy and physiology, Lavater and Gall warrant far more attention than they customarily receive.

(i) Lavater's 'Physiognomy'

Johann Kaspar (or Caspar) Lavater (1741–1802), a Swiss pastor, represents a pious precursor – progenitor, even – of German *Naturphilosophie*[5]. His central, simple tenet is that character is reflected in form, form being the outward expression of a creature's inner spiritual essence. The opening aphorisms of his *Aphorisms on*

Man (1789) are:

> 1. Know, in the first place, that mankind agree in essence, as they do in their limbs and senses.
> 2. Mankind differ as much in essence as they do in form, limbs, and senses – and only so, and not more.

As well as human character Lavater does not baulk at extending his meditations to monkeys, horses, elephants, birds, even insects. 'The ostrich', he assures us, 'knows not what compassion means.' While physiognomy had enjoyed great vogue, in Italy especially, in the sixteenth and seventeenth centuries, Lavater's approach was radically different from those of della Porta, Ralph Hill and Cardano, for whom it was essentially a matter of fortune-telling, often with a strong astrological component[6]. Their interpretations had invariably been atomistic, not holistic, in character – large nostrils, hairy eyebrows, a mole on the cheek, blood-flecks in the whites of the eye, lobeless ears and the like would each be taken to signify some particular virtue or, more often, vice. During the eighteenth century belief in the reliability of appearances had waned – partly because the message of the new sciences was read as an exposé of the covert corpuscular nature of things, partly as a result of a broader cultural preoccupation, in literature and fashion alike, with their deceptiveness. It was a period in which artificiality of self-presentation reigned supreme, the heyday of wigs, garish make-up, masked balls and fans.

The publication of Lavater's ideas coincided with a cultural reaction against this arch reluctance to present the self in everyday life, a reaction marked by a new stress on authenticity and self-disclosure[7]. When Lavater revives its fortunes, physiognomy itself wears a new aspect. While individual features may have diagnostic value, the individual is a spiritual unity, not a mere collection of traits. We are dealing with particular instances of universal principles extending throughout Nature, Divine principles which unite form and essence, soul and body. 'Harmony' is now the watchword ('sin and destruction of order are the same': *Aphorisms*, p. 8). His physiognomical enquiries are founded in, and guided by, a deep religious conviction of the Divine orderliness of the cosmos, and the soul's participation in this. Nevertheless Tytler recovers an extensive Europe-wide interest in physiognomy in the century preceding Lavater, becoming progressively closer to his own approach. De la Chambre's *L'art de connoistre les hommes* (1660) long remained popular, while eighteenth-century physiognomical works include Jacques Pernetti's *Lettres philosophiques sur les phisionomies* (1746), A.J. Pernety's *Discours sur la physionomie et les avantages des connaissances physionomiques* (1769), and James Parsons's *Crounian Lectures on Muscular Motion* (1747)[8]. Nor was Lavater unique in his interest in the German-speaking world. His fellow physiognomists F.C. Nicolai and G.C. Lichtenberg both adopted ambivalent stances towards Lavater's own hugely successful writings on the topic. As we shall see later, the Romantic metaphysics underpinning Lavater's work is diametrically opposed to the theoretical thrust of Gall's phrenology.

Lavater's influence in Britain, as throughout Europe, was considerable, aided by the fact that his childhood friend, the Romantic painter Henry Fuseli, had settled in London where, for example, he managed the publication of the *Aphorisms* (1788). His son Henry Lavater was also training in medicine in Britain in the late 1780s. For Lavater, physiognomy was a hobby rather than his main vocation. This latter lay in his copious religious work, which constitutes by far the greater part of his 130 publications. He died in 1802 from the effects of a bullet wound received during a fracas with occupying French soldiers in Zurich in 1799. To the modern reader he is excruciatingly pious, but even allowing for the unremittingly hagiographic nature of his anonymous 1849 biography, he appears to have been greatly loved and respected by his contemporaries, and had a vast range of correspondents and friends among the European intelligentsia. His most revealing work is the *Secret Journal of a Self-Observer, or Confessions and Familiar Letters* (1795), originally published without his permission. It would indeed be interesting to know how far the intense and agonized spiritual introspections of Lavater, combined with his emotional sensitivity to Nature, contributed to the rise of Romanticism. The evidence is suggestive, and Tytler's positive conclusions in this respect are convincing, as is his contextualizing of Lavater within the broader framework of eighteenth-century German thought, as part of the reaction against Rationalism and French materialism. An interesting, fairly close connection here is the direct inspirational influence on Lavater of the Francophone Swiss naturalist Charles Bonnet, whose *Palingénésie philosophique* (1769) he actually translated. Bonnet was in the forefront of anti-materialist biology, a leading advocate of the 'Chain of Being' linking the lowest beings to the highest spiritual entities.

Lavater's aphorisms are generally, to modern ears, pretty dull, it must be confessed, but there are occasional flashes: 'The freer you feel yourself in the presence of another, the more free is he: who is free makes free' (no. 85), or 'Who trades in contradictions will not be contradicted' (no. 134); but Blake valued these *Aphorisms* highly (he even engraved the frontispiece, as well as annotating his own copy) as displaying true Christian humanity, adapting the aphoristic format in his own *Marriage of Heaven and Hell* (Swedenborg being another major influence: Bronowski, 1954).

All this is, at first sight, far from the apparent superficiality of the physiognomy for which Lavater is now – albeit faintly – remembered, but indicates that Lavater's role is more complex than generally acknowledged. The massive (and massively popular) compendium of *Physiognomische Fragmente zur Beförderung des Menschenkenntniss und Menschenliebe* (4 vols, 1775–8), in any case, constitutes a survey of 'individual differences' on a scale without precedent, however haphazard the sampling. Gloriously illustrated, compulsively browsable, it reinforces the view of humans as a psychophysiological unity, challenging its readers to view one another with compassionate sensitivity (the full English title of the 1797 translation of *Essays on Physiognomy* rendering the German *. . . calculated to extend the Knowledge and the Love of Mankind*). Derivative works such as *Lavater's Looking-Glass* (1800) followed, and the ground was broken for phrenology[9]. In 1824 Francis Howell published *The Characters of Theophrastus; translated from the Greek, and illustrated by Physiognomical Sketches*, apparently the first scholarly translation of Theophrastus into English. The translator's short final essay, 'General Remarks on the Study of Human Nature', is curiously contemptuous of the

> flitting systems advanced by the dialecticians, the medico-metaphysicians, the infidel theologians, the physiognomists, craniologists, and phrenologists, and by those designated by the unmeaning term *materialists*, – who have appeared in quick succession during the past sixty years in Germany, France, and England. (p. 255)

But as his inclusion of 'physiognomical sketches' shows, he is nevertheless writing in a market-climate created by Lavater and Gall[10].

Physiognomy also inspired plays, both satirical and supportive (see Tytler, 1982, pp. 386–7) but, more seriously, it raised the possibility of practical applications for a science of character; the *Essays* standing to hand for consultation in hiring new servants or assessing new business acquaintances. Indeed, it cannot be stressed too much how great a craze for physiognomy Lavater launched across Europe – one which apparently continued unabated into the 1820s. At all levels of society, it seems, he inspired (along with Gall) a rage for *looking* at people (both others and oneself) in a new and attentive way, in order to discern the inner character from the outward form. Later, as is well known, Charles Darwin's nose nearly cost him the *HMS Beagle* trip by not pleasing Captain FitzRoy, a Lavater aficionado. For all the contemporary philosophical rhetoric about a 'Science of Man', Lavater's physiognomy was the first public appearance of something which actually looked like an empirically based study of human nature[11].

In any case, there is another, as yet shadowy, side to the psychological, if not Psychological, story of Lavater's significance: his doctrine of a universal correspondence between essence and form reconverts Nature back into the fully animated being which Natural Philosophy had rejected in the previous century. Nature itself becomes psychological as well as physical; its forms become signs of the inner spiritual, moral character of the variety of beings which comprise it. This greatly excited such contemporaries as Herder, who confessed to wanting to prostrate himself before Volume II of the *Physiognomische Fragmente*. For Lavater, pious Lutheran minister of St Peter's, Zurich, the implicit Pantheism was held at bay by intense religious orthodoxy, but not for his Romantic successors. (It was precisely this unremitting piety which eventually led to a breach with his one-time close friend Goethe.) As we have seen in discussing the Romantic view of language (see above, Chapter 2) for the first time since Hobbes and Wilkins had unwittingly hamstrung the process, identification with Nature as a route to psychological exploration could, by the end of the eighteenth century, again proceed unhindered. Lavater provides us with an example of someone following precisely this path.

This is not to claim that Lavater launched Romanticism (though the force of his covert nudge has, perhaps, been underestimated), but rather to draw attention to his writings in general as both signifying and facilitating the final stage of its emergence into popular culture.

In 1771 Henry Mackenzie, a very dour Scot by all accounts, had published a best-selling novel, *The Man of Feeling*, the hero of which embodied the contemporary cult of 'sensibility', shedding tears at the least excuse, and exhibiting a painful sensitivity to all human suffering. This cultivated sentimentality, or 'sensibility', had served throughout the late eighteenth century in lieu of full-blooded emotion. The passions, tamed by Reason, were to be permitted a periodic catharsis; ready tears were the stigmata of the cultivated, deeper melancholy was a matter for the doctor. It is easy to see, reading Lavater's *Self-Observer*, how his often lachrymose religiosity could strike a sympathetic chord with this *mentalité*. But it is a deceptive, if not entirely false, resonance. In Lavater's effusions we seem to be dealing with something beyond cultivated sentiment, a heading into deeper waters of emotional struggle, where spiritual authenticity is genuinely at stake. He is engaged in transforming the cult of 'sensibility' into a more full-blooded Romanticism (but for a full account of Lavater's literary connections, affinities and effects, Tytler's study should be consulted). Of course he was no Kierkegaard, but neither, as Blake spotted, was he a complacent pedlar of consolatory platitudes. Lavater's writings, coinciding with the upsurge of humanitarianism on issues as varied as slavery and cruel sports, coinciding also with the rise of companionate marriage based on ties of genuine affection and a revival of Evangelical religion (e.g. Methodism), seemed to express many of the anxieties and yearnings of the late-eighteenth-century English middle class. His physiognomy offered a Science of Man at once empirical and evangelical, applicable and devout.

Fascination with physiognomy persisted throughout the following century. It was a multifaceted interest, gelling in with the early craniologically orientated anthropology of Blumenbach and his successors, notably in France. A second burst of enthusiasm for physiognomy accompanied the rise of degeneration theorists from the 1860s onwards, notably in the work of the Italians Cesare Lombroso and Paolo Mantegazza (both of whom were translated into English). In 1838 the eminent psychiatrist Sir Alexander Morison published a seriously motivated work entitled *The Physiognomy of Mental Diseases*.[12] The notion that the mad were physiognomically distinct remained popular, boosted by degenerationism and the advent of photography.[13]

More scientifically respectable than Lavater, Sir Charles Bell's *The*

Anatomy and Philosophy of Expression first appeared at the height of interest in physiognomy in 1806, while the enlarged third edition (1844) was lauded at the beginning of Darwin's *The Expression of the Emotions in Man and Animals* (1872) as having 'laid the foundations of the subject as a branch of science' (p. 2; see below, pp. 357–9). As well as Tytler's book dealing with the novel, the broader cultural impact of physiognomical thought has recently received attention from Mary Cowling (1989) in relation to nineteenth-century art. Reverberations of Lavater's physiognomical version of a 'Science of Man' thus seem to continue down to the advent of Psychology itself, in anthropology, psychiatry and physiology. The ubiquity of Lavater's influence unfortunately tends to be masked by the more visible career of the phrenology movement (itself originally referred to as a physiognomical system), but his absence from histories of Psychology remains one of the most remarkable of all the lacunae we have been noting.

(ii) Gall's 'Phrenology'

Franz Joseph Gall (1758–1828) was born in Germany and died in Paris after a singularly hectic career as doctor, physiologist and medical showman. Otto Temkin (1947) and Robert M. Young (1970, 1972) have gone a long way towards rectifying the traditionally dismissive accounts of his contribution to Psychology. Young sees in him the source of the concept of 'function':

> If one traces the concept of 'function' as applied to psychological and social phenomena back from its late-Nineteenth and Twentieth Century uses, one finds its source in the writings of Gall and his followers. (1972)

Before the appearance of his 'Craniology' (as he originally called his system) Gall made genuine advances in the understanding of brain anatomy[14], but the theoretical foundations for his Craniology preceded his neuroanatomy, and the two aspects of his work remained substantially in parallel rather than mutually interacting. He found himself opposing leading contemporary physiological writers like Cabanis and Bichat, particularly for their sensationalist reductionist approach. In any case, they were unable to explain individual differences. Superficially, Gall, like

Lavater, believed in the primacy of holistic organization, in a pervasive unity of plan, but his elaboration of this was radically different. While Lavater believed in a pervasive spiritual unity expressing itself in all parts of the organism, Gall's account was in terms of interacting functional parts, lacking any superordinate integrating principle. Whilst attacking the reductionism of the materialist *idéologues*, his own system was also fundamentally materialist in character. He is thus profoundly opposed to Lavater's mysticism and preoccupation with the spiritual homogeneity of the organism. What we inherit is a distinct cerebral endowment which determines the unique pattern of expression of our functional (i.e. adaptive) instincts. Young observes that this switches the 'innate ideas' problem from being an epistemological issue to being a biological one. In the event, Gall identified 27 fundamental faculties, of which 19 were shared with other animals.

Gall's closest associate, J.G. Spurzheim (1776–1832), preached phrenology across Europe and North America and co-authored the phrenological *magnum opus*, *Anatomie et Physiologie du Système nerveux et du Cerveau* (1810–20). Lavater's work had already created a cultural climate receptive to phrenology, and during the ensuing decades the fortunes of the two were closely linked, even though their advocates were frequently at loggerheads, and many who rejected one would accept the other. To tease out their differential contributions is extremely difficult (though Tytler has attempted to do so). As far as the history of Psychology is concerned, Gall's influence has overshadowed Lavater's – owing, of course, to its more evidently scientific pretensions and close connections with developments in neurological research during the early nineteenth century, which come to a head with Flourens's effective 'refutation' of phrenology in 1842. The work of Robert M. Young and Roger Cooter presents us with two complementary interpretative angles on phrenology which I will consider in turn. Young's work concentrates on the impact of Gall's thought on nineteenth-century psychophysiological research and theorizing, with particular attention to the two primary founders of British Psychology, Herbert Spencer and Alexander Bain. Cooter examines the social, cultural and ideological significance of phrenological thought in Britain.

As will be recalled, eighteenth-century physiologists such as

Whytt and Haller had succeeded in partly emancipating physiology from a preoccupation with the mind–body problem, while steering clear of Cartesian mechanism. Using the concepts of sensibility and irritability and moving away from a crude hierarchical model, they had opened the door for a more functional approach to physiological issues which would focus on the organism's interaction with its environment. It is in this context that Gall's phrenology becomes profoundly significant, and Young, as we have seen, makes him the effective initiator of functionalist Psychology. Gall's starting point in formulating his phrenological theory was his recognition of a need to establish precisely what functions the brain serves. Formally espousing the then still radical claim that all psychological functions were served by the brain, he refused to accept *a priori* the traditional faculty labels for these functions (such as Will, Reason, Emotion, and the like) because these had not been arrived at empirically.

From childhood on, Gall had felt able to recognize an association between certain aptitudes and distinctive cranial features. Exploring these linkages systematically, he believed he had found an empirical route to discovering the basic faculties. His rationale for this was that since our various physiological functions are served by distinct organs, cerebrally located psychological functions would be similarly served by specific regions of the brain. The greater the individual's endowment with a particular faculty, the larger the organ in question would be; thus (and here was the weak part) the shape of the cranium would reflect the relative sizes of the underlying functional 'organs'. One essential virtue of this approach would be that it would enable us to explain individual variations in temperament and ability for which the generalized traditional faculties could not account. Furthermore, this had the edge over Lavaterian physiognomy in terms of the ease with which the theory could be applied; where physiognomy involved an ultimately intuitive assessment of inner spiritual character, phrenology provided a straightforward algorithm for reading off character from cranial conformation. While the traditional faculties of the German philosophers do not entirely disappear, they are considered as 'general attributes' common to all people which play only a secondary role in determining character by affecting the operation of the 'determinate faculties'. Gall's approach may also be seen in the context of turn-of-the-century skull-orientated physical anthropology as being developed by J.F. Blumenbach on the basis of P. Camper's work on quantifying skull-shape, notably his notion of the 'Facial Line'.[15]

Gall's 'Craniology' (the term 'Phrenology' was coined by T.I.M. Forster in 1815) appeared at a time when a rather deep impasse was developing in relations between physiology and mental philosophy. On the physiological side it was becoming increasingly apparent that behaviour was determined in large part by native endowment, but this raised the spectre of 'innate ideas', anathema to the Sensationalist and Associationist philosophers dominant in France and England, with their *tabula rasa* image of all mental contents originating in individual experience. The conventional way of circumventing this as far as physiology was concerned, was to claim that the mind, or soul, was located in the cortex which, they believed, did not possess the property of irritability common to the rest of the nervous system; it could thus retain a certain 'blank slate' character. Following the discovery of the distinction between sensory and motor nerves by Charles Bell and François Magendie, the analysis of neurological functioning gained new momentum, but was not carried as far as the cerebrum itself. The image of the brain as exhibiting a fundamental division between the cerebrum and the subcortex represented, in physical terms, a continued desire to keep higher psychological functions – consciousness itself, the will, reasoning and memory, etc. – separate from the sensory-motor system as such. The cerebral cortex was held to be a generalized site for the 'Mind', a *sensorium commune* in Prochaska's terms. How 'acts of the Will' occurring at this level could actually connect with the motor nerves remained obscure. Gall, in locating the various psychological faculties at discrete sites in the cortex, was mounting a fundamental challenge to neurological orthodoxy, since his faculties included many which involved adaptive behavioural interactions with the environment (such as acquisitiveness and love of children).

As Young stresses, however, Gall's original theory, while establishing the need to view the psychological, biological and adaptive behavioural levels as a unity, remained conceptually stalled. The stumbling block was his commitment to a traditional, static, 'Chain of Being' concept of Nature. Within this framework the origins of the faculties or instincts themselves remained a matter of God's skill as a Divine Engineer, unamenable to further analysis. The incompatability with Associationist mental philosophy remained as patent as ever. For their part, the philosophers, especially later Associationists such as John Stuart Mill, were also becoming aware of the difficulty in rendering their philosophical doctrines compatible with the rapidly developing body of neurophysiological knowledge. In 1842 the French neurologist M.J.P. Flourens published his refutation of Gall, basing his case on the findings of his pioneer ablation experiments (going back to 1822–3). These he claimed, demonstrated that the cerebrum operated as a unity, as the seat of the 'Will', and endorsed the view that an analysis of nervous function in terms of sensation and irritation could not be carried beyond lower brain-structures such as the medulla. Accepted by Magendie and endorsed by the influential German physiologist Johannes Müller, Flourens's 'disproof' of the localization of function hypothesis remained accepted wisdom until Broca's discovery of the 'speech area' (1861) and the work of Fritsch and Hitzig (1870) which demonstrated that cortical stimulation could, after all, initiate locomotor movements.

Flourens's findings did not, however, solve the difficulties, and – in reverting, as far as the psychological side of things was concerned, to traditional non-empirically derived faculty categories – was a regressive step. Although phrenology lost esteem among physiologists, its defeat was not total, and a large number of scientists continued to give it credence. The respective methodological merits of Gall's Baconian data-gathering and Flourens's vivisection experiments were far from clear-cut; Gall, to be sure, failed to appreciate the importance of falsification, but neurophysiological experimentation was as yet crude and itself susceptible to a host of criticisms.

In the event, Young argues, Gall's central role in determining the character of Psychology was mediated via Alexander Bain and, even more, Herbert Spencer, both 'noteworthy' psychologists who were, *contra* Flugel, fully 'party' to Gall's 'indiscretion'. Bain, though a convert to Associationism, sought to integrate Psychology and contemporary physiological knowledge, and under the latter accepted, and incorporated, a high degree of localization of function. This is evident throughout his first book *The Senses and the Intellect* (1855) and even more so in his *On the Study of Character, Including an Estimate of Phrenology* (1861). He was a friend of George Combe, the most important British phrenologist, and in his early years steeped himself in phrenological literature. In the end Bain's attempted integration of phrenology with Associationism failed, owing to his inability to grasp firmly the functionalist perspective. As a result he remained committed to a basically orthodox project of explaining psychological phenomena in terms of the individual's learning history. Spencer was more successful. Young's thesis is that Spencer's achievement was to break the impasse between Associationism and phrenological functionalism by means of his evolutionary theory. Even more than Bain, Spencer had been involved with phrenology in his early years, publishing articles in both the *Phrenological Journal* and Elliotson's *The Zoist* in the early 1840s. While gradually breaking away from the phrenological party line, he developed a rationale for localization of function which was directly to influence, even inspire, the later-nineteenth-century British neurologists Hughlings Jackson and David Ferrier, via whom it descended to Sir Charles Sherrington.

Spencer's key move was to convert Associationism from a doctrine which applied in *tabula rasa* fashion to the individual to a central evolutionary concept, the basis for an 'evolutionary Associationism'. Accepting the so-called (if erroneously) 'Lamarckian' notion of inheritance of acquired characteristics, Spencer argued that reiterated associations (e.g. a learned association between a particular behaviour and an outcome) resulted in neurological changes. These were then passed on to descendants, in whom the association would become an instinctive one. Spencerian evolution involves a constant progressive cosmic move towards greater differentiation and complexity. As time goes on the 'internal relations' within the lineage of organisms leading to man have come to reflect, with ever-improving fidelity, the 'external relations' in the outside world to which it is having to adapt; the faculties are really no more than various forms which this matching of internal to external relations has taken in the course of evolution. There is in fact a continuum from the simplest reflex, via instincts, memory, and imagination to reason. As the organism becomes more complex, so increasingly differentiated 'internal relations' become embodied in different organs and neurological networks.

On this basis, localization of function can be explained as the outcome of a long evolutionary process of functional adaptation, but with association continuing to operate as the central mechanism. This, of course, is rather different from the Darwinian 'Natural Selection' model, but a review of the respective roles of Spencerian and Darwinian accounts of evolution in the subsequent development of Psychology cannot be undertaken here.

If Gall is the source of the ideas of 'function' and, at one remove, 'adaptation', then his significance for Psychology is far greater than simply being the author of a *faux pas*. William James (1890), at least, was far from contemptuous of the doctrine: 'These correlations between mind and body are . . . so frequent that the "characters" given by phrenologists are often remarkable for knowingness and insight' (vol. I, p. 28). While we have so far looked at Gall's influence in terms of psychophysiological theory, the significance of the phrenology movement extends far more widely as a major factor in creating a receptive climate for Psychology as a biologically based discipline. Also, while Young has stressed the Associationist context, the Scottish connection has remained in some respects unexplored. Notwithstanding Gall's claim to be discovering faculties empirically, his list bears remarkably close affinities with the lists of 'Active Powers' identified by Reid and Stewart, who were also salient figures in Bain's intellectual background (see above, p. 171).[16] There can be little doubt that the prior presence, and wide popularity, of the Reidian faculty analysis in Scotland prepared the ground for a favourable reception of phrenological thought following Spurzheim's first British tour in 1814. Not all Scottish thinkers were sympathetic. Reid's editor, Sir William Hamilton, poured contempt on phrenology in the light of his own researches on brain-size and conformation which revealed, among other things, that:

> . . . by a comparison of all the crania of murderers preserved in the Anatomical Museum of this University [Edinburgh], with about nearly two hundred ordinary skulls indifferently taken, I found that these criminals exhibited a development of the phrenological organ of Destructiveness and other evil propensities smaller, and a development of the higher moral and intellectual qualities larger than the average. Nay, more, the same result was obtained when the the murderers' skulls were compared . . . with the individual crania of Robert Bruce, George Buchanan, and Dr David

> Gregory. (reprinted in W. Hamilton, 1859, pp. 410–1, originally *c.* 1836–7)

Similar vials of scorn were emptied on the doctrine by Prichard (1835). He first assaults Gall's reliance, as he sees it, on analogies between human 'actions and sentiments' and the 'characteristic habitudes of the brute tribes':

> Shall we conclude that Perry and Franklin sought the regions of the north impelled by the instinct of the migratory rat, and that Magellan and Da Gama traversed the southern oceans directed by an influence analogous to that which moves the flight of swallows? (p. 468)

So much for comparative Psychology! More to the point, however, Esquirol's large collection of lunatic crania and casts is, he has been assured by Esquirol himself, 'entirely adverse to the doctrine of the phrenologists'; as, he understands, is the even bigger collection of Foville (p. 477): 'I entertain a strong persuasion that the time is not far distant when the whole theory will be abandoned' (*ibid.*).

Such empirically based protests availed little. Bain's friend George Combe's best-selling *The Constitution of Man* (1828), which represents the conversion of phrenological thought into a fully fledged popular moral philosophical system, is now believed to have played perhaps the most significant role of any publication in preparing public opinion for Darwinian thought by promoting the acceptance of studying 'Man' in a naturalistic, quasi-evolutionary fashion. Its sales of 200,000 compare to about 50,000 for the *Origin of Species* (1859), and the contemporary furore surrounding it exceeded that generated by the latter. It is perhaps symptomatic of the orientation of many historians of Psychology that in the *Journal of the History of the Behavioral Sciences* a paper on Combe by A.A. Walsh was entitled 'George Combe: A Portrait of a Heretofore Generally Unknown Behaviorist' (Walsh, 1971), this label being justified by Combe's emphasis on 'education and external control of instinctive (reflexive) behavior', his belief that 'human behavior . . . was amenable to change' and his use of 'objective non-introspectionist methods' (p. 275). The elision of 'instinctive' and 'reflexive' here is clearly unacceptable, given that Behaviorism's key feature is its environmentalism. But in invoking Combe we are beginning to move towards the ideological connections between British and US phrenology, which Roger Cooter has explored in great depth. Both Walsh (*ibid.*) and Bakan (1966) had also previously drawn attention to the fact that although Gall's initial position may be seen as pessimistic regarding the possibility of individual change – we are determined by an inherited permutation of facultative strengths and weaknesses – phrenology as a movement rapidly became identified with reform and optimism about the meliorative value of such a Science of Man. To Cooter's amplification of this we now turn.

The widespread reluctance of modern Psychologists to acknowledge the extent of phrenology's influence is perhaps due in part to the sheer crudity of the phrenological account of the mind. It is seen as simply reifying and concretizing a range of human capabilities, dispositions and traits of quite different logical status, and converting them into explanatory principles. Although, from what we have said, such an image is clearly erroneous as far as Gall's own thought was concerned, it nevertheless has a degree of face validity when we turn to phrenology as popularly advocated. For Combe it was a dogma to be adhered to with religious fervour (Hunter, 1991). What Cooter has achieved is an invaluable reconstruction of the cultural and social context in which phrenology flourished. This allows us to recapture the nature and ideological ramifications of the appeal of this new science of human nature. What we are in danger of missing in retrospect is precisely how fresh and, indeed, liberating Gall's message was to a particularly important section of the British population in the early decades of the nineteenth century. The factors we see as most negative about it – its apparent simplicity and anti-intellectualist rejection of academic philosophy – were the very features which attracted the growing number of young professionals and skilled artisans being generated by the new industrial culture.

Here was an account of the mind rooted in down-to-earth empirical science – an account, furthermore, which could be readily applied by anyone willing to spend a little time mastering the simple rules of phrenological interpretation. Applied to oneself it would facilitate diagnosis of one's weaknesses and strengths, one's talents and aptitudes, applied to others (in a world, increasingly, of strangers) it enabled one to assess their trustworthiness, motives and temperament. Backed by a seemingly scientific physiological rationale, phrenology was just what every keen young male needed to survive and fulfil himself in the unpredictable social hive of the first Industrial Revolution: 'By a single consultation with a practical phrenologist, at the touch of an easily tutored hand, all of these agonizing problems could be solved' (Cooter, 1984, p. 176).

In the long run, phrenology's message proved ambiguous; on the one hand it provided a new 'modern' secular framework for construing human nature as naturally law-bound (strengthening the Scottish Moral Philosophers' previous extension of 'law' to matters of morality and social behaviour), reinforcing self-responsibility and the possibility of self-improvement. On the other hand its focus on the individual and the 'naturalness' of the existing bourgeois social order tended to undermine the credibility of socially couched radical critiques of the system and traditional 'class solidarity' notions. Ideologically, phrenology can thus be read as a central factor in establishing broad social consent to the individualistic values of nineteenth-century British culture by presenting as a 'neutral', 'scientific' (hence non-negotiable) truth the 'naturalness' of this system:

> Like reality itself, the science [phrenology] existed metaphysically without manifesting the alternatives to itself. Its metaphors of function, growth, harmony, order, and so on not only did not appear as the products of social consciousness but, insofar as they remained merely assumptions behind physiological 'facts', did not appear as metaphors at all. (Cooter, 1984, p. 192)

Cooter is far from wishing to argue that this was consciously intended by any individual group; on the contrary, his analysis elucidates very clearly the complexity of the process by which phrenology came to serve this interest. More significantly for us, the fragmented image of human nature offered by phrenology intensified the very alienation which its consolatory message of self-fulfilment promised to alleviate. Phrenology, in fact, provides an exemplary instance both of the Marxist notion of consciousness reflecting social structure and the physiomorphic argument that novel public phenomena become internalized as novel models of the mind.

From the Marxist perspective, the map of the divisions of the mind's labours provided by the phrenological chart constitutes a microcosmic mirror of the structure of society itself. From Spurzheim onwards the 'egalitarian' relationship between faculties present in Gall had been reorganized into a hierarchy, with 'Moral Sentiments' and 'Intellect' supreme (Combe, 1860 [1828]), in addition to which Spurzheim had added the faculties of 'Conscientiousness', 'Time' and 'Order' to Gall's list, while Combe added 'Concentrativeness': 'The concepts of time and work discipline were thus biologized through the very *qualities of character* that phrenology held nature as revealing' (Cooter, *op. cit.*, pp. 116–17).[17] Popular phrenological charts 'symbolically' depicted each faculty with an appropriate vignette: a pious preacher for 'Veneration', a fat gourmand for 'Alimentiveness', and the like; the net effect was to inscribe into the image of the individual mind itself a Dickensian array of good, bad and ugly social types. It may, of course, be queried whether anyone actually experienced themselves in quite such a fragmented fashion, but the implied correspondence between a 'natural' social structure comprised of contemporary social roles and a 'natural' psychological structure comprised of strictly analogous roles or functions is manifestly obvious. And just as social prosperity depends on harmoniously integrating these according to 'Natural Laws', so too does individual well-being similarly depend on maintaining lawful and harmonious order among the faculties of the mind.

From the physiomorphic perspective, the following passage from Cooter is, I find, especially provocative:

> Since human experience was quantified and forced into logical categories in the phrenological head, we can also think of it as functioning in ways analogous to the mechanized factory dealing with its raw material and labor. Indeed, the way reality is presented in the phrenological head bears a resemblance to the way the factory interior is illustrated in Andrew Ure's classic *The Philosophy of Manufactures* (1835): There, too, symmetry (in phrenology all the organs were duplicated), order, sense of mechanical complexity rationally understood, as well as purposeful function through division of labor emerge as the conspicuous features. As much as in the factory interior, the phrenology head was an advertisement for a less confusing and more automated reality in which character itself reduced to digits on a graft [*sic* – should be 'graph']. (*ibid.*, pp. 111–12)

While Cooter goes on to stress that it would more correct to see the dominant phrenological metaphor as an organic one stressing 'growth and development, . . . biology, adaptation, structures, and functions' (*ibid.*) rather than a mechanical one, I am unsure how distinct these metaphors actually were. By 1800 there had been considerable two-way traffic between these images; biology had itself become more sophisticatedly 'mechanized' (as we saw in discussing eighteenth-century neurophysiology) and social organization, if not machines themselves, biologized, particularly with respect to the 'division of labour' notion. Factory environments were both novel and the very settings in which many of those to whom phrenology appealed spent their working lives. Given this, the way in which the factory was organized, the functions and relationships manifested within it, would inevitably provide those living within them with a set of public schemata with which to construe their own self-experience. This being so, the popular phrenological account of human nature may well be read as representing, among other things, a physiomorphic assimilation of the factory as a complex functioning system. In other words, the factory provides a public, shared model of complex functioning available for use in construing the complex functionings of the brain/mind.

It is indeed ironic that the 'mechanization of the mind' was ultimately achieved by phrenology, the founder of which was radically opposed to the tradition supposedly most inclined to adopt this view. But it is a mechanization of a rather different kind to La Mettrie's and Diderot's; phrenology's paradigm machine is the full-blown factory system in which mechanical minutiae are less significant than the overall structure of the production process, a structure characterized by hierarchical power relations, divisions of function, and ongoing development, change, adaptation and innovation in the light of economic conditions and technological knowledge. And thus must the successful artisan himself strive to be – allowing his Moral and Intellectual Faculties the final authority over the operation of his constituent subordinate faculties, if he is to develop and adapt in a changing world.

The Marxist and physiomorphic perspectives are clearly complementary here – indeed, as far as phrenology is concerned, the psychological process of physiomorphic assimilation can be seen as the primary mediator of social structure (primarily the factory) into psychological structure. While I would not claim that physiomorphism can always be cast in this role, in this case, where the 'novel' is itself a visible socioeconomic innovation, the two kinds of account dovetail neatly.

Excepting France, the fate of phrenology in Europe was less successful. But even in France, where Gall left a number of eminent disciples and its status in the medical profession remained, until mid century, higher than any it achieved in Britain, it failed to extend its influence much beyond Paris. As in Britain, phrenology's central intellectual weakness was that in spite of the paramount importance it ascribed to brain functioning, its advocates themselves failed to engage in any further physiological researches into that very topic, their doctrinaire reliance on Gall's original work on cerebral anatomy resulting in a progressive decline in credibility. The movement's permanent impact in France seems to have been primarily in psychiatry, many of the leading French psychiatrists of the 1840s–1860s (Morel and Falret, for example) having begun their careers in the phrenology movement. As in Britain, there was a rapid expansion of applications of phrenology into such areas as education, criminology and anthropology during its golden age from the mid 1820s to late 1840s, while Auguste Comte himself was a keen admirer of Gall. But by 1858 M. Lélut, a leading critic, is happily writing phrenology off as impossible, false and ridiculous. While, at its height, phrenology undoubtedly had a far more significant presence in leading French scientific circles than it ever had in Britain, it never achieved a comparably pervasive ideological and cultural presence, and its decline appears to have been more rapid.[18]

In Germany, notwithstanding Hegel's praise and a brief vogue in the mid 1840s (with a journal, *Zeitschrift für Phrenologie*, being published in Heidelberg from 1843 to 1845), phrenology could not seriously compete with the flourishing university-based philosophical systems and physiological researches being promulgated in the wake of Kant. In Spain it was proscribed as atheism, although its leading exponent, Mariano Cubi i Solar, was an indefatigable campaigner and finally produced what is surely the biggest phrenological text: *La Frenolojía i sus Glorias* (1853–57), with 1,159 pages.[19] Italy's tradition of physiognomical writing ensured a more sympathetic intellectual reception, the leading Italian phrenologist being L. Chiaverini, but again its popularity was apparently limited and short-lived. Lanteri-Laura (1970) sees Lombroso as a direct heir to phrenology, but this masks a number of differences between physiognomy and phrenology, and between the ideological character of Lombroso's work and that which phrenology assumed elsewhere. The USA was a different story. Phrenology was introduced early on by Spurzheim himself, and its subsequent career as a popular psychological doctrine was colourful, especially when it was adopted and promoted by O.S. Fowler as part and parcel of a crusading and pious self-improvement philosophy (Bakan, 1966). These differing fortunes reinforce Cooter's analysis, since – to put it simply – phrenology's popular appeal appears to have been an inverse function of the level of industrialization.

Our final verdict on phrenology, then, must be that it played a very significant role in the evolution of Psychological thought. First appearing in the context of the more adaptationist and functionalist physiologies of Prochaska and Cabanis, it advanced functionalist approaches to the mind, which it located totally in the brain, and served as both a goad and an inspiration to psychophysiological research. But more broadly, it served to mediate a major change in the way in which human nature was popularly conceived, providing a modern, secular, and ostensibly applicable account reflecting and formally structuring the psychological character of its audience. Many phrenological terms and expressions enjoyed fairly wide currency throughout the late nineteenth century; people would talk of 'organs' being well or poorly developed, and might employ phrenological terms such as amativeness, combativeness, and the like in lieu of the simpler alternatives. In both its disciplinary and its cultural aspects, phrenology anticipated Psychology in often remarkable detail. While its conceptual legacy has faded within the discipline, its iconic legacy has persisted, even revived, phrenological heads and variations on them being a standard item in the repertoire of late-twentieth-century advertising and book-jacket design, while the busts themselves are now priced well beyond the reach of the average psychologist! Finally one notes that *new* books on phrenology began appearing during the 1980s as an – admittedly minor – strand of 'New Age' publishing. In fact it probably has more amateur adherents now than at any time since World War I. Mock on, Sir William Hamilton, 'tis all in vain!

2 Mesmerism

I have indicated elsewhere how Mesmerism may be construed as a very clear instance of the physiomorphic assimilation of a novel physical phenomenon (Richards, 1989a). The eighteenth century had seen an increasing interest in the growing number of electrical phenomena being discovered, but only hazily comprehended, by Natural Philosophers. Electricity was an 'imponderable fluid', an 'effluvium' or 'subtle matter', the nature of which was proving extremely elusive, nor was the connection between electricity and magnetism clearly established until Ørsted in 1820. Electrical and magnetic evidence nevertheless suggested that the Universe, after all, contained forces more akin to those espoused by the Hermeticists and Paracelsians than was compatible with the simple cogs-and-levers mechanism already rapidly waning in physiological theory (see above, pp. 196–9). Mesmer's move in promulgating his notion of 'Animal Magnetism' involved a quite explicit elaboration of the notion of the human being as a magnet, with the Mesmerist's goal being to align patients correctly with the cosmic flow of this force. His doctrine had distinct echoes of astrology, as the title of his 1764 doctoral thesis, 'The Influence of the Planets on the Human Body', indicates. It was, even so, couched in Natural Philosophical terms as being a further extension of the Newtonian cosmology. While Mesmer's is the most significant example of the psychological impact of magnetic and electrical phenomena, it was not, as we shall see shortly, without physiological predecessors in linking nervous function with electricity.[20] C.L. Hoffmann, Professor of Medicine at Halle University and Unzer's teacher had attempted earlier in the century to explain the operation of the *anima sensitiva* (or sensitive soul as distinct from the rational soul) in terms of an ethereal fluid, diffused throughout Nature, by means of which the soul acted on the body; blood received this from the atmosphere, whence it was extracted by the brain and sent along the nerves. Such ideas were obviously in the air.

Although Mesmer originally practised in Austria, it was in France that his ideas came to prominence in the early 1780s, simultaneously with at least two other varieties of electric (rather than magnetic) therapy: one advocated by Nicolas-Philippe Le Dru, the other by P.J.C. Mauduyt de la Verenne. The rationale for these was a general belief in a meteorological factor in determining health, and more specifically, as a corollary of this, the importance of atmospheric electricity as demonstrated by Benjamin Franklin and Jean-Antoine Nollet. The French Royal Society of Medicine eagerly promoted research into the relationship between climate and health. Le Dru and Mesmer were both to be damned by the Society's investigating committees, but Mauduyt (a respectable member rather than an outsider) remained untarnished[21]. Mesmer's advent in Paris also coincided almost exactly with the appearances of 'sex therapist' James Graham's magnet-encased 'celestial bed' in London,[22] and of Perkinism in the United States (this latter, invented by Dr Elisha Perkins, was a painkilling technique involving stroking patients with a pair of gold and silver 'tractors', its efficacy being explained in terms of 'animal electricity')[23].

More generally, electricity offered neurophysiologists a new way of conceptualizing the way in which nerves operated (although a clear grasp of the electrical nature of nerve conduction had to await later advances in the understanding of both electricity and neural biology). Hartley's mention of it has been noted already. Max Neuberger (1981, p. 195, n. 38) reels off a list of late-eighteenth-century thinkers who were equating the 'nerve agent' with electricity, including Joseph Priestley, Erasmus Darwin, Charles Bonnet, Prochaska, Cabanis and Thomas Young. In Britain Richard Mead was speculating along these lines as early as the 1740s[24]. Electric shocks entered the mad-doctor's armoury during this period, and the term 'electrifying', first used by W. Watson in 1745 (and B. Franklin in 1747) acquired a PL meaning by 1752 (Lord Chesterfield).[25] As electricity was the rarest and subtlest of fluids, it could also be argued (by Le Dru, for example) that it could somehow cleanse nerves (which he still believed to be tubes) clogged by unduly viscous nervous fluids (Sutton, 1981). Nor, of course, did the therapeutic use of electricity and magnetism disappear with the demise of Mesmerism; the following century saw their increasing use in treating (e.g. by 'galvanization') psychopathological conditions such as hysteria and, especially in the USA, 'neurasthenia'[26]. Mesmerism's immediate impact was felt most strongly in France, Germany and Austria. What was its effect in Britain?

The story of Mesmerism in Britain falls into two phases; the first, short-lived, phase is contemporary with Mesmer's own activities. Helped neither by its French provenance nor by the character of its advocates, it had fallen into disrepute by around 1810. Prichard (1835) critically discusses 'Animal Magnetism' at the end of his *A Treatise on Insanity*, but the second major phase of interest was stimulated by a visit to Britain by Dupotet in 1837 and is associated with Mesmerism's use in medical anaesthesia by Elliotson and Esdaile in the 1840s and early 1850s. Elliotson's journal *The Zoist* was the major forum for this movement. This phase also saw the rise and fall of Spencer Hall's 'Phrenomagnetism' – an attempt to combine Mesmerism and phrenology. The most important text from this period was James Braid's *Neurypnology* (1843), which introduced the term 'hypnotism' and provided a physiological explanation of Mesmeric phenomena as a form of sleep[27]. Apart from Esdaile and Elliotson's anaesthetic work and Braid's crucial theoretical contribution, the story of Mesmerism/animal magnetism/hypnotism in Britain is something of a sideshow in comparison with events in France, especially after around 1860. Both phases none the less prove instructive regarding the way in which new psychological ideas can be received, as well as yielding insights into the British intellectual climate immediately before the appearance of Psychology. In addition, the whole story has a highly entertaining side.

Our knowledge of the first phase remains scanty, although Jonathan Miller (1973) and Roy Porter (1985b) have made important preliminary forays. The term 'mesmerize' itself is first recorded in English in 1802 (although the more general PL sense does not appear until 1862). Before this, 'animal magnetism' (or 'magnetism' alone) is always used.[28] Mesmerism first came to wide attention with the publication in 1785 of William Godwin's translation of the hostile French Royal Society of Medicine report (1784), in his introduction to which he makes the interesting argument that since the magnetic theory is false, then, in the phenomena themselves, we are seeing a purely mental phenomenon – errors such as the magnetic theory are more interesting than truth, since they enable us to 'see the human mind naked'.[29] The principal advocate of 'Animal Magnetism' in Britain would appear to have been John Bell. In his pamphlet *An Essay on Somnambulism or Sleep-walking, produced by Animal Electricity and Magnetism* (1788; published in Dublin) he is styled 'Rev.' and described as 'Member of the Philosophical Harmonic Society of France . . . and the only person authorised to teach and practise that science in Great Britain, Ireland, etc.'. In 1792, now styled 'Monsieur le Docteur Bell', he published a somewhat longer (80-page) work, *The General and Particular Principles of Animal Electricity and Magnetism &c. in which are found Dr Bell's Secrets and Practice as delivered to his pupils.* This has a 'certified copy' of his admission to membership of the Philosophical Harmonic Society of France, with a list of signatures including de Puységur's. In the earlier work he explains how he was introduced to the 'Science' by a Father Harvier of the Augustin Convent in Paris, and introduced to Puységur. The later text includes instructions on how to magnetize a tree, a shilling or guinea, a harpsichord, a room or a bed, a pond, a bath and a tub of water. Bell's doctrines are those of Puységur (founder of the Philosophical Harmonic Society), which differed from Mesmer's only in being less committed to the details of the Mesmeric theory and more orientated to practice. It was Puységur who, in 1811, 'discovered' the use of 'passes' to induce the Mesmeric trance – the hand movements now so central in the stereotype of the hypnotist's procedure. Mesmer and his follower Puységur remained on friendly terms. What is curious, then, about Bell's two works is that he never actually mentions Mesmer.[30]

Other eighteenth-century English publications include John Martin's booklet *Animal Magnetism Examined* (1790), an anonymous tract, *The mysteries of animal magnetism displayed* (1789), John Pearson's *A Plain and rational account of the nature and effects of animal magnetism*, and a pamphlet, *A True and Genuine Discovery of Animal Electricity and Magnetism* (1790) – plus Samuel Stearns's response to the last, *The Mystery of Animal Magnetism Revealed to the World* (1791).[31] John Haslam's *Illustrations of Madness* (1810) is also important in providing a lengthy account of the case of the psychotic James Tilly Matthews, whose delusions revolved around varieties of Mesmeric persecution. Martin is primarily concerned with discrediting the magnetizers as ignorant and unscientific, in dispute among themselves, and contrary to religion ('religion and magnetism are at everlasting variance' p. 20) even hinting in the latter part of the booklet at some satanic source for the Mesmerist's powers.

Distorted by Martin's antipathies as the information is, we can nevertheless obtain some idea of the activities of magnetists or Mesmerists at the end of the century. Dr de Mainauduc figures as the one to first bring magnetic doctrines to Britain in 1785, although he learned these from Dr d'Eslon rather than from Mesmer – who had refused to help him. He proposed establishing a 'Hygioean Society' to be incorporated with that of Paris, to which end he sought twenty 'ladies' who would each contribute 15 guineas. This did not meet with great success. Half a dozen 'London Magnetists' are listed on page 10, including Dr Yeldal ('the most famous') and Mr de Loutherbourg, who attracted 3,000 to a meeting in Hammersmith. Reading between the lines, it appears that the majority of London magnetizers adopted more traditional occult explanations, invoking Fludd, Paracelsus, Helmont and Agrippa as their authorities rather than, as Mesmer did, contemporary Natural Philosophy. It was obviously a topic open to opportunistic quackery, with magnetists such as Mr Holloway offering to sell their secrets, raising money ostensibly as subscriptions for the publication of their lectures, and generally milking the gullible public. We have insufficient evidence, though, to convict them all of charlatanry, and some, such as Mr Cue, did venture into print.[32] Martin hints also at the dangers women might be exposing themselves to during the magnetic 'crisis'. He does not claim that the phenomena are fraudulent, but argues for mechanistic – or what we would now (adopting Coleridge's term) call 'psychosomatic' – explanations, favourably citing Falconer's *Dissertation of the Influence of the Passions upon Disorders of the Body*[33]. Within a few weeks Martin's attack elicited a response under the anonymous authorship of 'The Analyzer': *The Examiner Examined in Six Letters to the Rev. John Martin on the subject of his letter entitled Animal Magnetism examined* (1791), but we learn little more from this, since it is pitched as a systematic demolition of the logic of Martin's arguments and his ignorance of the subject, rather than producing new data.

Stearns's 58-page pamphlet is frankly hilarious. The author was a doctor and 'Astronomer to His Majesty's Provinces of Quebec & New Brunswic: also to the Commonwealth of Massachusetts, and the State of Vermont in America'. Ostensibly sympathetic, the tone is by turns satirical and bemused, but Stearns clearly accepts that *something* genuine is going on. According to Pearson:

> . . . the body may be compared to an Electrical Machine; the arms, the conductors; the fingers, the pointers. . . . Hold the fingers of both hands for some time towards the invalid's pericardium, and

> you will soon perceive all the effects of Electricity in the patient. Continue the motion till it is filled with the electrical fluid, which will flow with great velocity from your fingers, in proportion as your mental faculties are engaged . . . (p. 4)[34]

The rules which the 'Operator' must follow are then spelled out: he must be filled with benevolence for the subject, maintain 'constant intention within him', exert 'the strong internal faculty of volition', for example (pp. 5–6). There may occur an 'incorporation of atmospheres' leading to 'a strange connection' between Operator and subject. What flummoxes Stearns, however, is the sheer versatility of the claims made for Animal Electricity and Magnetic Effluvia:

> . . . that it is not only emetic and cathartic, but anodyne, antispasmodic, diaphoretic, antiseptic, vulnerary and nervine; that it opens obstructions, expels morbific matter, eases pains, allays spasms, promotes sweat, cools fevers, resists putrefaction, digests, incarnes and cicatrizes wounds, ulcers, abscesses, &c. restoring the injured parts to their former life and vigour; and in a word, that all the virtues of simple and compound remedies are contained in it. (p. 10)

If claims for this panacea are true, Pearson's wisdom in issuing the pamphlet may be questioned. Stearns lets rip on a Mandevillean fantasy of how the collapse of the medical profession, and unemployment for both the clergy (nobody will need to pray for recovery from illness) and candle-makers and chimney-sweeps will all ensue (people will transmit magnetic warmth to each other). Robbers, meanwhile, will flourish by throwing their victims into a Crisis and stealing their possessions. How can the phenomena be explained? The three options appear to be Imagination, Supernatural, and Motions of Operator's Hands. One senses that Stearns really favours the first, but he rules none out, while insisting, in the case of the second, that such powers would come from the Almighty and not from Satan. Next he spends some time playing off the Magnetizers against the Shaking Quakers, a sect which had arisen in north-west New York State in 1779 and was given to ecstatic dancing, induced trance states and miraculous healing. Regarding these effects, Stearns queries:

> . . . may we not impute it to the violence of the Electrical and

> Magnetic Effluvia? which must be put in motion by their dancing, turning round, falling down, clapping their hands etc? (p. 48)

The Shaking Quakers claimed to be able to see into heaven and hell in their trances, while European Magnetizers had claimed that in certain trance states subjects could see into their own internal organs in great detail:

> But I think the Shaking Quakers have not yet arrived to the knowledge of this branch of the Science; and though they are before us in looking into the invisible world, yet it seems they have not arrived to our art, of looking into the *corpus humanus* (p. 51)

Stearns also reports on two visits to a 'grand theatre of Animal Magnetism' in December 1790. He ends with a pair of light-hearted recipes for Magnetical Pills (including Balsam of Self-Abstraction, Roots of Attention, Bark of Intention, Seeds of Volition and Syrup of Confidence) and an Elixir for patients embarking on a Crisis, or Elixir Magneticus Mirabile ('Take of the Chymical Oil of Fear, Dread and Terror of each . . . 4 ounces' and 'rectified Spirits of Imagination . . . 2 pounds). He leaves his reader with a message of encouragement to 'cultivate and improve it [i.e. the Science] to the best advantage' and not to be disheartened by derision. With a plug for his forthcoming *Tour from London to Paris* – 'the completest account of the Revolution in France, of any hitherto published. Also a New Constitution, founded on the Principles of Justice and the Laws of Humanity; with A Description of the Road to Liberty' – he exits as merrily baffled as he entered.

How far Mesmerism or 'Animal Magnetism' penetrated into British popular consciousness at this time is obscure; some kind of craze apparently occurred in London between 1785 and the mid 1790s, no doubt leaving a legacy in the childhood memories of those who reached middle age three or four decades later to witness the revival. Some such penetration is perhaps evidenced by its incorporation into the psychotic fantasies of Haslam's patient Tilly Matthews (Haslam, 1810) who, as mentioned above, believed himself the victim of a Mesmeric plot.[35] The impression one gets of this phase is that few genuine adherents of Mesmer's own theories were practising in Britain, and that we are dealing with a fairly short-lived craze for something called 'Animal Magnetism' of which nobody had any clear idea except that it was somehow an exciting, newly discovered (or rediscovered) occult force by means of which individuals could exert power over one another's minds and bodies. It also elicited religious condemnation from those, such as Martin, who effectively saw it as latter-day witchcraft.

The second phase of interest was initiated by Dr John Elliotson of St Thomas' Hospital, London, in the 1840s, in conjunction with an India-based colleague, Esdaile. For these doctors the primary value of Mesmerism was as an anaesthetic technique and it is arguable that but for the advent of nitrous oxide ('laughing gas', initially used only 'recreationally'), ether and chloroform, scientific research on hypnotism would have been pursued considerably further than it was in the nineteenth century. Elliotson's journal *The Zoist* (1843–56)[36] contains many impressive reports from James Esdaile (and India-based correspondents who had witnessed his activities) of the efficacy of his work at Hooghly, particularly on scrotal tumours and elephantiasis, including the removal of a 50lb tumour of the testes (1846, no. XV, p. 413), but also on numerous other conditions including urinary blockage (*ibid.*, p. 309), breast cancer, chronic rheumatism and enlarged lymphatic glands (1848, no. XXI). A favourable government report on Esdaile was apparently published in 1847. In all these cases (numbering well into three figures) patients reportedly underwent successful painless operations while in a Mesmeric trance. *The Zoist*, edited and dominated by Elliotson, served as a forum for reports on Mesmeric phenomena and its use in medical contexts, as well as reviews of books on the subject. Unfortunately for these medical Mesmerists, the 1840s also, as noted above, saw the arrival of pharmaceutical anaesthetics. These rapidly established themselves as the preferred method, primarily by virtue of the ease of their routine application but also because, being physical rather than psychological in character, they were more congruent with orthodox medical attitudes. The success of such rival techniques deprived Mesmerism of its principal practical role, and although it continued to command a certain level of popular interest, scientific curiosity waned and it soon became associated with spiritualism and other mid–late-Victorian occult movements. For the scientists, Braid's physiological account served both to confirm the validity of the phenomenon (which he renamed 'hypnotism' or 'nervous sleep') and to demystify it by providing an alternative non-magnetic explanatory theory.

Dr James Braid's *Neurypnology* appeared in 1843, and was initially kept at arm's length by Elliotson and the orthodox Mesmerists. His interest was first aroused by attending a 'conversazione' at which the French Mesmerist M. Lafontaine (held, says Harte [1902, p. 82] to be 'the last of the great magnetisers'), had given a demonstration in 1841, the book itself stemming from a favourably received 'conversazione' of his own given at the 1842 British Medical Association meeting in Manchester. Braid's work first attempts to sever the links with 'animal magnetism', considering hypnotism

> . . . to be merely a simple, speedy, and certain mode of throwing the nervous system into a new condition, which may be eminently available in the cure of certain disorders. (1899 edn, p. 86)

None the less, Braid is wary of rejecting Mesmerism outright, and a *modus vivendi* with the magnetizers (of whom he knew several) was established in which both sides agreed that Braid had independently discovered a new way of inducing sleep-like states, but that the range of phenomena generated by their respective procedures was different, and the similarities between Braid's hypnotic trance and the Mesmeric trance was superficial. Braid thus quotes with approval a letter from a 'celebrated lecturer on animal magnetism', Mr H. Brookes, very much to this effect, which concludes: 'in fact you are the original discoverer of *a new agency*, and not of a mere modification of an old one' (*ibid.*, p. 90). Later, Braid explicitly states that his method cannot produce all the effects reported by Mesmerists (particularly the clairvoyant ones), and although we might detect an underlying scepticism, he is careful not to reject these outright. The dissonance reduction tactic on both sides, then, is to attempt to present themselves as dealing with different phenomena rather than offering rival theories of the same thing. The distinction was long maintained by true Mesmerists.[37] At this stage Braid and the Mesmerists have too much common cause in the face of medical hostility and incredulity to want to fall out, while Braid himself is too reliant on the Mesmerists for access to interesting phenomena to want to alienate them. Even so, Braid is in no doubt that his hypnotic method is easier, quicker and more reliable, than those of the Mesmerists, and thus more suitable for medical exploitation.

For Braid, the hypnotic trance is a purely neurological phenomenon which he summarizes as follows; he is, he writes, proposing

> That the effect of a continual fixation of the mental and visual eye in the manner, and with the concomitant circumstances pointed out, is to throw the nervous system into a new condition, accompanied with a state of somnolence, and a tendency, according to the mode of management, of exciting a variety of phenomena, very different from those we obtain either in ordinary sleep, or during the waking condition. (*ibid.*, p. 216)

The manner in question involves requiring the subject to fixate on an object (he tends to use his lancet case):

> . . . at such position above the forehead as may be necessary to produce the greatest possible strain upon the eyes and eyelids, and enable the patient to maintain a steady fixed stare at the object. The patient must be made to understand that he is to keep the eyes steadily fixed on the object, and the mind riveted on the idea of that one object. (*ibid.*, p. 109)

This paralyses the 'nervous centres in the eyes and their appendages' (*ibid.*, p. 99) resulting in a 'derangement of the state of the cerebro-spinal centres, and of the circulatory, and respiratory, and muscular systems' (*ibid.*, pp. 101–2). A two-stage process ensues: first the patient is highly excited and their senses become extraordinarily acute, then follows a 'cataleptiform' state in which they are quite insensible, and during which they can be switched at will back and forth between the two states by a puff of air on the face. Braid explores the differences between ordinary sleep and hypnotic trance in detail, discussing also the differences between natural and hypnotic somnambulism.

As is typical of Mesmeric expositions, we are introduced to a succession of illustrative cases and demonstrations involving impeccably reliable and respectable witnesses and subjects, often irreproachable wives of acquaintances (who profess ignorance of anything pertaining to the topic), with naive servants making the occasional entrance. Müller, Liebig and other authorities figure in lengthy footnotes. While there is no doubt that Braid's neurological theory was original, there are hints of a move in this direction in Prichard (1835) who, while out of sympathy with the magnetic theory, accepts the reality of some of the reported phenomena and believes it to have drawn attention to some important issues. Prichard's discussion carries him into a fairly extended survey of somnambulistic phenomena, quoting numerous continental authorities such as Abbé Faria, a practitioner who rejected the magnetic theory, and Dr Johann Steiglitz of Hanover, who explained Mesmerism in terms of a suspension of brain and spinal cord activity:

> . . . the nervous structure connected with the ganglions, and appropriated generally to the functions of physical life, assumes vicariously the office of the brain, and becomes a new sensorium. (Prichard, 1835, p. 432)

This is reminiscent of Prochaska's belief that there may be some degree of connection between nerves below the *sensorium commune* level[38]. Prichard was unusually well informed regarding continental work – Leigh (1961) labels him a 'xenophil' – so one should not, perhaps, read any direct influence on Braid from figures such as Steiglitz. Since Prichard's discussion occurs in a psychiatric text, it is by no means certain that Braid was familiar with it (neither Prichard nor Steiglitz is cited in any of the works included in the A.E. Waite edition).

In Chapter 6 Braid ventures into new and riskier territory, for he has become increasingly impressed with the activities of T. Spencer Hall and begun experimenting with phreno-magnetism, rechristening it phreno-hypnotism. As before, numerous 'experiments' and demonstrations are invoked to illustrate his case: that in the hypnotic trance patients may be manipulated into evincing behaviours characteristic of the various phrenological organs by stimulating the appropriate region of the head. Braid's view of phrenology is not uncritical, and he naturally disputes Hall's 'magnetic' explanation, arguing that the procedures work by stimulating the subcutaneous nerves which ultimately connect up with the organ in question, rather than by direct magnetic stimulation of the brain through the skull. While Braid is adamant throughout that hypnotism cannot be used to induce people to act contrary to their moral principles – he even suggests that they become more moral – there is an unacknowledged contradiction between this dogma and the findings reported here, in which stimulation of 'acquisitiveness' induces theft and 'combativeness' aggression.

Part Two of the work reports 68 medical cases in which hypnosis has proved efficacious[39]. Where Esdaile used Mesmerism primarily as an anaesthetic technique, Braid's cases claim a direct curative effect of hypnosis on a variety of conditions (only three involve the use of hypnotism as an anaesthetic). The biggest category (14 cases) are cases of paralysis, mostly the consequences of strokes (but some sound as if they could have been psychosomatic); 12 report cures of sensory defects – poor eyesight, deafness – and 10 concern rheumatic conditions. Headaches (mostly migraine, as far as one can judge), epilepsy, heart palpitations, tics and 'tonic spasms' comprise most of the remainder (35 cases were female, 32 male, one unspecified). Braid continued to publish pamphlets and journal papers on the topic, the last appearing in 1855, but does not seem to have developed his theory significantly further. In 1847 he published two papers in the *Medical Times* evaluating the respective merits of Mesmeric/hypnotic anaesthesias and ether, and conceded the superiority of the latter. He also conducted further experiments to support a claim, made in *Neurypnology*, that magnets and electrical stimulation had no effect on hypnotic phenomena – this being occasioned by the publication of Baron von Reichenbach's eccentric researches on magnetism, in which the contrary was maintained.[40]

How are we to construe Braid's work? In coining 'hypnotism' (from the Greek *υπνος* = sleep) his is obviously one of those relatively rare cases from the pre-modern period where we can unproblematically ascribe and date the introduction of a new Psychological concept. Yet this is slightly misleading since for Braid it was a purely medical, physiological term, and he goes to some lengths to counter arguments that the phenomenon was a result either of imagination on the 'subject's' part or will-power on that of the hypnotist (while admitting that imagination may play a part if the subject has previously been hypnotized). Whilst *persona grata* with both the medical fraternity and Mesmerists, Braid failed to stimulate other British doctors or neurologists into exploring hypnotism any further than he himself had done, and remains an isolated figure. Unlike Liébeault in France, he never acquired a popular following. It was not until the 1890s that serious interest in hypnotism revived in Britain in the wake of the great upsurge of attention it was receiving in France, Braid's physiological account then served to counter the continued use of the notion of 'Animal Magnetism' in France (see below) with a seemingly more down-to-earth and scientifically orthodox explanation. Ironically, then, Braid's concept of hypnotism finally won the day over Mesmerism and animal magnetism precisely because it was fundamentally non-Psychological. That is not to say that these rivals were themselves explicitly Psychological – after all, animal magnetism was conceived of as a quasi-physical force. Yet in practice they held the Mesmerist's will-power and personal character to be factors in determining the efficacy with which he could manage this force, while the manner of Mesmerism's effect was also psychically direct (if not exactly psychic in the modern sense), unmediated by ocular nerves and cerebrospinal nerve roots. It was Liébault and his associates, known as the Nancy School (in opposition to Charcot's Paris School), who developed a genuinely psychological account in terms of a principle of 'suggestibility', although earlier investigators such as Abbé Faria, Bertrand and Noizet had espoused a similar position. Finally, the implicit and explicit negotiations between Braid and the Mesmerists provide an interesting and discrete case history of the social construction of knowledge claims which would reward further study.

It was in France that the Mesmeric tradition eventually proved strongest, although there too its popularity abated during the early nineteenth century. In contrast to Britain the link between Mesmer and the *fin-de-siècle* revival of interest centred on Charcot was, if not entirely continuous, at least only briefly interrupted. Notwithstanding Mesmer's condemnation, his follower de Puységur continued to promote the doctrine, and by the early decades of the nineteenth century it had considerably revived, with some fairly powerful advocates such as Deleuze, Mesmer's biographer, and Dupotet, who conducted experiments on Mesmerism in Paris hospitals in 1820. Against opposition it continued to be defended in the ensuing years by Rostan, Georget and Foissac.[41] Others, such as Bertrand, rejected magnetism, invoking the action of the Mesmerizer's feelings and the imagination of the Mesmeric subject.

In Prussia the practice of magnetization was restricted to physicians by royal order in February 1817. The German magnetist Kluge identified six degrees of Mesmeric trance from a waking stage characterized by feelings of lightness and rising temperature to the sixth 'Allgemeine-Klarheit' stage, 'where things hidden in futurity or in the distance of space are subjected to his survey'.[42] They were obviously catching up on the Shaking Quakers. Other noted German practitioners in the 1830s and 1840s included Ennemoser, Hensler and Siemers. The German interest in Mesmerism, until around 1840, should be understood in relation to the prevailing philosophical climate in which increasingly mystical varieties of post-Kantian Idealism and Romanticism were widely popular. These almost always involved some belief in a cosmic evolutionary process in which a striving, evolving consciousness was engaged in transcending matter and heading for fusion in the realms of Absolute Spirit. What could be easier, then, than to see Mesmeric phenomena as evidence of the latent powers of consciousness, testimony to the as yet unrealized potential of the human mind?

It is only in France, I think, that a direct connection between the Mesmeric tradition and the character of its national Psychology can be seen. This followed Liébeault's successful therapeutic usage of hypnotism at Nancy in the 1860s and his associate Bernheim's wider promotion of interest in the phenomenon, which grew at an accelerating rate to peak around 1890. By the late 1880s hypnotism had become linked with the notion of suggestibility, and both were becoming construed in an evolutionary (often degenerationist) framework bolstered by hierarchical models of neurological organization. As well as the psychiatrist Charcot – and, of course, his pupil, Pierre Janet – most French psychologists of this period (Gabriel Tarde, Alfred Binet, Theodore Ribot, Charles Féré and Gustav Le Bon) become involved in one way or another with this nexus of concerns, which appears to offer a route towards accounting for madness, double consciousness, crowd behaviour, national and racial character, and social deviance of all kinds. By this time the cultural meaning of hypnosis in France has undergone a great change. Unravelling the dynamics of this transformation as it played itself out over the century is a task which remains to be undertaken.

Conclusion

Both phrenology and Mesmerism offer us the opportunity to observe the way in which ideas regarding the psychological change. Both sought to present themselves as scientific, both involved refashioning the psychological to reflect changes in the external world, and both discovered – or created for themselves – a social role akin to that of modern Psychology. We have also seen how they were both engaged in some degree in the construction of that discipline. Phrenology's greatest impact was in Britain and North America, where economic and social conditions rendered its simple, practical, inspirational doctrines especially attractive to large numbers of striving middle-, lower-middle- and upper-working-class people uninterested in speculative philosophy. At the same time its scientific plausibility was, for a long time, just about high enough to maintain a genuine interest in it by psychophysiologists, and provide an intellectual point of departure for Spencer and Bain, neither of whose social origins were particularly elevated. Mesmerism or 'Animal Magnetism' spread more evenly throughout Europe, but exerted most long-term influence in France. Its appeal was more, perhaps, to a psychological than a social constituency – that is, to the neurotic, the chronically sick, and the bored. But it also appealed initially to those who were in intellectual rebellion against materialism and the rule of Reason – that is, to Romantics, *Naturphilosophes*, and occultists. Again, the weight of evidence in support of the phenomena, if not the theories at first proposed to explain them, was sufficiently strong to ensure that at least some natural scientists – and, more particularly, some physicians – would remain interested.

Both have left iconic legacies for our culture in the phrenological head and the penetrating eyes of the hypnotist, symbols for the mapping of the mind and the mastery of the will, power over the self and power over others.

PART THREE
1800–1850:
Three Routes to Psychology

Introduction

Straddling, as we are, the juncture of the eighteenth and nineteenth centuries, it is important to take stock before carrying this account further. By the beginning of the nineteenth century the eventual appearance of Psychology is clearly on the horizon, but – to pursue the metaphor – there are numerous roads which appear to be leading in that direction. And appearances can be deceptive. Some of these roads may sooner or later merge, some may peter out or change direction, and it is also possible that where they do apparently converge on 'Psychology', this convergence may turn out to be an illusion, a rhetorical construction of disciplinary historians. We have so far talked of the discipline finally being constituted in the 1850s, but it may be more correct to talk of a number of enterprises, sharing the same title but actually distinct, doing so over a rather longer time-span.

In the chapters which follow, we trace three routes to Psychology during the decades up to 1850 and identify the most important ideas which each introduced. These are: (a) the German Route; (b) the British Route, and (c) the French Route. How, and how far, these eventually merged will be dealt with in Part II of this work. Such a division in terms of national rather than, say, disciplinary terms demands some justification. Certainly there is considerable cross-traffic between countries, a trading of ideas, findings and methods. Even so, the routes taken towards Psychology appear to be more largely determined by their respective cultural traditions and climates than by international within-discipline dynamics. Within each country the founding of Psychology is a multidisciplinary affair, but the nature of this disciplinary interaction varies. In Britain and Germany there are distinct philosophical and physiological sources, but these fuse in Germany earlier than in Britain. In Britain the growth of evolutionary thought is a far more salient factor than in either France or Germany, and conditions the character of the physiological input (as indicated in the discussion of phrenology above).

As a result, the issues – and hence the conceptual innovations – dominating the proto-Psychological works of British, French and German writers differ considerably.

Kurt Danziger (1990), focusing on the history of experimental Psychology, has identified the differing national traditions in terms of methodological orientation. In Germany, Wundt's primary paradigm was physiological research of the kind which had been making dramatic advances in the early nineteenth century in the work of people like Johannes Müller, E.H. Weber and Hermann Helmholtz. In Britain, what Danziger terms a 'Galtonian' methodology (after Francis Galton) was initiated rooted in a social statistics tradition, while France was more dominated by a medical 'clinical' case-history orientated approach (Charcot being his paradigm example). Eventually the 'Galtonian' approach would win out over the others in experimental psychological research. While this analysis sheds light on the origins of methodology (Danziger's primary aim), as far as psychological ideas are concerned it is less appropriate, and in discussing these various national routes, a broader consideration of the contextual, mediating factors continues to be necessary, while we will also be noting texts which appear to have been largely ignored hitherto.

7
The German Route: Between Matter and Metaphysics

D.B. Klein (1970) remarks that 'British empiricists rather than post-Kantian philosophers should have been the pioneer experimental psychologists' (p. 500). One reason why they were not is straightforward enough – in 1800 Germany and Austria had at least thirty universities, England had but two, Oxford and Cambridge, both only beginning to awaken from a prolonged intellectual slumber, besides being restricted to Anglicans. In Scotland (with four) the Reidian anti-Associationists were dominant. Troubled Ireland's Trinity College Dublin could hardly redress the imbalance. Germany thus had a well established academic tradition with all that implies: opportunities for full-time intellectual work, networks of professional influence, university-centred publication, ongoing debate, and continuous teacher–student lineages of thought. Furthermore, it was undergoing considerable change during the period we are concerned with[1]. The majority of eighteenth-century German psychological writers after Leibniz (a diplomat-cum-librarian) were university based, and continued to be so (although non-university based thinkers such as Goethe could be highly important).

Nor was the English situation much improved by 1850 (only three more had been founded: London University, King's College, London, and Durham, in 1826, 1829 and 1831 respectively)[2]. It is in fact hard to see where the establishment of an English experimental Psychology could have happened even had anyone been minded to found it. This glaring disparity underlies a more immediate cause of Germany's lead: the fact that by 1800 German philosophers had developed a far more sophisticated conceptual repertoire for construing the psychological. (Nobody felt this more strongly than Coleridge, whose continental sojourn brought home to him the relatively parochial nature of English thought.) Conversely it is equally important to bear in mind that Germany was far behind Britain industrially and technologically – the number of steam engines, for example, was minute compared to those in Britain and France until the middle of the century; in 1812 there were only two small ones in the whole of Prussia[3]. The implication of this for our purposes is that there was a corresponding poverty in technical mechanistic concepts which could be co-opted metaphorically to provide genuinely novel 'scientific' models of psychological phenomena[4]. The first part of the chapter will be concerned with exploring this topic. We will then turn to the rather distinct – though eventually convergent – philosophical and physiological strands in early-nineteenth-century German thought. Froebel's educational doctrines and German psychiatric theories, essential aspects of German Psychological thought, are then addressed in the final parts of the chapter.

1 The German Conceptual Repertoire

German philosophy during the Enlightenment may be seen as continuously wrestling with the legacy of Leibniz (discussed in Chapter 1). Committed to an active, holistic concept of the mind, as opposed to the more passive reductionist, atomistic British and French doctrines stemming from Locke, German philosophers were required to identify and address the nature of mental processes which Lockean philosophers barely acknowledged, or saw as unproblematical products of a simple aggregative process. Christian Wolff (1679–1754) is generally accepted as the first to render Leibnizean thought more psychologically coherent in his two works *Psychologia empirica* (1732) and *Psychologia rationalis* (1734). Since Wolff, unlike Leibniz and Locke, was university based (at Halle), this sometimes earns him the soubriquet of 'first academic psychologist'. Two of Wolff's conceptual innovations largely determined the subsequent agenda of German philosophy regarding psychological matters: his differentiation of 'Psychology' into 'Empirical 'and 'Rational' varieties, and his identification of interacting mental 'Faculties' by analogy with physiological processes such as digestion and blood circulation. Two other, more specific technical ideas which he introduced were 'redintegration' and 'psychometry'. We will consider these in turn.

Wolff's division of Psychology into Empirical and Rational varieties represents a distinction between the task of enquiring in an empirical scientific fashion into the 'facts' of inner experience and the philosophical task of logically deriving a set of metaphysical first principles within which the very possibility of Rational enquiry could be guaranteed. In Wolff's work neither has priority, they are quite complementary. Since the latter involved going beyond experience it was a move which in itself raised epistemological problems and was eventually rejected by Kant for whom no knowledge beyond experience was possible. If, therefore, Wolff's approach may be read in one respect as a first step towards differentiating Psychology from philosophy, his immediate successors rejected it, and the division it adumbrated failed to materialize. Furthermore, his concept of Empirical Psychology, though 'scientific' in principle, did not in practice lead him to engage in modern type experiments; as Brett (1912) said, he 'named and defined empirical psychology, though he made no significant contribution to it' (1953 edn, p. 401). Rather, its methodology remained basically intuitive and introspective, adhering to the notion of an 'inner sense' allowing us to observe mental events, just as 'outer sense' enables us to observe the world. Only J.N. Tetens (1736–1807) appears to have undertaken any genuine empirical research into a psychological phenomenon – the duration of sensations – in Enlightenment Germany. As Villa (1903) remarked:

> In Germany, with the advent of other great philosophers, intellectual activity became absorbed by metaphysical questions, and Psychology became again one among the philosophical sciences with no special importance of its own . . . (p. 15)

In some respects the German situation resembled that in Britain, where throughout the eighteenth century there is a persistent rhetoric about the central importance of a Science of Man or of Human Nature which nevertheless continually fails to materialize, or remains constrained within philosophical agendas. The nearest Germany comes to such a science is in *Anthropologie*. To understand how the German philosophical tradition of proto-Psychogical thought developed, we must first look more closely at Wolff's system.

(i) Christian Wolff

Wolff is best known for his resurrection and reformulation of the

Faculty account of the human mind. This was not inconsistent with the unity of the soul, since the faculties he identified and hierarchically arranged were not thing-like but manifestations of a primary integrative capacity or power of the soul, the *vis repraesentiva*. In view of this, Cassirer (1932) prefers to call Wolff's position a 'functional' rather than 'faculty' Psychology, faculties being 'only the various tendencies and expressions of a single basic force, that of representation' (1955 English edn, p. 121). Symbolism, especially language, played a major role in the integrative process, since symbols served as 'representatives of or surrogates for experience' (Klein 1970, p. 470). Murphy and Kovach (1972) are typical in seeing Wolff's faculties as similar to – if not directly leading to – those of Reid and Stewart. Both, they claim, ultimately rest content with systematic cataloguing, and fail to move beyond this. This, however, is not entirely consistent with Cassirer's reading. The number, arrangement and naming of the faculties underwent numerous shifts as each philosopher in turn sought to provide their own version. The details of these permutations of Reason, Will, Feeling, Sensation, Desire, Memory, and the like are less important than the kind of discourse such constant shuffling generated among German philosophers. Inconclusive though their labours were, before Kant, the writings of Moses Mendelssohn, Baumgarten, Lessing, Lambert and the rest served to articulate and explore a wider range of psychological issues than their British and French contemporaries. To quote Cassirer again:

> Thus the doctrine of the faculties - and herein lies its systematic value - always endeavours to treat psychology not only as a doctrine of the elements of consciousness, that is, as a doctrine of sensations and impressions, *but rather as a comprehensive theory of attitudes and behavior.* (*op. cit.*, p. 127, emphasis added)

Eventually it was Tetens's tripartite identification of Knowing, Willing and Feeling that won out in providing a starting point for Kant. While accepting the need for an empirical approach, the Germans saw Associationism and reductionist Sensationalism as fundamentally flawed by a failure to appreciate the essentially active character of the mind and the need to account for the highest achievements of the human spirit[5].

The relationship between Wolff's pedagogically motivated and thorough system and Leibniz's philosophy is complex. Wolff adopts the doctrines of the unconscious and apperception, and the active unitary soul, but converts the monads to more orthodox atoms and shifts from Leibniz's parallelism to a more conventional mind–body dualism. While it loses the subtlety of Leibniz, his system was ideally fashioned to serve the needs of the new university-based philosophy, retaining Leibniz's core vision of the mind as part of a dynamic and organic cosmological process, a process which its own structure reflected. At the same time he is able to assimilate many of the insights of the Lockeans.

It is characteristic of the use Wolff makes of the Associationist account that he identifies as its main inadequacy its inability to provide an explanation for the phenomenological realities of recall and memory. It is the holistic nature of memory which attracts his attention – the way a single event can trigger recall of an entire biographical episode. This is, of course, a clear example of the integrative *vis repraesentiva*, and he introduces the term 'redintegration' to refer to it. A holistic 'law of redintegration' is thus added to the principles of association. Klein quotes Dessoir's 1912 'version of Wolff's formulation: "Every idea tends to recall to the mind the total idea of which it is a part"' (1970, p. 471). The concept of 'redintegration' remained in the discipline's technical vocabulary, resurfacing in Sir William Hamilton and then, in the present century, in the work of the US psychologist H.L. Hollingworth[6]. Klein further credits Wolff with introducing the concept of 'psychometry', measuring psychological phenomena, but apart from Tetens's isolated excursions into putting this into practice there is no evidence that Wolff played a significant role in inspiring the mid-nineteenth-century advent of psychometrics.

(ii) Immanuel Kant (1724–1804)

The culmination of the philosophical tradition initiated by Leibniz and Wolff comes with Immanuel Kant. Kant's significance for Psychology is peculiarly ambiguous, for while rejecting the very possibility of such a discipline being a 'science' (which, for him, involves measurement and the identification of the general mathematical laws governing the phenomena being studied) he provided a thorough analysis of the 'laws of understanding' in the context of his own metaphysical system. Nor did he reject the value of empirical investigations into human behaviour, even if they could never serve as a basis for a natural science. And this very tension between the supposed logical impossibility of a scientific Psychology and the acknowledged value of empirical enquiry into the psychological served to challenge his successors to find ways of outflanking Kant's veto. Conceptually the most important feature of Kantian thought for us, apart from reiteration of the active nature of mind, is his elaboration of the 'Categories' and Faculties in terms of which this activity is conducted. It is around these latter that he structures his analyses of Pure Reason [*reinen Vernunft*] in the *Critique of Pure Reason* (1781) and its operation in practice (in the *Critique of Practical Reason* [1788] and *Critique of Judgement* [1790]). The other works containing his psychological thought are *Anthropologie in pragmatischer Hinsicht abgefasst* (Anthropology from a Pragmatic Point of View; 1798) and *Metaphysische Anfangsgründe der Naturwissenschaft* (Metaphysical Foundations of Natural Science; 1786).

Kant's 'Psychology' may be summarized as follows: the nature of the Soul itself is rationally unknowable for we cannot move beyond the bald assertion 'I think' (itself an empirical proposition) to discover anything about the 'essence' of this 'I'[7]. We can discover the attributes of this Ego only via the manner in which it serves as the active 'vehicle of all concepts'. While sensory experience is the basis for all knowledge, the processing of sensory information is actively performed by the mind using *a priori* principles which do not themselves derive from experience – the higher mental functions are thus separate from sensation and low-level associative processes. These *a priori* principles include the 'categories' of space, time, causation and substance. In other words, the world we experience – the phenomenal world – is constituted by our mind, while the world as it is 'in itself' – the noumenal world – is beyond Reason's grasp. This applies even to knowledge of the Soul itself; the Soul is knowable phenomenally via the operation of our 'internal sense', but its noumenal nature again forever eludes us. Grasping this last point is absolutely essential for an understanding of Kantian thought.

The operations of the mind are of three kinds, which may be considered at the philosophical or psychological levels. These correspond to Tetens's three faculties of Knowing, Willing and Feeling but as Leary (1982a) stresses, Kant distinguishes them far more clearly than Tetens and 'must be given credit for firmly establishing the tradition of tripartite functional analysis' (p. 26). At the philosophical level Knowing is considered as Pure Reason or Understanding, Willing as Practical Reason, and Feeling as Judgement, psychologically these manifest themselves as Cognition, Will or Desire, and Feeling respectively. Imagination is a subsidiary cognitive process. The faculty of Feeling is in some respects intermediate between Cognition and Will, operating in terms of basic feelings of pleasure or pain, which may be of three kinds: sensuous (e.g. physical pain and pleasurable sensations, real or imagined); intellectual (pertaining to ideas and cognitions) and moral (pertaining to desires).

Notwithstanding the complexity of Kant's own 'philosophical Psychology', he was adamant that a true science based on the evidence of the internal sense, our only direct access to psychological phenomena, was impossible. These phenomena have no spatial or substantial properties which would render them amenable to quantitative study, while the very act of introspection alters – and is ultimately uncontrollable in its relation to – what it is observing. The best he can recommend for empirical Psychology is to abandon introspection and adopt an anthropological approach based on observation of people in the world supplemented by travelogues, biographies and history etc. From this enterprise we may glean some empirical regularities of behaviour, but it cannot be dignified as a proper 'science'. All this is rather prophetic; one cannot help remarking immediately that William James endeavoured to promote precisely the kind of introspective stance which Kant is here refuting as impossible.

The final point to be made on Kant at this juncture is that, as Leary elucidates, there is a central tension in his position between the notion of humans as essentially free active beings (which seems to be guaranteed by the ultimately active and constitutive nature of the Soul) and the necessity of adopting a deterministic account of human nature in so far as it can be an object of rational knowledge (which stems from the fundamental *a priori* category of 'cause' in terms of which we have to construe our experience). The Free Will versus Determinism debate dates back far beyond Kant, of course, but precisely because even Kant appeared unable to transcend it (while succeeding in transcending nearly everything else) it continued to haunt Psychological thought with even greater intensity, signifying one of its core dilemmas.

(iii) Post-Kantian Philosophers

Two papers by David Leary (1978, 1982a) have clarified Kant's pivotal role in German Psychological thought. The picture which emerges is of two different kinds of reaction, each playing a distinctive role for the discipline. The Idealist response of Fichte, Schelling and Hegel endeavours to reassert the possibility of a genuine transcendental knowledge of the nature of the Soul – a task which Kant had held to surpass 'all powers of human reason'. The Empiricists, by contrast, tried to demonstrate that a genuine mathematized empirical and/or experimental science of consciousness was after all possible, this lineage being represented by J.F. Fries, J.F. Herbart and F.E. Beneke. Towards the middle of the century there were several attempts at integrating the insights of the two streams in an undogmatic and scientifically informed manner, notably in Hermann Lotze's massive *Microkosmos* (1856–64). This *Idealrealismus* position, especially as expounded by Lotze at Göttingen during the 1840s, exerted a particularly powerful influence on early psychologists as varied as William James and Lotze's pupil Hermann Helmholtz. While unravelling the tangled web of early-nineteenth-century German thought (which was dominated by the issues Kant had raised) is beyond our present scope, the major conceptual innovations which resulted may, drawing on Leary's work, be identified.

From the Idealist side the focus on consciousness led eventually, in Hegel, to a shift in concern from individual subjectivity to concern with Mind as a unitary Absolute (favourite Idealist word!) Reality. While this seems initially uncongenial to scientific enquiry, it revitalized the earlier Romantic concerns of people such as Herder with the collective dimension of psychological life, providing a rationale for *Völkerpsychologie*, which eventually mutated into Social Psychology. Ideologically, the idea of a national 'Spirit', vehicle of a progressively striving collective Will, would eventually prove calamitous to German culture, but the immediate effect was less evidently noxious and had a number of subsidiary pay-offs for Psychology. It brought into focus the nature of the individual Ego and its development, and more generally raised the issues of personality and Will. Ironically, it also led writers on

Völkerpsychologie such as Dilthey to adopt proto-Social Constructionist positions stressing the importance of cultural (as well as instinctual) factors in determining the psychological. The question of the status of Psychology as science or humanity (or, more correctly, *Naturwissenschaft* or *Geisteswissenschaft*) remained a theme in German Psychological thought, with Dilthey, for example, continuing to reject experimental Psychology, and Wundt himself drawing a boundary between the two facets of the discipline. Stimulated by contemporary conceptual developments in physiology and a growing body of geological and palaeontological information, the Idealists drew increasing inspiration from an evolutionary vision of the Universe as the product of a dynamic Absolute spiritual principle, with Man as its most advanced product. This led them to take a growing interest in the geological and zoological evidence, raising the possibility of developmental and comparative studies. In the *Naturphilosophie* of Schelling and Oken, and in Hegel's Philosophy of the Absolute, this scientific Romanticism reached its most fervent pitch. Although it was very different from Darwinian theory, this vision continued to affect the way in which evolutionary thought was construed in Germany[8] – 'Darwinian thought was often assimilated in Germany through an essentially naturalized idealist framework' (Leary, 1982a, p. 35).

Post-Kantian Idealism, while essentially Rationalist in spirit, none the less provided a conceptual basis for what we may term the 'Humanist' side of Psychology, notably Social Psychology and personality, as well as developmental and comparative Psychology[9]. But it must be stressed that Idealists remained opposed to the notion of Psychology as an autonomous discipline separate from philosophy. It is also fair, I think, to claim that even if they did raise social, comparative, personality and developmental issues, it was in the Empiricist Darwinian climate that they finally struck root in Britain, the USA and France. For experimental Psychology, Idealism also played a role in providing the theoretical framework in which Fechner conducted his psychophysical research. This is ironic, given the major role which this research actually played as a model methodology for the kind of experimental research which Idealism opposed.

The Empiricist responses to Kant of Fries, Herbart and Beneke were varied in nature; Fries's approach was fundamentally a philosophical critique of Kant's dismissal of the notion of a scientific empirical Psychology in which he took issue with the 'mathematization' criterion. He argued, *contra* Kant, that 'rational principles' could indeed be derived from experience, claiming that Kant's own 'analysis of the a priori forms, categories, and ideas of the human mind' had been arrived at on this very basis (Leary, 1978). Of the three it was Herbart (who studied under Fichte at Jena) whose theoretical work is now considered the most prescient. This is primarily contained in three works: the two editions of *Lehrbuch zur Psychologie* (Textbook of Psychology; 1816, 1834) and *Psychologie als Wissenschaft* (Psychology as Science; 1824–5)[10]. Herbart's model ultimately hinges on two central technical concepts: 'apperception' and '*Vorstellungen*'. By 'apperception' Herbart, following Kant, means something akin to attention – if something is apperceived it is being focused on, clearly grasped, as opposed to being vague and peripheral. At any given moment there exists a constantly fluctuating 'apperceptive mass' – a mass of material constituting the core of our conscious experience. It is not quite the same as 'consciousness', it is whatever we are clearly attending to, thus something of which I was 'vaguely aware', and hence conscious, would not be part of the 'apperceptive mass'. This 'mass' consists of *Vorstellungen*, which it is tempting to translate as 'Ideas' – it is related, however, to the German word for 'to present', and covers all mental contents from sensations to abstract concepts.

An easy – albeit crude – way of envisaging Herbart's model is to see consciousness as a stage on which these *Vorstellungen* are constantly making entrances and exits, but this suggests a very atomistic picture, which is not quite what Herbart wants to convey. By entering into the apperceptive mass, *Vorstellungen* are placed into a context which enables them to combine, or even fuse, with one another; it is here that they acquire their meanings. Nor are *Vorstellungen* passive, they are actively energized, they have force and a tendency towards self-preservation[11]. This is very different from the British Associationist account, to which Herbart's bears a superficial resemblance. As the theatre stage metaphor implies, there is an 'off-stage' – an unconscious, and a threshold which *Vorstellungen* cross, when sufficiently energized, to enter the apperceptive mass. They can also of course be in conflict with each other, and some may be ousted from consciousness – repressed or *verdrängt* (hence '*Verdrängung*' or repression, the very terms Freud later used). Herbart held that his model provided a basis for mathematization of the whole process – by assigning values to the strength or intensity of the various *Vorstellungen*, etc. Thus instead of dismissing the mathematization criterion he accepted it and attempted to demonstrate that it was a condition which could indeed be met.

It is widely accepted that Herbart played a major part in promoting the notion of an unconscious level of mental life; although this was already present in Kantian and Idealist metaphysics Herbart moves towards rendering it – in principle, anyway – amenable to naturalistic enquiry. More specifically in this context, his influence on Freud has been a matter of considerable debate[12]. His continued development of the concept of 'apperception' and his introduction of the idea of the 'limen', which became central to psychophysics, constitute Herbart's major conceptual innovations at the theoretical level. Dunkel (1970) also notes that Herbart was opposed to the idea of presiding faculties, though not, presumably, to Kant's functionalist version of them. His reaction against Kant (whom he succeeded at Königsberg) was, in fact, on a fairly limited front in that he accepted the central doctrines that the soul as such cannot be known, and that Psychology could not be experimental.

What is usually ignored in recent histories is that for the nineteenth century Herbart's major claim to fame was not his theoretical Psychology but his Educational Psychology. (Indeed, the British Library Catalogue lists numerous English translations of his educational work, mostly during the 1890–1910 period, but not one of his Psychological ones.) The relationship between these two sides of his work is not easy to disentangle. His educational theory is certainly concerned with the necessity of providing contexts and frameworks to facilitate the growth and organization of the child's knowledge – an approach which involves the idea of strengthening, and appropriately fusing, the child's repertoire of *Vorstellungen*. On the other hand, it also represents a direct continuation and development of the tradition of Rousseau and Pestalozzi (whom he knew), while in its concerns with the cultural context of development, the developmental process and particularly the creation and shaping of the child's will, its agenda has affinities with the Idealist programme. Herbart's pedagogical ideas were developed before his major philosophical works, and his experience in the educational field formed the experiential basis for the Psychological system propounded in the latter. Dunkel nevertheless concludes that it would be wrong to see him as turning to Psychology only in 1816, or to imply 'that his psychological theory was cobbled up simply as a justification for his pedagogy'[13]. John Davidson (1906) argued that Herbart's pedagogy was fundamentally inconsistent with his Psychology and philosophy, and that his practical pedagogic position is Leibnizian rather than Kantian. His earliest pedagogical writings date from the first decade of the century[14]. While we cannot explore Herbart's educational thought in any depth here, we should note that his image of the child is of neither an idealized innocent nor an untamed sinful savage, but someone with a variety of instinctive impulses and desires which have to be mastered and controlled by acquiring a will. For Herbart himself, at least, the philosophical and pedagogic facets of his work were complementary, the principles of the latter being rooted in the former. Although it initially had limited success, Herbartian Educational Psychology later enjoyed a considerable vogue, especially in the USA in the 1890s[15].

Beneke has fared less well. His *Die neue Psychologie* (The New Psychology; 1845), while sceptical of premature attempts at mathematization, was a programmatic call for a genuinely experimental discipline (though he never undertook the experiments he proposed). Even so, he saw himself as heir to the Kantian 'critical' tradition: 'Beneke closed the circle which began with Kant. With Beneke the conception of psychology which had been originally criticized by Kant had been revised to the point where it now met the conception of science which had guided Kant's critique' (Leary, 1978, p. 119).

It must not be thought that this brief survey exhausts the number of German writers on '*Psychologie*' during this period. Morell (1853), virtually the only British would-be Psychologist espousing a basically *Idealrealismus* position, cites numerous figures now forgotten (except, in some cases, by Boring) by Anglophone Psychologists: Christian Weiss, Heinrich Steffans, Drobisch, Exner, Waitz, Baader, Schubert and Braubach. Since all of these appear to be espousing some variant of one of the positions discussed above, their continued omission from the present text should not, I hope, prove too misleading.

It was not via philosophers alone, however, that the German empirical tradition was carried. The influence of Kant, the 'Sage of Königsberg', extended throughout all aspects of German thought, scientific as much as philosophical. He was (and to some extent remains) the common point of reference for German intellectual culture as a whole. For Psychology, the other route by which his influence was mediated was physiology. It is essential to stress this, since the arrival of 'scientific Psychology' with Fechner and Wundt was the product of a final meeting of the two lineages – an outcome to which *Idealrealismus* thinkers such as Lotze[16] had long aspired.

2 German Psychophysiology

The relationship between physiology and philosophy had long been closer in Germany than elsewhere. Stahl himself had finally allowed his metaphysics to swamp his physiology, while Unzer took pains to reconcile his views of cerebral functioning with Baumgarten's philosophical system. Kant's influence reinforced, but did not initiate, this intimacy. Between the turn of the century and Helmholtz's measurement of the speed of neural transmission in 1850 Germany continued to lead (though not to monopolize) European neurophysiological research. For Psychology this has a twofold significance: first, methodologically, it provided a research paradigm for experimental Psychology; secondly, neurological work on the senses (extended, to a slight degree, to behaviour as well) provided German experimental Psychology with much of its initial content, whether in the form of Fechner's extension of E.H. Weber's work on tactile discrimination and judgement, Wundt's research on reaction time[17], or Helmholtz's extensive researches on perception. The transformation of these aspects of physiology into Psychology was facilitated by the close connection between philosophy and biology which was maintained until a generation of more positivist materialist scientists came to the fore around the middle of the century. Even Helmholtz remained Kantian in his epistemological views. Philosophers such as Helmholtz's teacher Lotze could move easily between grand metaphysics and the findings of experimental physiology, between theories of the cosmos and theories of perception. A central figure in this was Müller, to whom we now turn.

(i) Johannes P. Müller (1801–58)

Müller's significance for Psychology is complex. As the father-figure of experimental physiology he initiates the German research tradition leading directly to Wundt and Helmholtz (who studied under him). The general character of subsequent German Psychology was thus greatly indebted to him, particularly methodologically (Danziger, 1990). With respect to the history of ideas, however, he is rather more transitional, using his new physiological research to address more traditional questions arising within the context of Kantian philosophy, always his point of departure. His work on perception, for example, attempts to reconcile Kantian nativism with the evidence for perceptual learning (especially with regard to space). His solution in this case is to differentiate between a 'general capacity' for spatial perception and learning how to deploy this capacity. Concentrating on the latter, he can then address the functional physiology of the external eye-muscles and optic nerves[18]. His most influential doctrine, derived in part from Sir Charles Bell (see below, Chapter 8), was that of 'specific nerve energies'. As Murphy and Kovach (1972) point out, there are certain affinities between this doctrine and phrenology, the difference being that in Müller's case the functional specialization is located peripherally rather than in the brain which, – following Flourens's work – Müller accepted lacked regional specialization. This doctrine held that the nerves themselves were specialized in terms of the kind of information they conveyed – sensations of light, sound, touch, motor-impulses, etc. He considered, but (wrongly, as it eventually turned out) rejected, the notion that the sites where modal differentiation occurred were the terminals in the brain. Müller also continued to ponder the mind–body problem, retaining an insistence on a 'mental principle' (localized in the brain) distinct from a pervasive 'vital principle'.

What we are seeing in Müller's work (most influentially in his two-volume *Handbuch der Physiologie des Menschen* (1833–40)) is an omnivorous and largely eclectic synthesis of physiological information gathered from all quarters which can serve as an authoritative central reference and starting point for physiological researchers throughout Europe. In the process, the involvement of the physiological with the psychological became ever more obvious, and as a result the incorporation of physiological into Psychological thought became patently inescapable. Nevertheless, crucial for the discipline's history though Müller may be, his conceptual innovations were limited and of short-lived duration.

The influence of E.H. Weber (1795–1878) is at once more

circumscribed and more directly specifiable, deriving from the concepts and methodologies he had introduced in his physiological researches on the senses, the most important of which, on the sense of touch, were published in 1834 and 1846. (Boring's extensive accounts of this work [1942, 1950] need not be repeated here.[19]) It is Weber who introduces the concept of 'just noticeable differences' (j.n.d.'s), and gives substance to Herbart's 'limen' or threshold concept. It is also in Weber's extension of physiological work to research on touch, taste and smell sensitivities that we find the first clear examples of experimental work which is Psychological in all but name[20]. It was left to the more mathematically sophisticated Fechner to convert this into a fullyfledged 'psychophysics' during the 1850s by devising a way of quantifying sensation itself. Only with Hermann von Helmholtz (1821–94) do we see physiology succeeding in largely extricating itself from the coils of metaphysical philosophy, and then only by espousing an adamantly positivistic reductionist philosophy of science of its own. Even so, Helmholtz remained an admirer of his *Idealrealismus* mentor, Lotze. Since it was under Helmholtz that Wundt began his research career the physiological entanglements of mid-century German Psychology extend to the very laboratories in which it was born. Helmholtz's major achievements, however, belong to the post-1850 period and are beyond our present remit.

The anti-metaphysical reaction in German, when it finally came, involved the adoption of an even more reductionist position than that which had characterized late-Enlightenment French *Idéologie*. This, according to Doerner (1981), is explained by the fact that in France (and Britain too) materialist Natural Philosophers had remained engaged with the underlying philosophical debates in which their work was grounded. This kept in view the sociopolitical dimensions of issues which this philosophy, as an avowedly liberating doctrine (especially in France), sought to address. German philosophy, by contrast, had successfully resisted both materialist Empiricism and the adoption of an expressly social reforming role. On the contrary, operating, as German philosophers did, in the setting of autocratic State-run feudal principalities, they invariably supported the status quo, and their radicalism took the form of a more introverted exploration of the individual (with Romanticism, and the cult of the lone Romantic hero, being the most extreme expression of this). This was productive, as we have seen, in terms of psychological ideas, but it meant that the anti-metaphysical backlash of the mid nineteenth century would take an extreme form, largely unleavened by Enlightenment humanitarian concerns, and fundamentally conservative politically. Ideologically, service to an authoritarian State remained the prevailing imperative.

3 Froebel's Educational Psychology

Education was one arena in which Romantic ideals exerted an important, and arguably more positive, influence. We have already noted the influence of Rousseau and Pestalozzi on Herbart. Another educationalist who pursued this tradition – albeit in a more high-flown, some claimed mystical, fashion – was Friedrich Froebel (1782–1852). His best known work, *The Education of Man*, first appeared in 1826, and was followed by more practical pedagogic works such as *Mother Songs* (1843; see also Froebel, 1862–83) and *Pedagogics of the Kindergarten*. The common Romantic image of education as akin to gardening found its most literal expression in the term 'kindergarten', a term Froebel introduced in 1840. Froebel's – now unacknowledged – legacy in popular culture, in addition to the kindergarten, is probably his widely misunderstood doctrine of 'free expression', still sometimes heard as a negative catch-all phrase to refer to 'progressive' approaches to education.

It would not be putting it too strongly to see in Froebel the real beginnings of the European tradition of empirical study of child development which led to Piaget. In 1914 E.R. Murray published a book, *Froebel as a Pioneer in Modern Psychology*, in which a plausible case is made out for the 'modern' character of Froebel's understanding of child development, which had, the author claimed, been overlooked by everyone except John Dewey[21]. There are, admittedly, problems with this thesis: (a) a demonstration of anticipation is different from a demonstration of influence; (b) the 'moderns' whom the author takes as a reference for comparison are Stout, Ward, McDougall, Lloyd Morgan and the now forgotten developmental psychologist Irving King. Of these, only Lloyd Morgan (possibly) would now be seen as typifying the mainstream 'modern' tradition. And (c) the case rests, in places, on a certain amount of retrospective reinterpretation. Even so, when one discovers that Froebel postulated a 'sucking-in stage' where the child 'makes the external internal', one cannot help but be impressed! The five areas in which Murray sees Froebel as most clearly anticipating modern (i.e. 1914 British) Psychology are:

> 1. his doctrine of the 'tri-unity' of action, feeling and thought as inseparable aspects of conscious life – this is easy to relate to G.F.Stout's 'noetic synthesis' notion;
> 2. his intense empirical study of early mental activity and definition of the will – again Stout's is an obvious contemporary point of comparison in the case of 'will';
> 3. his conception of earliest consciousness as an undifferentiated whole;
> 4. his recognition of the importance of action in feeling as well as perception (i.e. in emotional as well as perceptual maturation);
> 5. his 'supremely complete' account of instinct.
>
> (adopted from Murray, *op. cit.*, p. 10)

Froebel's broad position is a fairly orthodox *Naturphilosophie*, one involving an evolutionary process of striving towards perfection, and a triad of Love, Life and Light corresponding to humanity, Nature and God respectively, manifested psychologically as feeling, doing (the will) and thinking. When it comes down to details, however, Froebel has considerable insight and empathy, seeing the child maturing actively in interaction with its environment and stressing the constructive nature of its mental activity. The advent of language enables the child to begin organizing its experience in ever more complex ways. The child, in imitating, is to be understood not just as reproducing a stimulus, but as seeking a new experience. And the role of 'expression' is central, because in expression:

> The child . . . strives to make his inner life outwardly objective and thus perceptible, and so to become conscious of it, to see it mirrored in the outward phenomena. It is for this reason that the child tries to do himself whatever he sees done. (Froebel, quoted in Murray, *op. cit.*, p. 51)

For Froebel the 'tri-unity' of action, feeling and thought is not mere metaphysical doctrine but has direct relevance to education and child-rearing. It implies that they cannot be developed in isolation, that it makes no sense to try and separate the teaching of, say, perceptual skills from thinking ones, or to separate either from the development of emotional responses. Thus in his own teaching practice he strove constantly to combine all three, and saw education's task as ensuring their full, balanced and integrated maturation. From the earliest stages of infancy the child *actively* differentiates, from an initially undifferentiated continuum of experience, the 'three great perceptions' of space, time and objects, as well as of itself and others. The mother, interacting with the child, should (and instinctively does) incorporate all three aspects of consciousness in her games and caretaking activities – teaching it simultaneously to see new things, to respond emotionally to them and to relate them to other things (thinking).

On occasions, as with the 'sucking-in stage', we seem, on Murray's account, to find Froebel on the verge of various modern doctrines – the sight of an object immediately triggers an activity towards it in a way reminiscent of the Gibsonian notion of 'affordances'; there is even a hint of Vygotskian 'scaffolding' to his recognition of the importance of the mother talking to her baby before it can understand language, while the cycle of receiving and reacting on 'impressions' and actively organizing and reorganizing consciousness is distinctly proto-Piagetian. For all his stress on innate needs and instincts, Froebel understands that the forms in which these will manifest themselves depend on the child's environment and the nature of the stimulation it receives. It is clear that Froebel avidly sought observational accounts of child behaviour, and tried to base his Psychological doctrines on these, albeit within the framework of a fairly mystical religious metaphysics.

Like Herbart's educational ideas, Froebel's methods became widely disseminated later in the century, the first kindergarten in England being founded in Fitzroy Square, London in 1854, one in Dublin in 1862, and the Froebel Society of London – which published a journal *Child Life* – in 1874. *The Education of Man* was translated into English by W.N. Hailmann, 'Superintendent of Schools at La Porte, Indiana', and published in New York in 1887.

The popularity of Herbart and Froebel in the USA at this time raises the question of their influence on the supposed 'founding' of child Psychology there under G. Stanley Hall at Johns Hopkins University in the 1880s (and later at Clark University). At the very least they would have had some role in preparing the cultural ground for Hall's project, while it is hard to imagine that during his sojourn in Germany Hall did not encounter their ideas. For Hall they were both, however, in some opposition camp[22]. What we see as the 'permissiveness' of Froebel's system must be viewed in the counterbalancing context of the general authoritarianism of bourgeois German domestic life; transferred to North America, it perhaps slid only too easily into parents living for their children, as Hall sarcastically observes in passing[23]. The rejection of Froebel as mystical and sentimental seems to have prevented his genuine insights from being appreciated, scattered as they often were in practical books for teachers, mothers, and kindergarten workers. Some of his ideas obviously filtered through unascribed as part of conventional pedagogic wisdom, but Murray's attempt to resurrect him as a prophet of modern child Psychology was – not surprisingly, given its inopportune publishing date – unsuccessful. If G.S. Hall's early hostility also assisted Froebel's long exclusion from the canon, a reappraisal of the case therein mounted would nevertheless appear to be overdue.

4 German Psychiatry

The evaluation of psychiatric thought presents serious problems. The traditional histories of Zilboorg (1941) and Alexander and Selesnick (1966), while strong on factual information appear naive in their interpretational stance in the wake of Foucault *et al.*; on the other hand, especially in the German case, taking on board the complexities of the cultural situation as expounded by Doerner (1981; German 1969) is simply impractical. To talk of Reil and Heinroth as a 'romantic reaction', as Alexander and Selesnick do, is obviously unacceptable, but to explain fully why Reil's Romanticism was not a simple 'reaction' of spiritual sensitivity to some dominant materialist status quo would involve us not only in explaining that there was no such status quo in Germany (and why), but also in explicating such propositions as:

> In Reil, the essential motive of Western psychiatry, in the reflexive self-consciousness of a bourgeois society producing its own sufferings, developed out of the contrast to the savage, to man in his natural state, still largely identical with his own body. (Doerner, 1981, p. 201)

Two contextual points must nevertheless be stressed. First, in Britain and France pressures for reform in the management of lunacy were embedded in the wider reform programmes being advocated by a newly empowered bourgeoisie. Insanity thus presented a major challenge to reformers infused with a sense of the possibilities of change at both individual and social levels. Hence the management priority shifted from coercive external control to developing a potential for internalized self-control (see below, pp. 351–2). By contrast, as Doerner argues in considerable detail, the German middle classes never experienced or achieved social and political power until much later in the nineteenth century. The priority in treating the insane thus remained at the level of public protection from the threat they presented to social order or, in so far as their cure was given priority, their utility to the State as a labour force. Secondly, stemming from this, whereas leading British and French reformers were actively engaged in treating the 'lunatic poor', German writers on madness tended to have little direct involvement in actually managing and treating the conditions about which they wrote. Additionally, it is vital to understand that in Germany at the turn of the century psychopathology was considered to be as much, or even more, the province of the philosopher than of the physician – it was the philosopher who was the expert on the Mind and the vicissitudes of Reason. Even Kant was prepared to hold forth confidently on madness, and argued that the job of expert witness in court cases involving insanity rightly belonged to the philosopher. This situation, too, was uniquely German. As ever, then, but with a special intensity, German psychiatric theorists are operating in terms of Kantian or post-Kantian philosophical frameworks, a factor to which we will return.

In the end it is perhaps more important for us to understand the German psychiatric tradition than either the French or the British ones, since it is this lineage that eventually produces Freud, Jung, Kraepelin and Kretschmer – produces, in fact, almost all the clinical Psychologies that have been most influential on modern Psychology in general – including, in Jaspers and Binswanger, its existential wing. Can we find any clues in this period as to why German psychiatry would eventually prove so conceptually prolific?

In attempting to answer this I shall focus on three figures only, all of whom are generally considered to be major contributors to psychiatry's development in Germany during the first half of the nineteenth century: Johann Christian Reil, Johann Christian Heinroth and Wilhelm Griesinger. Furthermore, I shall be concerned primarily with their theoretical ideas rather than their ideas regarding therapy (excepting Reil, in whom they are central).

(i) Johann Christian Reil (1759–1813)

Reil's *Rhapsodien über die Anwendung der psychischen Curmethode auf Geisteszerrüttungen* (Rhapsodies about the Application of Psychotherapy to Mental Disturbances) of 1803 is the most extreme statement of the Romantic view of mental illness. Considered the founding text of German psychiatry (the term *Psychiaterie* was introduced by Reil), it espouses a fundamentally psychological approach to madness. Physical factors, while implicated, are seen more as the consequence than the cause of madness – or at least, as far as the brain is concerned, as curable by psychological change. The unifying concept in all this was the universally pervasive *Lebenskraft* or 'life-force', of which consciousness was the highest manifestation. Physically, madness involves disruption of the nervous system, the senses or the brain, a disruption which renders the soul rudderless as the synthesis of consciousness is lost. But madness is also a product of modern society's alienation from Nature, the internal physical disruptions reflecting the disruptive, unnatural conditions of modern life; hence the physician's task is somehow to re-establish Nature within the patient. The consequent emphasis Reil places on treatments calculated to change the lunatic psychologically (by re-establishing inner balance, negating contradictions and re-establishing the rational synthesis of consciousness) earned him high praise from historians such as Zilboorg and Alexander & Selesnick: for the former his therapeutic methods were ahead of their time; while for the latter his system is part of the valuable Romantic reassertion of the need to address inner conflict as well as the conflict between 'man' and the external world.

Doerner's picture, by contrast, is somewhat sourer. Unlike Battie and Pinel:

> he never made an effort to acquaint himself firsthand with the

> deranged poor, to join their side, as it were, before making theoretical pronouncements about them. He had practically no experience with the mentally deranged when he wrote his basically poetic, literary anthropology. (1981, p. 200)

Reil was indeed a humanitarian in spirit, but Doerner is less forgiving than his predecessors regarding the exotic forms of 'non-injurious torture' which he proposed as therapeutic methods. In some of his passages we enter a world of megalomaniac Gothic fantasy as the therapist ruthlessly assails the lunatic's recalcitrant soul with counterbalancing insane fantasies of his own:

> Hoist the patient by a tackle block to a high vault so that he, like Absolom, may hover between heaven and earth; fire a cannon near him, approach him grimly with white-hot irons, hurl him into raging torrents, throw him in front of ferocious beasts . . . or let him sail through the air on fire-spewing dragons. A subterranean crypt, containing all the horrors ever seen in the realm of the ruler of hell, may be advisable, or perhaps a magic temple, in which, amid solemn music, the enchantment of a charming sorceress conjures up one glorious vision after another out of thin air. (quoted in Doerner, *ibid.*, p. 205)

(In 1968 we'd have been queuing up to get in.) In Britain the 'moral therapist' Francis Willis based his method on 'a wholesome sense of fear', deemed necessary to re-establish in the patient a contact with reality, but the cold douche, the stern eye, the spinning chair and the like were no match for Reil's (mostly unrealized) theatrical prescriptions. More economical and down-to-earth methods such as immersion in tubs of live eels, whipping with nettles and 'walking across flimsy bridges' also figure in his repertoire. There is a mingled sense of desperation and sadism in all this – the patient's own pathetic plight offers the therapist a pretext for uninhibited projection and acting out of his own soul's embattlement with the forces of unreason.

Even if Reil's direct encounters with the mentally disturbed were minimal, he discussed many forms of psychopathology which remained largely unattended to until much later, such as split consciousness and what are now termed 'psychoneuroses', as well as coming close to recognizing the role of guilt in their aetiology. Nor were all his proposed therapies cruel; anticipations of psychodrama and sex therapy might also be found, while his utopian plans for the ideal mental hospital stress beautiful and peaceful surroundings, in line with the goal of harmonizing the patient with unconflicted Nature.

Reil's emphasis on psychological methods and the psychological nature of madness was more thoroughgoing than that of his predecessors. His exuberant therapeutic fantasies also at least established the notion of some creative *engagement* with the insane rather than an objectifying distancing. But for Reil the meaning of madness remains a philosophical challenge; it is a phenomenon laden with metaphysical implications. When he wrote the *Rhapsodien* his Romanticism was still balanced by a need to address the physical, derived from his considerable expertise as a practising anatomical researcher and physician. Later he became a full convert to Schelling's Idealist *Naturphilosophie*, and wrote no further significant works on insanity. Even if his successors backtracked from his excesses, Reil's work remained an acknowledged landmark for German psychiatry, and we may surely, albeit in confused form, discern a concept of the psychotherapist's task which Freudian psychodynamic theories brought to the forefront of that tradition a century later.

(ii) Johann Christian Heinroth (1773–1843)

The psychological nature of madness soon received even greater emphasis in Heinroth's *Lehrbuch der Störungen des Seelenlebens* (a rough translation would be 'Textbook of Disorders of the Soul') (1818). The two features of this which it is appropriate to stress here are (a) his notion of madness as having its source in 'sin'; and (b) his nosology, which influenced James Cowles Prichard's concept of 'moral insanity' (see below, pp. 353–4). Heinroth's system is deeply embedded in a pious, and politically conservative, Christian metaphysics. In internalist history terms there is an unavoidable temptation to interpret it, as Alexander and Selesnick do, as structurally anticipating Freud. His tripartite division of the mind as comprising a lowest hedonistic level of instinctual forces, a central ego and a higher level of 'conscience', the '*Über-uns*', maps only too neatly on to the id, ego and superego of psychoanalysis. But we must remember that this division is ubiquitous, in various forms, throughout German thought at this time (cf. Froebel's 'tri-unity' above, pp. 307–8). What is distinctive about Heinroth's model is the orthodox religious framework in which the division is construed. Consciousness, he holds, evolves upwards through these three successive levels, towards a final submission to the dictates of the last, which is the 'sole path to God'[24]. Madness results from a blockage of this ascent, a blockage which can originate only in the individual's rejection or infringement of the demands of this Divinely guided, fully rational conscience – in a word, sin. This refers not so much to overt sinful acts as to a felt inner disobedience, again easily translatable into 'sense of guilt'. The analogies with psychoanalysis, even if genuine, are superficial – the Freudian superego is not exclusively rational, and abasement to its dictates can itself be a source of pathology; nor is it the intrapsychic representative of a transpersonal divinity. More broadly, the psychoanalytic locus of rational control and integration is the ego, not the superego, nor does it accept *Naturphilosophie*'s notion of a pervasive upwardly striving spiritual dynamic. Finally, the essence of sin for Heinroth is selfishness rather than sex.

In practice this model yielded little by way of therapeutic innovation other than an even more rigorous tightening up of the orthodox procedures aimed at securing the therapist's physical and psychological omnipotence over the patient. Taken in conjunction with his views on society at large and his politics, Heinroth's is clearly a highly authoritarian 'law-and-order' Psychology, in which sin itself becomes pathology. Ironically this has some pay-offs in fudging the erstwhile clarity of the sanity–insanity boundary and in its insistence on the need for a holistic account of personality functioning and structure.

Heinroth's analysis also provides the basis for a systematic nosology, since disorders can occur at each of the three levels. Since they can take the form of either depression or excitation this yields six basic categories, although his further subdivisions identified thirty-six[25]. Disorders of the lowest level, relating to passions and feelings (presumably stemming from 'sins' committed regarding these), therefore take the form of either dejection and melancholy or violent emotions; disorders of the ego or will are typically either 'moral imbecility' or *Tollheit*, rage and frenzy, while those of reason itself, stemming from directly intellectual sins, yield imbecility or mental illusions and monomania. He also offered a six-stage 'evolutionary history of mental disorders' corresponding to these, starting from excitatory disorders of the passions in the 'heroic age' and finishing with depressive disorders of the intellect – foolishness and idiocy – reflecting 'the present degenerate, licentious, physically and morally enfeebled modern era'[26].

Heinroth's Christianized version of post-Kantian Idealism was culturally appealing, and he became the first German to acquire an academic professorship as a specialist psychiatrist. If his direct experience of treating the insane was more extensive than Reil's, it was nevertheless 'not very intensive' according to Doerner,[27] and before the publication of his book it was in unreformed prison and orphanage contexts.

An enduring legacy of Heinrothian ideas is hard to identify, although his model may have served as a kind of latent template for structuring the thinking of later psychodynamic theorists of a quite different kind. If so, its influence was well hidden; Freud cites neither Heinroth nor Reil in the *Studies on Hysteria* or the *Interpretation of Dreams*, nor is he mentioned in a number of works at hand by Jung and Janet. Ernest Jones derided the Romantic psychiatrists' 'unbalanced megalomaniac emotionalism'[28]. The surface picture of events is rather that post-1850 there was a wholesale condemnation of Romantic psychiatry in Germany, as the profession adopted ever more physicalist and medical-classificatory approaches in an atmosphere of therapeutic pessimism. Freud's initial training under the latter regime and the critical role of his encounter with French psychiatry reinforce this version of events. If there is a contrary subtext it pertains not to specific doctrines but to a persisting awareness of the possibility of some kind of therapeutic project focusing on the dynamics of the individual mind. Assuming that the reaction against Romanticism was as intense as the Ernest Jones quote suggests, this in itself signifies acknowledgement of some shared focus of concern. Might it not, then, be interpreted as a rejection of the terms in which Romanticism couched and implemented the project of 'psychotherapy', rather than the project itself? But if the Romantics, as appears to be the case, initiated that project, this surely leaves them with a large residue of credit.

(iii) Wilhelm Griesinger (1817–68)

The next generation did not directly abandon the analysis of the psychological character of madness, but in Griesinger's *Mental Pathology and Therapeutics* (1845, 2nd edn 1861, English transl. 1867) this analysis is seen as necessary in lieu of physiological knowledge:

> A classification of mental diseases according to their nature, that is, according to the anatomical changes of the brain which lie at their foundation – is, at the present time, impossible. (Griesinger, 1867 edn, p. 206)

It would be an error, however, to see Griesinger's position merely as transitional towards a later physiologically orientated orthodoxy. Doerner credits him with formulating 'the first comprehensive theoretical and practical paradigm of psychiatric science in Germany'[29], but from his extended ensuing attempt at pinning down Griesinger's significance, he emerges as an ambiguous, protean figure who has been interpreted in quite different ways until the present day. This ambiguity was apparent almost from the start, Griesinger was attacked as overly positivist and materialist by the metaphysically orientated establishment and overly philosophical by more positivist and reductionist physiologists. His psychiatric career continued after the publication of *Mental Pathology*, although this remained his most important publication, and he succeeded in introducing radical changes in the institutional practice of psychiatry within Germany, abandoning forcible restraint, integrating psychiatry into neurological medicine in general, and by this extending its 'catchment area' to categories of middle-class neurotic patient who had hitherto eluded attention.

The appearance of Griesinger's book coincided with and reflected a growing hostility among younger members of the profession towards an establishment they saw as infusing into madness an unwarranted philosophical significance. This was part and parcel of the wider mid-century disentanglement of German natural science from the post-Kantian metaphysical frameworks in which it had previously been conducted. Forms of liberation are necessarily conditioned by those of oppression, and the situation in mid-nineteenth-century Germany was rather the reverse of that which has obtained in the present century. If the contemporary enemy has been felt to be a dehumanizing, objectifying, mechanistic approach to madness which denies the authenticity of individual phenomenological experience and what we might broadly term 'spiritual' strivings towards wholeness, the enemy in mid-nineteenth-century Germany was an oppressive insistence on the moral and spiritual significance of the lunatic's plight. In that context 'liberation' involved a demystification of madness, an earthing of the therapist's attention to the pathetic and banal nature of most psychopathology, and the need for practical terms in which to address it.

In the event, Griesinger performs a successful balancing act. He accepts in principle that madness is physiological but given our ignorance of physiology, we have to approach it psychologically. This approach must, however, be purged of the moral metaphysical dimension which had until then dominated it. The psychological manifestations of mental disorder thereby come under much closer empirical scrutiny, and the classification of madness is in terms of psychological symptoms.

Griesinger believed that underlying madness was a single dynamic process, that its most extreme forms were but the last, and incurable, stage of a process which began with milder, curable forms of mental distress. The 'two grand groups' of mental illness are, first, those characterized by 'morbid production, governing, and persistence of emotions and emotional states'[30] and, second, disorders of the intellect and will 'which do *not* (any longer) proceed from a ruling emotional state, but exhibit, without profound and emotional excitement, an *independent*, tranquil, *false mode of thought* and of *will* (usually with the predominant character of mental weakness)'[31]. The former precede the latter, which in turn are their consequences and 'terminations'. There is, then, a single 'morbid process'. It is widely accepted that in his elaboration of this Griesinger identified what later acquired the term 'manic depression'. His nosology differentiates between 'anomalies' of 'disposition, desires and will', of 'intellect' and of 'sensorial functions, movements and conduct'[32]. This, of course, reproduces yet again the familiar triad, although emotions as such seem to have been promoted from the lowest level to join the will at the middle one. Conditions produced during the first stage – melancholy, mania and monomania – are curable, rarely being accompanied by organic alteration; whereas chronic mania and dementia, characteristic of the second stage, involving 'secondary lesions', are generally incurable. The first form in which the morbid process manifests itself is 'hypochondria', marked by mercurial feelings of bodily distress; this is succeeded by various degrees of 'melancholia'.

By 1867 his British translators were billing Griesinger as 'essentially the representative and the acknowledged leader of the modern German School of Medical Psychiatry'[33]. While his importance for German psychiatry is obviously paramount, it is more difficult to identify his specifically Psychological significance[34]. There are certainly connections to Freud in that Griesinger was crucial in providing the psychiatry of the German-speaking world with the university-based framework in which his training was undertaken (as well as bringing middle-class neuroses into the open). This framework was both theoretical, in its commitment to a neurological aetiology of mental illness, and institutional, in that it brought psychiatry under the aegis of university-centred neurological medicine (or, more accurately, Griesinger's medical 'imperialism' assimilated neurological medicine into psychiatry). But by Freud's time Griesinger's initial vision of a harmoniously integrated psychiatry in which psychological understanding and physiological knowledge mutually reinforced each other had largely faded and been replaced by the positivistic reductionism of neurologists such as Freud's teacher Brücke, a graduate, as it were, of the Helmholtz–Du Bois-Reymond school of physicochemical materialists who, in their academic youth, had sought to sever German science from metaphysics.

From the viewpoint of the historian of Psychology, the impact of early-nineteenth-century German Psychiatry appears very much delayed. Decker (1977) paints a sombre picture of the psychiatric status quo as Freud encountered it: it has become a therapeutically impotent medical subdiscipline preoccupied with attempting to classify varieties of mental illness and disease in physiological terms resembling the classification of physical disease. The boundaries between sane and insane have became rigidly ossified again, and the relevance of studies of the 'normal' (Psychology) to the understanding of the abnormal, and vice versa, is not recognized. Only rarely, and rather late, does an orthodox German psychologist such as Gustav Störring (1907) or a psychiatrist (e.g. Kraepelin) attempt to bridge the gap between Wundtian Psychology and contemporary psychiatry. Such psychological ideas as German psychiatry produced during the early nineteenth century played little direct role in the founding of Psychology, but rather lay dormant until the issues they were addressing resurfaced at the beginning of the twentieth century. By this time, however, they seemed largely obsolete and misguided to those reconnecting the two disciplines.

Yet it remains true that it is in German psychiatry and clinical Psychology that the most profound tensions of modern Western psychology (in the subject-matter sense) were most patently manifested and most thoroughly articulated in the period up to the Second World War. The possibility of German-speaking psychiatry's simultaneous containment of Freud and Kretschmer, Jung and Kraepelin, Jaspers and the Jaensch twins, was created, I would argue, by the presence within it, from the first decades of the previous century, of a tension between its 'psychological' and 'physiological' wings. How can we account for this presence? Given the complex necessary sociocultural conditions detailed by Doerner, a more immediate, proximate explanation lies in the dominating role which these conditions led German philosophy to assume in relation to the whole of German academic and scientific life. Before the 1840s at the earliest it was inconceivable that any German researcher, in whatever field of the *Geisteswissenschaften* or *Naturwissenschaften*, could fail to set his (invariably) work within the context of one or other of the Kantian and post-Kantian systems. This being so, the construal of madness, or unreason, was initially inseparable from philosophical construals of reason, while the construal of physiological pathology was similarly inseparable from philosophical construals of the cosmic meaning of organic life. By mid century the presence within German psychiatry of a 'Romantic' strand was as ineradicable as the presence of that strand within German culture as a whole, even if this was only at the level (as in Freud) of an early emotional – and motivating – empathy with Goethe and Schiller rather than Reil and Heinroth.

Modern Psychology naturally sees the labours of Wundt and Fechner in an epoch-making light, but it is essential to remind ourselves that their Psychology was a project on a relatively minuscule scale compared to psychiatry and philosophy, and even to philology, a discipline practised in a mere handful of universities even in 1900, with no professors and no degrees and subservient to departments of philosophy. That being the case, its aspirations towards natural science status could be realized only in close alliance with basic physiological research focusing on the elementary micropsychological phenomena which formed the subject matter of psychophysics, carefully demarcating its concerns *qua* experimental science from those of the established *Geisteswissenschaften*. Precisely because it sought to address the central subject of philosophy, consciousness, 'scientifically', it had systematically to avoid the minefield of live metaphysical issues, saying as little as possible about the mind–body relationship, the meaning of life, Man's place in the cosmos, reason, the will, or morality. When tackling these the psychologist would be careful to wear a quite different professional hat. Psychiatric ideas therefore had no place in the pioneer German experimental psychologist's conceptual repertoire. This contrasts with the British situation where, as we shall see, the discipline originated outside the academic institutional framework and on a far more eclectic base (which did *not*, though, include psychophysics).

In conclusion, then, the influential psychological ideas originating within German psychiatry during this period are of two contrasting kinds: at the micro-level there are clear preliminary identifications of specific syndromes such as manic depression (Griesinger) and multiple personality (Reil); at the macro-level there is the concept of the psychotherapeutic project itself, albeit in Romantic terms which later psychotherapists vehemently rejected. As for the vast intervening region of middle-range concepts and models, however, it appears to have left little by way of a visible legacy.

5 A Note on Völkerpsychologie

Alongside the appearance of experimental 'physiological' Psychology, the 1850s and 1860s also saw the origins of a distinctive German tradition of *Völkerpsychologie*; the canonical texts were the early volumes of Haim Steinthal and Moritz Lazarus's journal *Zeitschrift für Völkerpsychologie und Sprachwissenschaft* (1860–90). As is well known, Wundt also saw this as part of his brief, but was careful to differentiate it as belonging to the *Geisteswissenschaften*, distinct from scientific, laboratory-based experimental Psychology. The interests of *Völkerpsychologie* were similar in some respects to those of later Anglophone Social Psychology, but it would be erroneous to conflate the two; the German discipline embraced much philology and anthropology, concerning itself principally with language, ethnology, mythology, folk customs and folklore[35]. The roots of this, once again, lie in late-eighteenth-century and post-Kantian philosophy. *Anthropologie*, for instance, had established itself in the last quarter of the eighteenth century in the work of philosophers such as Herder and Kant, and been empirically pioneered by Baron von Blumenbach. Inspired in part by Herder's work, from the 1820s onwards the Grimm brothers, and then Franz Bopp, had succeeded in establishing philology as a major discipline. Karpf (1932) identifies the more immediate origins of *Völkerpsychologie* in the joint influence of Herbart and Hegel. These developments must, however, remain unexplored in the present volume, since a discussion their influence on Psychological thought would require us to go too far into the latter half of the century and beyond.

Conclusion

The strong institutional base of German academic and scientific life resulted in a far more consciously articulated and programmatic approach to the development of the human and social sciences generally than was possible elsewhere. The first half of the nineteenth century sees a plethora of publications with *Psychologie* in their titles, and from Kant onwards philosophers and educationalists produce a variety of blueprints for the putative discipline. These invariably involve some demonstration of the possibility of such a discipline within the terms of a metaphysical framework, and the derivation from this of essentially *a prioristic* accounts of the nature of mind as a possible object of investigation. Clear empirical research agendas rarely follow. These accounts are not so much Psychological theories in their own right as philosophical systems. Nevertheless, this prolonged tussle with the nature of mind and consciousness, their structure, their dynamics, their cosmic and evolutionary significance, and the means by which such issues might be addressed, produced a conceptual repertoire more extensive and subtle than those being deployed by contemporary British and French philosophers.

Since the reaction against metaphysics by natural scientists in the 1840s had to be conducted within the same institutional arenas as those occupied by their opponents (under whom they studied and alongside whom they taught), the eventual shift was more in the nature of a transformation of a single collective enterprise than a revolutionary replacement of one set of paradigms by autonomous and distinct alternatives. Their education and culture ensured that German scientists continued to remain philosophically informed, and even philosophically engaged, until the rise of the Third Reich. As a discipline, German experimental Psychology appears to arise as the outcome of the identification, within the confusing matrix of existing philosophical Psychologies, of a number of relatively discrete micro-topics amenable to research by the new experimental methods being developed in physiology. Even inserting a wedge-end this thin between physiology and philosophy was in practice problematical and was achieved primarily by the indefatigable policing of the boundaries of his infant discipline by the tireless workaholic Wilhelm Wundt. Given the wide spectrum of psychological interests within German academic and scientific culture at this time, what is most notable is over how extremely limited a section of this spectrum the new German Psychology managed to establish intellectual property rights. Personality, language, madness, education, cognition, child development and learning are all left aside, while even perception remains shared with physiology. All these topics were, however, being explored by educationalists, philologists, psychiatrists, philosophers or natural historians. But these other explorations of the psychological were often oppressed by the suffocating weight of philosophy's academic authority. Reconciliation between the explorer's ideas, findings and methods, and the metaphysical school to which he (without exception) owed allegiance was constantly required. Of those we have looked at, only the educational ideas of Froebel, and to a lesser extent Herbart, might be considered as an exception – and then, in Froebel's case, because the immediately practical nature of the work, and geographical isolation from academic centres of learning, enabled him to subordinate (at least to some extent) his *Naturphilosophie* to his data, rather than vice versa.

The image of Psychology's German début which I am proposing here differs from the one that is usually offered. In general it is seen as resulting from a meeting of philosophy and physiology, the two strands finally merging. By contrast, I would see it as arising initially almost unnoticed in the interstices of these established and continuing research projects. Historians of the discipline have tended to be overly Psychology-centric in the story they tell. The creation of German experimental Psychology had little effect on German philosophy, which continued to offer rival accounts of the psychological and harass the Wundtian project (e.g. Dilthey). The German philosophical tradition, for its part, would continue to affect Psychology through the work of Avernarius, Brentano, Mach and Husserl, while the focus on Wundt has led to a retrospective marginalization of the psychological work of slightly later figures such as G.E. Müller, W. Preyer, W.F. Volkmann and Carl Stumpf[36]. Clearly, the influence of the Psychological ideas developed in the first half of the century was not, in the first instance, mediated via Wundtian Psychology. Nor was German Psychology initially a response to socioeconomic management pressures, being tangentially involved at best in applying its findings beyond the laboratory.

Perhaps we have here one of those rare cases where the weight of explanation for a major development in the history of science does rest on a single individual, namely Wilhelm Wundt. A Doerner-like contextual analysis would undoubtedly reveal much about why German experimental Psychology emerged when and where it did. Yet it is difficult to see Wundt as initially representing any widely present movement heading inexorably towards the enterprise he actually inaugurated, either within or outside German academia. This is not to deny that the appearance of an empirical Psychology as such was an inevitable outcome of the intellectual and social dynamics in play, from Beneke and Herbart onwards philosophers had aspired towards it, while physiologists since Weber had been expanding their territory to include psychophysical and basic behavioural phenomena. In the anti-metaphysical mid-century climate, some kind of meeting of the two was only to be expected.

But there are two quite feasible alternative forms which the outcome of such a meeting might have taken in Wundt's absence. First, physiology could have continued to expand into psychophysics and behavioural analysis unopposed but without seeking introspectively to address the nature of consciousness. Secondly, the *Völkerpsychologie* movement might have expanded its ambitions downwards, so to speak, to capture the study of the psychological in general from philosophy, and evolved empirical methods to do so. In the first case German Psychology as such would not have appeared at this point, in the latter it would have assumed a far broader character. By astutely snatching the psychophysical from physiology and using it to implement the longstanding *philosophical* project for a science specifically of consciousness, Wundt also pre-empted the second move by operating on the *Naturwissenchaft* side of the great *Naturwissenschaft–Geisteswissenschaft* divide. That the verdict of history on the project he inaugurated, and continued to pursue in virtual isolation until the latter part of the century, has been so negative suggests that there was indeed perhaps something essentially idiosyncratic, if not eccentric, about the whole episode. Wundt's greatness (which I do not attempt to deny him) lay in the systematic way in which he was able to justify and develop the project, matters which we will have to leave aside here. My present suggestion is that in order to understand why it was in the form of Wundtian experimental Psychology that the discipline appeared in Germany rather than either of the other two routes being taken we will indeed, for once, have to focus on the man himself (and – who knows? – perhaps on his wife as well). Finally, these observations should, I must stress, be considered as provisional, pending a further exploration of the issues in Part II.

8
The British Route: The Nervous Empire

Introduction

In contrast with the physical sciences, John Stuart Mill observes, as late as 1843, that:

> . . . the laws of Mind, and, in even a greater degree, those of Society, are so far from having attained a similar state of even partial recognition, that it is still a controversy whether they are capable of becoming subjects of science in the strict sense of the term; and among those who are agreed on this point there reigns the most irreconcilable diversity on almost every other. (*Logic*, 8th edn, p. 546)

In this chapter we will consider the central ideas of some of these diverse parties and the process by which a degree of reconciliation sufficient for the emergence of a distinct – albeit still diverse – discipline of Psychology was achieved. First we must address the nature of this diversity. In many respects the British situation was more variegated than the university-centred German one. A sort of division of intellectual labour had evolved among those regarding the mind and human nature as their scientific or philosophical property. At one end of the spectrum were philosophers, who fell into three broad camps: the Associationists, Reid's heirs of the Scottish 'Common Sense' school, and those influenced by Kant and post-Kantian German philosophy. As representatives of these we may cite, respectively, James and John Stuart Mill, Dugald Stewart and both Sir William Hamilton and Samuel Taylor Coleridge. The boundaries between them are not always clear-cut; Sir William Hamilton's roots are in the Reidian tradition, for example, while Coleridge's intellectual influence on John Stuart Mill ought not to be underestimated[1]. The influential work of Thomas Brown has, we will see, affinities with all three. In addition there were numerous now forgotten writers such as John Abercrombie (1840, 10th edn) and Robert Mudie (1838) who espoused more hybrid and, often, more pious positions.

In science itself, the anti-Utilitarian philosophy of science of William Whewell (Master of Trinity College Cambridge) was immensely influential in the 1830s and 1840s (it was he who coined the word *scientist*, among many other new technical terms – an activity for which he had a particular flair). In reaction against metaphysics in general were, as previously discussed, the phrenologists such as – most eminently – George Combe, who sought to bring moral matters on to the scientific agenda. Not unsympathetic to the latter, and sometimes overlapping with them, were what we may call the proto-evolutionists and anthropologists such as William Lawrence, Robert Chambers and James Cowles Prichard. Nor should we forget that bolstering this perspective (though the immediate messages were often ambiguous) were a number of archaeological publications such as J.J.A. Worsaae's *The Primeval Antiquities of Denmark*[2] and, in the same year, A.H. Layard's *Nineveh and its Remains* – and behind them were the geologists, like Sir Charles Lyell, who were almost literally chipping away the traditional Judaeo-Christian cosmological framework[3].

At the hard 'scientific' end of the spectrum are physiologists concerned with psychophysiological matters, of whom Sir Charles Bell, Marshall Hall and W.B. Carpenter are the most notable, though far from the only, representatives. They were much less dominated than their German counterparts by metaphysical rationales for their work. It would none the less be false to see positions as located along a single philosophy–physiology continuum; psychiatry and educational theory continued to generate their own texts, while psychological issues were frequently tackled in genres such as medical works on gynaecology and infant care (including popular manuals), economics, education, criminology, art and aesthetics, linguistics (though the philosophical connection is very strong here) and, lest we forget, the novel. As far as non-human psychology is concerned, data on animal behaviour and the operation of 'instinct' were accumulating rapidly in zoology and natural history.

Ideas about human nature and our place in the universe were being reconceptualized on a number of fronts. The overall effect was to assimilate an increasing number of psychological issues into some kind of scientific framework – character and morality in the case of phrenology, sensation and movement in the case of physiology, madness in the case of psychiatry, and 'human nature' in general in the proto-evolutionary works of Lawrence and Chambers. Furthermore, as we saw in relation to phrenology, the need for such a move, with its promise of control and management of the phenomena so assmilated, was widely felt and acknowledged by those who were conscious of the problems facing the urbanized, industrialized society which Britain was rapidly becoming. Problems which a relatively stable village society could handle informally (e.g. subnormality) required managerial intervention in the new, demographically volatile conurbations.

If the grosser features of the situation are relatively easy to discern, the detail is often more difficult. Here we need to focus on the conceptual problems facing those involved in effecting these changes and conditioning their mutual relations. An outline of some main lines of tension will assist us in providing a more integrated examination of the diverse parties to which John Stuart Mill refers. Although they are often correlated, five dimensions of tension can, I think, be teased out as structuring the intellectual agendas of those addressing psychological issues during this period.

The first is that between – to put it at its simplest – the spiritual and the secular perspectives. This operates, of course, both between and within individual thinkers. While orthodox Christians may often remain dogmatically self-insulated from secular psychological perspectives, few among the generations coming to maturity after 1810 remained immune to the respective appeals of either (secular) science or (spiritual) Romanticism. Apart from Coleridge nobody, perhaps, in Britain attempted to fuse the two in quite such a fervent manner as we have seen German *Naturphilosophie* adopting, but even such a paradigm of secular thought as John Stuart Mill understood the need to pay Romanticism its due. Conversely, the essentially secular Phrenological movement felt bound to give the organ of spirituality an honoured bulge atop the skull, and, in Combe, to retain reassuring vestiges of at least a Deist, if not an orthodox Christian, cosmology. Much hinged, as we have seen already, on the notion of Natural Law, the emancipation of the concept from its Natural Religion connotations being a protracted process unravelling throughout our period. The Bridgewater Treatises constituted the final stand (at least of genuine scientific significance) of the stalwarts of the Argument from Design (the contributors did after all include Bell alongside Whewell and Buckland). Combe's merging of Moral with Natural Laws, discussed above, is a less orthodox attempt to hold the same line. In short, even the most materialist thinkers rarely (unlike the French *idéologues*) wished to serve iconoclastic reductionism, while at the other end of the spectrum few serious thinkers felt it possible to remain entirely disengaged from secular analyses of human nature. Neither party really welcomed the protracted erosion of the terms on which eighteenth-century British religion and science had been able to coexist.

Closely correlated with – but conceptually distinct from – the spiritual-secular tension is that between holistic and reductionist orientations. While both Christians and Romantics naturally viewed reductionism negatively, secular thinkers were divided. Associationists were keenly reductionist, and this was increasingly consistent with the position being adopted by positivist (or proto-positivist) physical scientists such as Ernst Brücke, Du Bois-Reymond and Carl Ludwig in Germany. Scientific progress seemed inseparable from the discovery of ways of accounting for macro-phenomena in terms of underlying micro-phenomena, and it was hard to see why a science of the mind or of human nature should be an exception. As we saw, Spencer's co-option of the Associationist principle as a central evolutionary mechanism provided a major theoretical basis for Psychology. Yet Spencer's position was hardly reductionist in any strict sense, for he does not claim macro-phenomena to be 'nothing but' aggregates of micro-phenomena; rather, they represent systems of 'relations' of sufficient complexity for new properties to emerge. John Stuart Mill also backtracked, in his footnotes to the 1869 edition of his father's *Analysis of the Phenomena of the Human Mind*, from more extreme reductionist positions, acknowledging emergent properties irreducible to those of apparent elements (e.g. the perception of a rotating colour-wheel as white). But the momentum of reductionism with respect to physiological phenomena was gathering pace and the issue would continue ever after to bedevil Psychology as it strove for both scientific credibility (which seemed to entail reductionism) and cultural credibility as a meaningful study of psychological phenomena (which seemed to entail holism). This tension is especially apparent in psychiatry, where the mainstream of the medical profession (e.g. James Cowles Prichard) are eager to advance physiological explanations against the psychological meanings of madness generated during the heyday of Moral Therapy.

Methodologically, this tension yielded a further, third, polarity between intuitionist approaches on the one side and Empiricist, analytical approaches on the other. Intuitionism retained a belief in sufficiency of the appeal to common experience as a criterion of a psychological proposition's validity, but again the scientific tide was running the other way; scientific truths were not obvious and had to be based on empirical 'facts'. Conceptually, the former continued to deploy an abstract philosophical vocabulary, while the latter (as in phrenology) tended to concretize and reify. It was not until towards the end of the century in the work of William James and Edmund Husserl, that modern phenomenological methods began to develop, especially in Germany – although Thomas Brown anticipates some of their problems.

Danziger (1990) argues that one particularly powerful methodological source for British Psychology was the social statistics tradition (going back ultimately to Petty and Graunt in the seventeenth century) which was being developed further by the Belgian Quetelet. By incorporating new mathematical concepts from probability theory (notably Poisson's notion of the normal distribution curve) this work provided a basis for the application and expansion of parametric statistical techniques within Psychology, first by Galton and Karl Pearson, and then across experimental Psychology as a whole. The salience of this methodology in Britain arose from the unparalleled importance which social statistics had acquired for bureaucratic and economic administrative purposes during the Industrial Revolution. Essentially a 'management' technology, its application to behavioural and psychological topics became inevitable as such issues moved up the administrative agenda. But this methodology was still in the future for the period under consideration, with the exceptions of lunatic asylum records and some efforts at establishing population norms for skull proportions within phrenology and anthropology. For the most part Empiricism remained a fairly unsystematic, eclectic but non-experimental matter of anecdotal gleaning and inferences from the latest physiological findings.

Fourthly, at a different level, a polarity between proto-evolutionary or historical and anti-evolutionary modes of explanation developed dramatically during the first half of the century. While Associationism was implicitly anti-evolutionary in view of its stress on environmental determinants of psychological phenomena, Spencer, as we have seen, was able to reconcile them. The main weight of anti-evolutionary thought was religious or philosophical – the most powerful opposition coming from Whewell, Paleyite Natural Theologians, and – albeit in a different sense – those influenced by the *Naturphilosophie* of Germans such as Oken. Within the evolutionary camp itself a further split was under way regarding the origin of human diversity. This is generally referred to as the monogenist–polygenist controversy. It was a core issue for all would-be human sciences, since it concerned the biological unity of the human race itself: were we a single species whose physical diversity was due to adaptations to differing conditions of life, or were some 'races' in fact different species? This debate would 'run and run' for the remainder of the century and beyond, reaching its greatest intensity from around the 1850s to the 1880s. Nor, of course, was it confined to Britain. Positions on this were determined by a complex mixture of religious, ideological and biological factors[4].

Finally, as a background to all these, was a pervasive, if far from clear-cut, political tension between conservatives and radicals. It would be misleading to translate this directly into modern Right–Left terms, since radicals included extreme *laissez-faire* thinkers such as Spencer as well as socialists like Robert Owen, while the conservative camp included Whewell, whose image of science verged on the Romantic[5]. The distinction is, rather, between those seeking reform and change in the context of some progressivist credo (be it humanitarian, evolutionary or socialist in character) and those striving to preserve existing social institutions, values and structures (whatever the basis of their antipathy to change). Translating this into differences in 'Psychological' thought is not easy, although secular thinkers such as the Utilitarians were of course radicals, polygenist evolutionary thinkers (e.g. James Hunt) were conservative (and pro-slavery) while, as we have seen, phrenology was quite ambiguous. Robert Owen can espouse an extreme environmentalism on the question of character-formation, but still sprinkle his texts with pious references to the Laws of God.

Early-nineteenth-century British proto-Psychological thought evolves, therefore, at the confluence of these tensions, which to a large extent operate within, as much as between, the psyches of those addressing psychological issues. And when this is the case, the result is as often an attempt at reconciliation as it is unambiguous espousal of a position at one end of a polarity. Bearing these tensions in mind, we can now consider a 'representative sample' of proto-Psychological thought in Britain during this period.

1 Philosophy

How far did the numerous philosophical positions being espoused at this time yield any genuinely new psychological ideas? As far as minor writers such as Abercrombie, Mudie and Upham are concerned, we have to admit straight away that they did not, and whatever role they played in creating a cultural climate congenial for the later labours of Bain and Spencer, their long-term intellectual impact has, as far as one can tell, been minimal. Given the virtually total neglect of this group by modern historians, one ought perhaps to be wary of too categorical a judgement. A scan through the Scots doctor John Abercrombie's *Intellectual Powers* (1840[1830]) does not provide grounds for optimism, even though he includes chapters on such psychological topics as the credibility of 'testimony', dreaming and insanity. He is firmly anti-metaphysical and eager to place 'the Science of Mind' on the basis of facts, but can dismiss the controversy about the nature of perception (as direct or indirect) thus:

> The mind can be compared to nothing in nature; it has been endowed by its Creator with a power of perceiving external things; but the manner in which it does so is entirely beyond our comprehension. (1840, p. 27)

Abercrombie writes as a physician, and is at his best when he is regaling the reader with medical anecdotes. Some move towards Psychology is discernible in his general orientation, but conceptually his text is unoriginal, resting mostly on Reidian orthodoxy and ending with a pious hope that the 'medical observer' may learn to 'cheer the bed of death with the prospect of immortality'. Abercrombie's book was highly popular as a source of information on current philosophical understanding of the mind (the 1840 edition was the tenth) and even Charles Darwin appears to have devoured it avidly at one point (he has many notes on it in the 'M' and 'N' notebooks).

The most significant conceptual developments during this period are those made by Thomas Brown, Sir William Hamilton, and John Stuart Mill.

(i) Thomas Brown (1778–1820)[6]

Brown's *Lectures on the Philosophy of the Human Mind* (1820) represent (a) a significant breakdown of the polarization between the approaches of the Reidian 'Common Sense' school and Associationism; and (b) an important further step towards a more clearly 'scientific' concept of the task of Philosophy of Mind as a branch of Natural Philosophy. It is in the context of the first of these, his attempted *rapprochement* between the two dominant British philosophical traditions, that his conceptual innovations occur. Although overtly he maintained loyalty to the Reidian school, his differences with Reid and Stewart, and his evident respect for much of Hume's analysis, clearly place him in an intermediate position[7]. Furthermore, his exposition of the nature of the science of mind in Lecture 2 has a distinctly Kantian flavour. While at first sight his innovations might appear to be only further technical variations on long-established positions, there is little question that they exerted a persistent influence on Psychological thought for the rest of the century (his *Lectures* was, after all, one of the most successful philosophy books of the period, going through nineteen editions). His 'Primary' and 'Secondary' Laws of 'Suggestion' in particular (especially the latter) can be readily translated into later Psychological terms, and served as a preliminary mapping of issues which exercised subsequent researchers in learning and memory (Klein, 1970). We can be reasonably sure that they had read Brown; William James quotes him *in extenso* three times in the *Principles of Psychology* (1890), twice in the key 'Stream of Thought' chapter and on each occasion with approval, while pre-First World War authorities typically include him, alongside Hamilton and the Mills, as a member of the philosophical quartet responsible for finally preparing the ground for Bain and Anglophone empirical Psychology generally[8].

Brown's novel psychological ideas comprise, first, the restriction of the expression 'association of ideas' to refer to a relatively limited range of phenomena, generally replacing it by the term 'suggestion'. When this is elaborated into the various 'Secondary Laws of Suggestion', it enables him to extend his analysis to a wider spectrum of psychological phenomena. Secondly, he thoroughly integrates 'feeling' and emotion into his account, something his predecessors had failed to do. It is the central concept of 'Suggestion' which demands our closest scrutiny, for not only is it the linchpin of his philosophy of mind, but it is also a concept which enjoys a somewhat colourful subsequent career. Brown rejects the expression 'association of ideas' on two main grounds. In the first place, 'association' had previously been limited

> to those states of mind, which are exclusively denominated Ideas [which] has, I conceive, tended greatly to obscure the subject, or at least to deprive us of the aid which we might have received from it . . . The influence of the associating principle extends, not to ideas only, but to every species of affection of which the mind is susceptible. (Lecture XXXIV, 1836 edn, vol. I, pp. 340–14)

The suggestion principle is thus much more general in character than mechanistic 'association'. He goes on to claim that a further advantage is that this principle 'consists not in its mere revival of thought and feelings . . . but in its revival of these in a certain order' (*ibid.*, p. 343). To this initial explanation he later, in Lecture XLIII, adds another, which is more revealing of his deeper motives. This arises in the context of a really rather ferocious attack on Hartley. The notion of 'association', we gather, seems to have implied a dependency of the mind on 'corpuscular motions'; its very use in this respect has been of 'material disadvantage'; it 'seems to invoke some connecting process, prior to suggestion, some co-existence of perceptions, linked, as it were, by a common tie' (*ibid.*, p. 438). Had greater attention had been paid to the 'more refined suggestions of analogy or contrast' instead of 'grosser contiguity':

> the readers of many of those romances, which call themselves systems of intellectual philosophy, would have viewed with astonishment, the hypotheses of sensorial motions, and currents of animal spirits, and furrows in the brain, and vibrations, and miniature vibrations, which false views of the mere time of association, in a connecting process of some sort prior to suggestion, have made them, in many cases, too ready to embrace. . . . It is chiefly in the southern part of the

> island, that the hypothesis of Dr Hartley has met with followers; and his followers have generally been extravagant admirers of his philosophical genius, which, I am afraid, seems to me to be the very opposite to the genius of sound philosophy. (*ibid.*)

He becomes even more contemptuous, sarcastically observing:

> If we wished to have a substance, that should damp and deaden every species of vibration, so as to prevent a single vibration from being accurately transmitted, it would not be very easy to find one better suited for this purpose, than that soft pulpy matter which is supposed by Dr Hartley to transmit with most exact fidelity, all the nicest divisions of infinitesimal vibratiuncles. (*ibid.*, pp. 439–40)

Clearly, any account which places Hartley and Brown unproblematically in a common lineage is seriously misleading, and while Brown's 'suggestion' is frequently portrayed as a sort of idiosyncratic personal synonym for 'association', it is in fact a quite major revision of that concept. For Brown, 'suggestion' both covers a wider range of phenomena and carries no connotation of prior, quasi-physical, systems of connections being built up. Though the 'Primary Laws of Suggestion' are 'resemblance' and 'contrast', which is not too far in spirit from Hume, suggestion is, if not quite a fully active (as opposed to passive) principle, at least one which operates in a way that is fully embedded in the whole complex motivational and emotional life of the individual.

What kinds of new phenomena are now incorporated, what are the 'more refined suggestions of analogy or contrast'? Two examples may suffice to indicate what Brown takes as occurrences beyond the competence of 'association'. The first is the fact that when we encounter a new object, to which no 'associations' can have ever been formed, it commonly reminds us of some object or objects we have encountered before. (This line opens up the whole topic of metaphor.) Secondly, perhaps with Wolffian 'redintegration' in mind, there are cases when 'an analogous object suggests an analogous object, by the influence of an emotion or sentiment, which each separately may have produced before, and which is therefore common to both' (*ibid.*, Lecture XXXV, p. 350).

In order to clarify Brown's arguments here, three earlier moves must now be mentioned: first, his adoption of the term 'affection' as a general term (replacing, for example, 'idea') for all particular states of mind, including emotions and feelings; secondly, the very central role which he ascribes, in glowing rhetorical terms, to memory, which he does indeed conceive of as an active principle; thirdly – and very importantly – his use of the term 'relation'. To elaborate on this last, the whole possibility of a Science of Mind hinges on our ability to undertake an 'Intellectual analysis' of mental phenomena. This:

> . . . is nothing more than the successive developement [*sic*], in application to the various mental phenomena, of this feeling of equivalence, or comprehensiveness, which . . . extends to almost every thought and feeling of which the mind is susceptible. . . . Analysis, then, in the Science of Mind . . . is founded wholly on the feeling of relation which one state of mind seems to us to bear to other states of mind . . . (*ibid.*, Lecture X, p. 102)

Thus the ability actively to deploy the relational concepts of resemblance and contrast in an Intellectual Analysis of what passes in the mind is the necessary condition for being able to have a Science of the Mind in the first place. Memory, 'the noble endowment . . . with which the Creator has blessed us' by enabling us to bring past affections before the mind, 'enables us to class the phenomena of our own spiritual being as we class the phenomena of the world without' (*ibid.*, Lecture IX, p. 92). But it is in terms of the principles of suggestion themselves that memory ultimately operates. In encountering a new object, we seek for a prior 'affection' of the mind which it resembles. In this transmutation of types of 'association of ideas' into forms of 'relations between affections', the dynamics of the mind have been fundamentally altered; 'suggestion' is always centred on the present – on discerning, both actively and passively, the 'relations' pertinent to the moment. The way is thus opened up to explore factors which affect the ongoing workings of suggestion, factors which go way beyond simple 'strengths' of 'associative bonds'. Brown identifies (in Lecture XXXVIII) nine such 'Secondary Laws of Suggestion' (see Table 8.1) which, as mentioned earlier, provided a starting point for much subsequent Psychological research, though he claims to be doing no more than 'to arrange facts that, separately, are well known'.

The concept of 'relation' continues to be deployed in Brown's

Table 8.1 Thomas Brown's 'Secondary Laws of Suggestion'

1. length of time during which the original feelings . . . continued when they coexisted or succeeded each other;
2. liveliness of original feelings;
3. frequency of renewal;
4. recency;
5. feelings are more closely associated as 'each has co-existed less with other feelings';
6. original constitutional differences;
7. differences in temporary emotion (gloom, cheerfulness, etc.)
8. changes produced by the state of the body (health, intoxication, etc.);
9. general tendencies produced by prior habits.

(Dennis [1948] reprints Brown's text on these fairly fully)

classification of the emotions, which occupies much of Volume II; these fall under the following headings: (1) Immediate Emotions (either not involving or involving 'moral affections'); (2) Retrospective Emotions (having relation either to others or to ourselves); and (3) Prospective Emotions comprehending our Desires and Fears (which, though not explicitly so subclassified, comprise self and other-directed types). It should be noted, before leaving this general account of Brown's 'Psychology', that before James and John Stuart Mill he makes the explicit analogy with Chemistry in describing the task of Intellectual Analysis, hinting, furthermore, at Mill *fils*'s argument that the properties of combinations cannot always be reduced to those of constituent parts (see *ibid.*, p. 103). As D.B. Klein clearly shows, the Mills derived the notion of 'Mental Chemistry' directly and explicitly from Brown[9].

In severing the Science of Mind from the sciences of matter (including physiology), Brown may be viewed as having made a retrogressive move. Yet this move enabled him to provide not only a more phenomenologically authentic and comprehensive account of mental phenomena than the Associationists had previously managed, but also a more dynamic and analytical one than his peers in the Reidian tradition (Stewart being his academic patron) had produced.

It remains, however, to address a final aspect of Brown's position which has been hitherto unremarked. If we read the *Lectures* with an eye to his views on the nature of psychological language an interesting unacknowledged contradiction emerges. This has two facets: first, there is the question of whether psychology (as subject matter) is fixed or mutable; secondly, the question of whether our 'metaphysical language' itself affects the mental phenomena it is being deployed to analyse. Regarding the first, in his initial efforts to establish the centrality of a Science of Mind to the sciences generally (continuing the orthodox Enlightenment rhetoric on this to some extent), Brown argues that the knowledge gained by the physical sciences is itself a product of the operations of the mind, and that its progress has been the product of improved understanding of the 'laws of the observing and comparing mind'[10]. In the case of Newton, while the world was the same for him as for everyone else, 'the successions of thought, in his mind, were . . . obviously different from the successions of thought in other minds' (*ibid.*, p. 20).

One high task of the Science of Mind is thus held out to be the possibility of improving the intellectual functioning of the mind itself, enhancing the powers of the 'intellectual instrument'. Brown's account clearly means that the efforts of philosophers and mental scientists can actually bring about widespread psychological change (he explains how their insights, initially understood by only a few, then spread throughout the population). Yet elsewhere he adopts a quite different position, talking of the mind's original 'created' character as susceptible to the 'affections' under investigation. This is particularly apparent in a passage which fuses the two issues under discussion here, and arises in the following way: he has been discussing the various schemes for classifying the phenomena of the mind, but is aware that the very existence of such variety raises problems, and is particularly keen to scotch reification of the categories produced by such schemes into thing-like faculties:

> . . . you are not to conceive, that any classification of the states or affections of the mind, as referable to certain powers or susceptibilities, makes these powers any thing different and seperate from the mind itself, as originally and essentially susceptible of the various modifications of which these powers are only a shorter name. (ibid., Lecture XVI, p. 162)

Now while this initially sounds straightforward enough, it actually conflates two issues: (a) an uncontroversial warning against reifying the 'powers', etc., which classifiers of mental phenomena identify; and (b) the persistence of mental phenomena unmodified independently of the terms in which they are identified. A similar contradiction arises earlier (p. 104) when he wants to say, simultaneously, that since Berkeley's work on perception we now 'regard perception very differently' *and* that perception 'was surely the same before' Berkeley (the point being made is similar to that made earlier about Newton). The argument he wants to make, of course, is that ignorance regarding mental phenomena can be 'rectified', just as ignorance about the physical world can. The bind he is in becomes clearer if we focus on the term 'regard': if we learn more about a physical phenomenon, we may well be said to 'regard' it differently as a consequence. But the phenomenon in question here is 'perception' – a mental phenomenon – and the 'regarding' cannot be said to be literal in character, but is rather a 'metaphysical' regarding and, as such, is itself an aspect of the mind.

Brown is thus apparently stuck in a dilemma: either his mental phenomena exist independently of the Intellectual Analyser and his categories, or they do not. If they do so exist, then the Analyser's efforts and categories can have no effect on them. If they do not, then any changes, etc., which the Analyser introduces are themselves constitutive of change. But since he clearly does not want to view the activity of intellectual analysis as other than a reflexive deployment of the mind's powers, and opposes reification, he cannot be adopting the first position. Yet to accept the second would subvert the whole project of a Science of Mind differing from the physical sciences only in terms of the subject matter on which the powers of analysis, etc., are being turned. 'What the *chemist* does, in matter, the *intellectual* analyst does in mind . . . distinguishing by a purely mental process of reflection, the elements of his complex feelings' (*ibid.*, Lecture XI, p. 107). In spite of fairly detailed discussions of the reflexive nature of the Science of Mind, Brown never resolves this dilemma; he cannot accept that Intellectual Analysis is in some sense constitutive, or that the categories we use in construing mental phenomena can actually affect or determine those phenomena – and this despite the fact that he is quite clearly aware of the dependence of 'metaphysical' language on material language (*ibid.*, Lecture X, p. 102). He even accepts that the very concept of analysis is not being used in this context quite in its literal sense (*ibid.*, p. 101), but thinks he can resolve this by terming it 'virtual analysis'.

Brown's *Lectures* are distinctive in attempting to set out an agenda for the Science of Mind independently of metaphysics (he considers the controversy between idealism and materialism irrelevant for such a science for example) and in integrating English, Scottish and – to some extent – German perspectives. But he remains unable to conceive of such a science as anything other than an exercise in introspective 'Intellectual Analysis', and fails to resolve the underlying contradiction this entails regarding the nature of mind itself as both changing itself *by* this process and yet immutable object of 'scientific' scrutiny. This is exacerbated because it is the former position which renders the 'Science of Mind' of such paramount value, while the latter position is necessary if it is actually to qualify as a science.

In fairness to Brown, we must ask if the discipline has ever genuinely resolved this contradiction. His labours were not in vain, the Secondary Laws of Suggestion as he enumerated them supplied Psychology with much of its later agenda. But Brett's verdict that he is 'alive to more possibilities than he can hold in his grasp'[11] needs perhaps to be augmented by the observation that he was also blind to some central impossibilities.

(ii) Sir William Hamilton and the Mills

We now turn to the other major figures in British philosophy during this period. While John Stuart Mill (1806–73) does directly address the nature of Psychology, their conceptual innovations in general are relatively limited. Sir William Hamilton (1788–1856) represents the final phase of the Scottish philosophical tradition begun by Reid, bringing to the task a far higher level of erudition in classics and contemporary European thought. The historical verdict on his efforts has been harsh. Hamilton's version of Idealism left little room for taking the rapidly growing wealth of physiological information on board in a constructive fashion. For Psychology he is of interest primarily in his adoption of the concept of 'redintegration' as an alternative to 'association', and as the target of a huge critique by John Stuart Mill, *An Examination of Sir William Hamilton's Philosophy* (1865; this in turn elicited a now forgotten counterattack from the Reverend James M'Cosh, *An Examination of Mr J.S. Mill's Philosophy* [1866]). Hamilton was the first to use the term 'redintegration' as a technical Psychological concept in English, although the word itself dated back to the Middle Ages and had a variety of chemical, mathematical and other usages[12]. Its philosophical use originated with Wolff (see above, p. 295), and Hamilton's usage does not differ significantly from his except in giving it a more crucial role, replacing rather than supplementing association. (John Stuart Mill's attack on him appeared too late for consideration here, although Daniel N. Robinson [1982] considers, rightly, that it is crucial for understanding the full range of Mill's Psychological thought. By 1865, however, the die has already been cast for the form which Psychology would subsequently take, and John Stuart Mill's direct influence on this stems primarily from the *System of Logic* [1843], to be discussed below.)

James Mill's *Analysis of the Phenomena of the Human Mind* (1829) distils rather than advances the classic Associationist position. The sensations in which ideas have their source are subject to Synchronous ordering and Successive ordering, and these provide the basic Laws of Association. In effect, James Mill (1773–1836) reduces these to two: what Hume would have called contiguity, and succession (which amounts to a single principle of contiguity operating spatially and temporally). He doggedly pursues this analysis as a basis for explaining all mental phenomena, including the will, although he concentrates on 'cognitive' aspects of the mind. Coupled with a Utilitarian view of motivation reducing to a simple Pleasure–Pain Principle, James Mill articulates the most spartan and rigorous of the various Associationist visions of human nature. It was a Pyrrhic victory, for when his son, along with Alexander Bain and various other scholars, produced a new, fully annotated edition in 1869, their commentaries amounted to a major withdrawal from many of the author's positions, even if they endorsed the aims of the project. Since James Mill believed, with Brown and Hamilton, that physiological matters were of little relevance to psychological enquiry, it might be thought that his work gave little direct impetus to the construction of the discipline. Ironically, one of his most avid readers was W.B. Carpenter, who took James Mill's philosophical position as a starting point in developing his psychophysiological thought later in the century[13].

It is to Book VI of John Stuart Mill's *System of Logic* (1843) that we must turn for a more considered treatment of the possibility of Psychology. This is an interesting transitional text in which John Stuart Mill attempts to establish the methodological principles on which such a science should be founded and the limits of what it can reasonably expect to achieve. As far as the discipline's task is concerned, he begins largely sharing Brown's view that it is about:

> the uniformities of succession, the laws, whether ultimate or derivative, according to which one mental state succeeds another – is caused by, or at least is caused to follow, another. (p. 557)[14]

(Although he concedes the relevance of physiology:

> I do not scruple to affirm that it [the Science of Mind] is in a considerably more advanced state than the portion of physiology which corresponds to it . . . [*ibid.*])

His confidence derives from his conviction that his father's Associationist account has indeed identified a number of 'general' Laws of Association, which have 'been ascertained by the ordinary methods of experimental enquiry' (*ibid.*). While these laws generate all mental phenomena, it must none the less be stressed that while this is sometimes done 'mechanically' (in which case there is a simple 'Composition of Causes'), in other cases their operation is analogous to that of 'chemical laws', in which genuinely novel outcomes – emergent properties, as we might now say – occur. Although this is often taken as signalling John Stuart Mill's moving beyond his father's 'mechanical' version of Associationism, both Brown and James Mill had in fact made the same point, although certainly the 'mechanical' dominates in James Mill's work. 'Complex Ideas', while generated by a blending of simple ones do not therefore necessarily merely consist of them (p. 558).

John Stuart Mill rapidly moves beyond this more or less party-line Associationism to raise other matters. There are, he holds, two kinds of 'law': 'empirical laws' gleaned from observation and 'causal laws' which explain the 'empirical laws'. These latter may be very few in number, but their operation can generate phenomena of great complexity (a fractal theory of the mind?), and it is invariably impossible to trace completely all the causal sequences actually involved in determining an event. This is true of all sciences, setting intrinsic limits to the predictability and uniformity of phenomena. Such a situation means that scientific enquiry proceeds at two levels: the level of empirical observation, yielding 'empirical laws', and another level at which we pursue the operations of the real 'laws of Nature' – the causal laws or principles governing the heterogeneous surface phenomena. Nevertheless, identification of these causal laws initially involves inductive 'experimental inquiry'. The Science of Mind is no exception. It is identification of the causal laws which is the great challenge, these alone can convert into true scientific knowledge the empirical knowledge encoded in that mass of familiar maxims, 'laws', and generalizations which centuries of informal observation of human behaviour have produced:

> Unless we have resolved the empirical law into the laws of the causes on which it depends, and ascertained that those causes extend to the case which we have in view, there can be no reliance placed in our inferences. For every individual is surrounded by circumstances different from those of every other individual; every nation or generation of mankind from every other nation or generation; and none of these differences are without their influence in forming a different type of character. (p. 564)

A real difference between John Stuart Mill's concept of the Science of Mind and his father's begins to emerge here, for the true goal of the enterprise is not simply a reductionist analysis but the more obviously relevant and practical one of determining how the causal laws revealed by such an analysis can be used to investigate the formation of 'character' at a holistic level; the 'laws . . . of the formation of character *being the principal object of scientific inquiry into human nature*' (p. 564, emphasis added). How is this to be done?

> Now to such cases we have seen that the Deductive Method, setting out from general laws, and verifying their consequences by specific experience, is alone applicable. . . . There are only two modes in which laws of nature can be ascertained: deductively and experimentally, including under the denomination of experimental inquiry, observation as well as artificial experiment. Are the laws of character susceptible of a satisfactory investigation by the method of experimentation? Evidently not; because, even if we suppose

> unlimited power of varying the experiment . . . a still more essential condition is wanting – the power of performing any of the experiments with scientific accuracy. (pp. 564–5)

This line of thought was to be crucial for the direction British Psychology was to take, for it leads directly to the insight that we can, by observation, observe only 'in what circumstances it is found that certain marked mental qualities or deficiencies *oftenest* exist' (p. 565, original emphasis). The next sentence is prophetic:

> These conclusions, besides that they are mere approximate generalisations, deserve no reliance, even as such, *unless the instances are sufficiently numerous to eliminate not only chance, but every assignable circumstance in which a number of the cases examined may happen to have resembled one another.* (*ibid.*, emphasis added)

Sampling procedures, inferential statistics and the whole Galtonian approach are adumbrated here. Not that John Stuart Mill is optimistic about such conditions ever being met – he patently isn't; nevertheless, the methodological problem is clearly stated here (and extensively elaborated) for the first time. For him the reverse procedure, the Deductive Method, is our sole recourse if we are to progress in founding a science of character – or 'Ethology', as he dubs it here[15].

> This science of Ethology may be called the Exact Science of Human Nature; for its truths are not, like the empirical laws which depend on them, approximate generalisations, but real laws. (p. 567)

While 'Psychology' is retained:

> . . . for the science of the elementary laws of mind, Ethology will serve for the ulterior science which determines the kind of character produced in conformity to those general laws, by any set of circumstances, physical or moral. (*ibid.*)

Psychology itself will proceed according to the 'observation and experiment' method; Ethology will be 'altogether deductive' (p. 568). The simple, general laws discovered by Psychology are, unlike those of Ethology, amenable to the former method by virtue of the simplicity of the facts which they govern. The truth of the matter is that John Stuart Mill can to some extent evade the methodological difficulties of ascertaining simple general causal laws because he believes that this goal has already been achieved by previous Associationists, particularly his father. The task ahead is to develop Ethology by systematically deducing from these laws their implications for the mind's response to environmental circumstance. We will remain for ever limited (as are many other disciplines) to predicting tendencies rather than specific cases, but this in itself will be of enormous practical value (e.g. for education). The final statement of the subject of this 'Ethology' is far removed from the Thomas Brown-like starting point:

> The subject to be studied is, the origin and sources of all those qualities in human beings which are interesting to us, either as facts to be produced, to be avoided, or merely to be understood; and the object is to determine, from the general laws of mind, combined with the general position of our species in the universe, what actual or possible combinations of circumstances are capable of promoting or of preventing the production of these qualities. (p. 570)

Finally, and very importantly, we may note that when he turns to social behaviour he explicitly states that this is produced by the summation of individual behaviours and that 'In social phenomena the Composition of Causes is the universal law' (p. 573); thus excluding emergent properties and affirming the ultimate centrality of the individual as the proper unit of analysis.

From the above it is evident that John Stuart Mill's concept of Psychology in many respects approaches the modern discipline more closely than anything we have yet encountered. He has largely abandoned the metaphysical problems of how the mind can study itself, and Book VI actually begins with an extended exorcism of the Free Will versus Determinism debate as due to a confused understanding of the meaning of the word Necessity[16]. Taking the Laws of Association as now established, he can move on to the task of formulating a programme for a potentially highly useful research project. He does not rule out physiology and heredity as irrelevant, but is happy that provisionally we need keep only a weather eye on the former and can assume the latter (instincts at any rate) to be modifiable 'to any extent, or even conquered' in humans by environmental or other 'mental' factors (p. 561). Methodologically, although 'artificial experiment' apparently remains logically impossible, the grounds for rejection are now practical rather than metaphysical (as in Kant), while the door is definitely pushed ajar for Galtonian style mass observation and identification of 'tendencies'. His 'Ethology' complements, for the first time, the core reductionist analysis of orthodox Associationism with a concern for the holistic level, and for what came to be called 'individual differences'. His explicit doctrine that the individual is the fundamental unit of analysis for understanding even the most social aspects of behaviour reflects, of course, the Liberal individualist credo of which he was a paradigm embodiment.

It is obvious, I think, if not spelled out in detail in the *System of Logic*, that John Stuart Mill's Science of Mind would in practice serve Utilitarian and social management ends. While his own efforts to develop further his Ethology seem to have petered out, David Leary (1982b) has argued that they were more keenly followed up in France, and that only after this detour was the project recommenced by Alexander Shand[17], whose initial inspiration they provided. Other British psychologists, notably W. McDougall and G.F. Stout, along with the anthropologists A. Radcliffe-Brown and Bruno Malinowski then adopted the resulting 'Theory of Sentiments'. The central weaknesses in John Stuart Mill's initial position were clearly his complacency about what Associationism had already achieved in identifying the 'universal laws of mind' and his indifference to the very biological factors which his friend Bain and others saw as vital ingredients of a scientific Psychology. But I am not sure that the immediate failure of Ethology in England was quite so clear-cut as Leary claims, since, as noted earlier, he does appear to foreshadow Galton in one crucial passage at least, which is not to deny the latter's different theoretical allegiance. Finally, as in the seventeenth century, albeit in another form, John Stuart Mill's Psychology must be understood in terms of an underlying political ideological agenda, albeit, as here, one fully integrated into an overtly epistemological treatise.

British philosophy in the first half of the nineteenth century was far from homogeneous. The Reidian and Lockean traditions were vigorously vying with one another, while ideas from German and French philosophers were eliciting increasing interest and being eagerly adopted by such thinkers as Coleridge and Hamilton. But the positions of the heirs of Reid and Locke began to blur as the debate continued. The latter's main spokesman, James Mill, was, after all, a Scot, and had attended Dugald Stewart's lectures as a student. In Thomas Brown's *Lectures* the two approaches came very close to final fusion. In this blurring, the distinctively Reidian positions of Scots philosophers were steadily eroded by the Associationists, whose concessions in the reverse direction were more limited (though they included adopting a more developmental orientation). Robinson (1982) is undoubtedly correct in suggesting that it was this move which 'successfully cut away' 'what we may judge to be missing in today's psychology' (p. 81) – that is, presumably, the spiritual or metaphysical dimension which persisted in Germany. Whether he is right to ascribe responsibility for this excision so exclusively to John Stuart Mill himself is another question. Exponents of continental ideas such as Coleridge and Hamilton and, later, Morell, while occasionally eminent, certainly made little widespread headway against what was increasingly a single broad Empiricist establishment. But the reasons for this go beyond the respective merits of the various philosophical orientations, or the advocacy skills of a single thinker.

The almost total erasure from the history of Psychology, except for the briefest of passing mentions (usually to its title), of J.D. Morell's 1853 *Elements of Psychology. Part 1* is significant here – as, perhaps, is the fact that he never produced Part 2. Morell, like John Stuart Mill, explicitly tried to advance the cause of a scientific Psychology, conceptually distinct from philosophy. His error was to steep himself in contemporary German and French work, from which he fashions a kind of English *Idealrealismus* account, including acceptance of the tripartite faculty classification and 'the Law of Progress' as a cosmic principle *à la* Fichte and Hegel. This yields an interesting table of the ways in which the faculties manifest themselves as they ascend through four stages of development. The book is unique in English proto-Psychology, and highly informative on contemporary mainland work, but exerted no apparent impact on the famous founding texts which followed ere the decade was out. He does nevertheless represent a position which enjoyed some contemporary popularity; others sharing it included T. Laycock and James Martineau.

Table 8.2 J.D. Morell's Classification of the Stages of expression of the Mental Faculties

	I *Intelligence*	II *Feeling*	III *Will*
1st Stage	sensation	pleasure & pain	parental instinct
2nd Stage	intuition	sentiments	passions
3rd Stage	representation	affections	art
4th Stage	thought	love	freedom

from J.D. Morell (1853)

The Associationist victors shared more than a common metaphysics; they were part of an extended intellectual network concerned with pursuing Benthamite schemes of Utilitarian social reform and *laissez-faire* economics. Their interests ranged from sanitation and education to the legal rights of women and parliamentary reform, and both the Mills were leading lights of contemporary campaigns on such matters. Their 'Psychological' writings represented but one facet of the overall vision of human life and society which they were promoting. In this context it is less surprising that authors operating either across a smaller portion of the cultural spectrum, such as Abercrombie, or in the context of ideological interests appealing to more restricted constituencies, should fail to carry the day. By virtue of its individualism, its de-emphasis on sociological critique and its message of self-improvement, the Liberal Utilitarian 'Associationist' camp benefited to a large extent from the same kind of cultural dynamics which we earlier saw Roger Cooter identifying as favouring phrenology. And we should remember that it was John Stuart Mill who converted Alexander Bain from phrenology to Associationism.

Did early-nineteenth-century British philosophy produce any new Psychological ideas? Only, I think, to a limited extent, although those it did produce were significant. At the most general level the idea of what a Science of Mind would be like has, in John Stuart Mill's work, moved far closer to the reality which was shortly to ensue – most notably, perhaps, in his notion of an 'Ethology' in which large numbers of cases would be used to confirm general trends deductively predicted from general laws. In addition, he has a clearer idea of the practical utility such a discipline would have. Thomas Brown's 'Suggestion', particularly as elaborated in the 'Secondary Laws of Suggestion', radically extended the scope of the Associationist approach, identifying numerous issues to which Psychology would later attend. Hamilton's 'redintegration', on the other hand, failed in the long run to establish itself as a productive concept in Anglophone Psychology.

Before leaving the philosophers I would like, briefly, to draw attention to Robert Owen's populist essays *A New View of Society: or, Essays on the Principle of the Formation of the Human Character, and the Application of the Principle to Practice* (1813–14) and *The Revolution in the Mind and Practice of the Human Race* (1849). These are rarely noticed in disciplinary histories, and neither, their titles notwithstanding, is really Psychological in character. But they do serve to provide an insight into the psychological background to the Mills' work, as well as complementing Cooter's thesis regarding phrenology.

Owen (1771–1858) was an out-and-out Utopian socialist, and a practical one at that, successfully sustaining the New Lanark community project for thirty years. He figures large in all political and economic histories of Britain during this period as a pioneering reformer. The relatively early *A New View of Society* comprises four essays dedicated respectively to William Wilberforce, The British Public, The Proprietors of the Principal Mill Establishments and His Royal Highness the Prince Regent. So much for his target audience! It is purely a succession of manifestoes. In Essay First he sets out a view of human nature to which he clung ever after with as much fervency as Combe did to his. All is really contained in the following two principles, printed in capitals in the original:

> That any character, from the best to the worst, from the most ignorant to the most enlightened, may be given to any community, even to the world at large, by applying certain means; which are to a great extent at the command and under the controul, [*sic*] or easily made so, of those who possess the government of nations. (p. 9)

There is but one single principle of action:

> The happiness of self clearly understood and fully comprehended, which can only be attained by conduct which must promote the happiness of the community. (p. 13)

This then is the grass-roots political level of the Utilitarian agenda which Bentham and the Mills were striving to pursue in more sophisticated philosophical terms. It entails a thoroughly environmentalist vision of human nature, and close attention to education. The terms in which Owen's rhetoric is conducted may be found in more elaborated form in the 1849 work, with Prefaces to Queen Victoria and 'her Responsible Advisors' and 'To the Red Republicans, Communists & Socialists of Europe' (whose violent methods he castigates – Europe having been gripped by revolutions the previous year).

I wish to draw particular attention to passages such as the following:

> To know how to manufacture the human character, is to know how to remove the chief causes of the miseries of the world . . . to uproot the cause of all inferior and injurious passions, which ignorance alone now maintains in the characters of all. (p. 75)

> . . . in short to know scientifically how to manufacture the material of human nature, – the most ductile of all materials, – in its endless capacity for varied knowledge, goodness and happiness, is to know how to change the present universal disorder . . . into a terrestrial paradise. (pp. 75–6)

> Children in small numbers can never be placed within the proper machinery to well form their physical, mental, moral, and practical characters, and make them well-formed men and women. (p. 79)

> All the children of the Township being trained and educated together, proper machinery for the formation of character may be created . . . (p. 80)

Phrenology, as we observed, internalized the factory as an image of human nature; Owen, in all innocence, goes one step further and sees human nature itself as the product of a quasi-industrial process in which social machinery manufactures character. The quality of the product depends on the intentions of the manufacturer and the design of the machinery. At present the former are conflicting and irrational and the latter is poor, but by promoting this very image he seeks to facilitate the achievement of the requisite reforms in both. Combe and Owen knew one another and openly disagreed on the solution to society's ills – Combe's individualist self-knowledge route clashing with Owen's (almost literal) social engineering. While at one level they are recasting the nature–nurture debate into its modern terms, they nevertheless both reflect the same underlying process of assimilating the salient features of industrial culture to human nature itself. Behind John Stuart Mill's cutting away of some ineffable metaphysical 'something' from British Psychology is the sheer momentum of this collective psychological change in *mentalité*, by which the yet unindustrialized Germans were so far largely unaffected.

2 Psychiatry and Madness

The century began with a crisis for proto-psychiatry. The rise of 'Moral Management' following William Tuke's establishment of The Retreat at York, publicized by his son Samuel's *Description of the Retreat* in 1813, threatened the established system on two fronts. First, the higher recovery rates achieved by this essentially non-medical approach undermined the medical profession's claims to therapeutic and theoretical expertise. Secondly, the philosophy of the new movement, stressing humane treatment, provision of extensive facilities, abandonment of physical restraint and acknowledgement of the patients' humanity ran counter to the whole eighteenth-century (and earlier) tradition as practised in the hundreds of private mad-houses throughout the land, from Bethlem (the most famous) downwards. 'Tradition' is perhaps the wrong word; the bestialized image of the lunatic provided a rationale for horrendous squalor, cruelty and neglect, copiously documented in works such as Scull's *Museums of Madness* (1979), which draws on the reports of the contemporary Royal Commissions and the extensive penumbra of pamphlets. Reforming zeal, on Scull's account, came from two directions: Evangelical Christians like William Wilberforce on one wing and secular Utilitarian Benthamites on the other. Vieda Skultans (1979) has challenged Scull's view of the pre-nineteenth-century situation as involving a cultural distancing from madness and a lack of medical interest[18]. Certainly there had been no lack of medical interest in melancholia, 'hypochondria', the spleen and kindred manifestations of the notorious English 'Black Dog' – on the contrary, there was a positive and chronic obsession with them.

But only in their extreme forms were these 'neuroses', as they would now be classified, viewed as madness. They were seen as the price the educated man of Reason paid for living in the English climate. Deluded lunatic paupers exhibited at Bethlem at weekends for a penny a visit were another matter. Whatever the truth regarding nuances of interpretation, there is now a broad agreement that events following the rise of Moral Management reflect an aspect of the underlying psychological change we have touched on in discussing phrenology and Robert Owen.

This is well summarized by Scull[19]. The Industrial Revolution, as ever, is at the heart of the story. This development involved two particularly profound changes of relevance to us here: the first was a growing realization that genuinely fundamental changes in the socioeconomic order were possible and, indeed, actually happening – a change that necessarily transformed people at the psychological level as they adapted to, and created, the new order. This, it is argued, contrasts with a previous attitude in which the world was 'not humanly but divinely anchored' and 'the possibilities for transforming man himself go largely unrecognized'[20]. The second change, stemming from the industrialization process and the pervasively competitive economic system itself, concerned the form of this psychological transformation: the need for a disciplined workforce in which norms of behaviour and attitude were internalized rather than maintained by external authority. It is in this setting that changes in the treatment of madness must be understood:

> The insistence on the importance of the internalization of norms, the conception of how this was to be done, and even the nature of the norms which were to be internalized – in all these respects we can now see how the emerging attitude towards the insane paralleled contemporaneous shifts in the treatment of the 'normal' populace.[21]

Moral treatment concentrated on enabling patients to learn *self*-control, and to conduct themselves according to the standards of their respectable bourgeois 'managers'. Since the mad are now seen as susceptible to transformation, restraint becomes not only inhumane but counterproductive. Cure, not close confinement, is the new priority. In the small-scale centres of moral treatment, the mad are taught to conform to the standards of respectable middle-class domesticity. But is this a job for doctors? The doctors certainly thought so, but the futility of their existing therapeutic armoury was obvious and undeniable. From the 1820s on, the tale is of a progressive *rapprochement* between reformers and doctors, mediated by some, like John Connolly, who were in both camps. Reforms are, slowly, achieved at the legal and regulatory level, from which both camps can derive satisfaction. Amelioration of conditions is accompanied by consolidation and extension of madness as lying in the medical profession's rightful domain. For a brief period, from the 1820s into the 1840s, there is an air of optimism. Reported recovery rates are high, and new public asylums are replacing the now notorious private mad-houses. Lecture courses on insanity start to be given to medical students[22]. But having co-opted the moral treatment reformers' case, the medical profession, never averse to empire-building (who was in the nineteenth century?) yield to cost-accountancy and begin compromising on central tenets of Moral Therapy regarding size and environmental quality. The result is ever larger, more prison-like and dehumanizing asylums. Only after 1840 does the kind of 'Great Confinement' Foucault saw in seventeenth-century France really get under way in England.

This development was bolstered by the rise of more pessimistic theories of madness, particularly the growing belief in the aetiological involvement of hereditary factors and, as the century wore on, the notion of 'degeneration', introduced by B.A. Morel in France in 1857. At the same time, ironically, the concept of 'Moral Insanity' enabled the emerging profession of psychiatry to discover (or collect), among the growing varieties of mental dis-ease and behavioural deviancy to which urbanized humanity was prone, ever more exotic species of pathology over which to exercise its proprietorial rights.

The number of works on insanity published in the first half of the century was extensive. From the translation of Pinel's *Traité* in 1806 onwards, the publication of psychiatric texts formed a major plank both of the medical profession's campaign to establish a monopoly in the treatment of madness, and of the reformers' humanitarian and Christian campaigns. Here I will glance fairly briefly at only two of these. The first is James Cowles Prichard's *A Treatise on Insanity and other disorders affecting the Mind* (1835), in which the concept of 'Moral Insanity' is introduced, the second is Thomas Laycock's *A Treatise on the Nervous Diseases of Women; comprising an inquiry into the nature, causes, and treatment of Spinal and Hysterical Disorders* (1840), in which the idea of psychosomatic disorder is anticipated.

(i) James Cowles Prichard (1785–1848)

Before proceeding to Prichard's 'Moral Insanity', we must consider the term 'moral'. Throughout much of the eighteenth century it had been roughly synonymous with 'mental', perhaps incorporating, but not confined to, the sense of 'pertaining to ethics' which it now exclusively possesses. It did, however, tend to refer more particularly to the emotional rather than the rational. Skultans argues that for advocates of 'moral treatment', 'there is a systematic ambiguity in the use of the term' in which the more modern sense 'is contained and sometimes hidden' within the older one[23]. Moral treatment involved the use of emotions to achieve its ends and stressed the emotional causes of insanity, but the religious character of the movement – particularly in the case of William Tuke, its effective founder – also led to a focus on bad habits and immorality in the modern sense as aetiological factors.

In Prichard's case the overt meaning of 'Moral Insanity' refers to types of insanity in which the disorder is emotional or behavioural in character, with 'an apparently unimpaired state of the intellectual faculties'. This, however, is the thin end of the wedge, since all the illustrative cases he gives depict such insanity as deriving from, and being symptomatized by, immoral behaviour. He defines 'Moral Insanity' as a perversion of 'natural feelings, affections, inclinations, temper, habits, moral dispositions and natural impulses' (p. 6). He broadly accepts the German Heinroth's classification of insanity into disorders of 'passion', of intellect and of will (with 'excitation' and 'depression' forms of each). Among the 'depression' forms of disorders of will we find 'moral imbecility'. Prichard sees that the identification of 'Moral Insanity' is problematical, since it readily blurs over into mere eccentricity. Using figures from Pinel and Esquirol, he later concludes that moral causes of insanity are more prevalent than physical ones[24]. The tabulations of 'moral causes' highlight the fusion of moral-as-emotional and moral-as-ethical; reverses of fortune, libertinism, 'domestic griefs', 'abuse of wine', disappointment in love and masturbation all appear.

An account such as this readily provides psychiatry with *carte blanche* for pathologizing behavioural deviance in general. The concept of 'moral imbecility' in particular later became especially pernicious, notably as providing a route by which unmarried lower-class women could be incarcerated if they became pregnant or sexually active – those in domestic service obviously being the most vulnerable. The modern concept of the 'psychopath' is also implicit in Prichard's concept of 'Moral Insanity', and this too has proved of dubious value because of the ease with which it can be used to pathologize unconformity for reasons of social and political control. From the Foucauldian perspective, of course, establishing and maintaining power relations is of the very essence of the diagnostic game. Undoubtedly, it is in works such as this that we see psychiatry establishing the range of its theatre of operations as an institutional instrument of social control. The way in which the term 'moral' slithers from being a descriptive to a prescriptive term between 1790 and the mid nineteenth century is a significant surface symptom of this process, with Prichard's 'Moral Insanity' marking the crucial transitional point.

(ii) Thomas Laycock's A Treatise on the Nervous Diseases of Women (1840)

My reason for selecting this is, as mentioned above, because I believe Laycock provides here the basis of a psychosomatic model of mental illness. He was also an important figure in the later development of British psychophysiology and the translator of Unzer and Prochaska. His approach is, from the outset, far more physiological than Prichard's. While 'hysteria and hypochondriasis' may well be due to such 'moral' – in Prichard's terms – causes as 'improper food, vicious habits implicating the sexual organs and debilitating the system', and the like, the immediate causes of such disorders are the effects they have on the blood and the nervous system. Laycock, in fact, places great emphasis on the blood and vascular system as being equally, or even more, involved in them than the nervous system. Not surprisingly, there are rich veins of patronizing sexism to be mined in Laycock's text:

> . . . but if the susceptibility of woman be a cause of her frailties, it is equally efficacious in giving lustre to her virtues; compassionate

> kindness, piety, honest sincerity, and constancy, appearing with the greatest perfection in the sex. (p. 76)

Reluctantly, we must leave these aside here. More relevant to us at the moment are the later passages, particularly Chapter X, in which, having provided a quite extensive and important 'state-of-the-art' review of the nervous system and neurological basis of consciousness, Laycock turns to the operation of the will. His central point is that while the effects of the nervous system *on* the brain and consciousness have received wide discussion, the possibility of effects in the reverse direction has been strangely neglected[25].

> It is singular that the action of the will on the sensorial fibres has excited so little notice. (p. 110)

Changes in the 'sensorial fibres of the encephalon' may

> originate internally as well as externally and excite movements: Tickling the fancy will excite laughter, as much as tickling the feet. In fact it may be hypothetically supposed that there is a surface on which sensorial fibres terminate, connected with ideas, and which is analogous to the sensitive fibres of the skin, or on mucous membranes. It becomes a matter of some importance to inquire how far the will can act on sensorial fibres in general . . . (p. 109)

In elaborating on this he invokes mesmerism:

> The phenomena of mesmerism (so called) are all illustrations of the power of the will over the brain. . . . [a]n act of the sensorial will becomes easier by repetition, and at last involuntary. After an individual has been mesmerized repeatedly, certain movements (passes) are no longer necessary to the excitement of the sensorial volition, it has become a habit, and it is produced by an insignificant associated circumstance. . . . It is thus that disinterested observers have been imposed upon; and thus hysterical girls can bring on convulsions, and any person ideas, sensations, and mental emotions, with more or less facility. (p. 111)

A little later Dubois's account of hypochondria and hysteria is cited, according to which hypochondria develops in three stages:

(1) only the mind is affected, the patient is 'harassed by imaginary diseases'; (2) changes 'in their innervation' are excited, which leads to (3) actual organic disease. Laycock stresses that he has 'followed a different line of investigation' to Dubois (and also to Bonnet), but arrived at a similar conclusion.

While Laycock is far from seeing psychosomatic symptoms as symbolic, in this section he is claiming that in the case of 'sensorial fibres' at least the input may come from the centre as well as the periphery, and general physiological consequences may ensue. There are numerous prophetic resonances: a lurking proto-theory of habit, even conditioning, and a linkage of 'psychosomatic' processes to hysterical symptoms may be detected in the last passage cited. Laycock's ideas here should be seen as part of the background of psychophysiological theorizing on which Bain was later to draw – a background to which we will be giving more attention in the next section.

Of additional interest to historians of Psychology are several other neglected works from this period which can be mentioned here only *pour encourager vous autres*: Thomas Burgess's *The Physiology or Mechanism of Blushing* (1828), Solly's *The Human Brain* (1836; extensively cited by Laycock), and R. M'Nish (or McNish)'s *The Philosophy of Sleep* (1830). Skultans (1979) has a brief discussion of the significance of blushing, for Burgess, as a indicator of a uniquely human 'spiritual nature', and the 'moral' meaning of the contemporary debate about whether or not 'Negroes' blush.

Early-nineteenth-century British psychiatric thought served, then, as a further vehicle and expression of those psychological changes in the concept of human nature which we have repeatedly seen pervading British culture during this period. Sanity is always defined in contrast to insanity, and changes in the meaning, range and perceived nature of the latter necessarily reflect similar changes in the former. This is not to deny the reality of mental distress or, indeed, the need for society to make the sane/insane distinction. But what must be insisted on is that we recognize (a) that the varieties of mental distress which fall on the insane side of the boundary vary considerably over time; (b) that the forms in which societies manifest the need for the distinction will similarly vary and reflect far more than simple medical understanding; and (c) that texts on insanity are necessarily texts on sanity also.

Current scholarship in the History of Psychiatry convincingly establishes the thoroughgoing penetration of hidden – and not so hidden – social, political, economic and sexual agendas into psychiatric discourse. The question is what remains when these are excluded. Very little indeed seems to be the answer, which need not surprise us because, after all, 'insanity' and 'madness' are social, not natural, categories – and the motives for constructing them are indeed social, political, economic and sexual, as are the majority of the subjective meanings of mental distress itself, even when physiological factors are involved. It is precisely when an unambiguously physical basis for a disorder (such as epilepsy) is discovered that the form of distress in question is removed from the 'madness' category. Psychiatric work during the early nineteenth century served also as vehicle and focus for psychophysiological, especially neurological, theorizing, for it was in this field that the vexed issues of the physical dimensions of will, emotion, rationality and consciousness had to be most directly confronted – which brings us to our next topic.

3 Physiology

The three figures of greatest significance for Psychology during this period were Sir Charles Bell, Marshall Hall, and James Braid[26]. It was the neurophysiological researches of Bell and Hall (along with those of their continental counterparts) which laid the basis for psychophysiological theorizing and enquiry for the remainder of the century, while Braid's physiological account of hypnotism, discussed above, played a major role in bringing the study of this and kindred phenomena into the scientific fold. From a conceptual point of view, the ideas introduced by Bell and Hall are of three kinds: (a) Bell's identification of the distinction between sensory (afferent) and motor (efferent) nerves; (b) Marshall Hall's concept of 'reflex action'; and (c) Bell's ideas regarding facial expression. First we will consider Bell's contribution.

Sir Charles Bell (1774–1842), one of the most eminent anatomists of his time, first announced the distinction between sensory and motor nerves in 1810, and in 1811 circulated a hundred copies of a monograph, *Idea of a New Anatomy of the Brain: Submitted for the Observations of His Friends*[27]. This discovery further entailed the notion of what Magendie later called 'specific nerve energies'; each component of the sensory nervous system generating its distinctive form of sensation. Thus Bell notes that if the retina's sensitivity to light took the form of 'a finer sensibility than the nerve of touch, it would be a source of torment'[28]. For Bell, it should be stressed: 'This law of the senses is arbitrarily or divinely ordered; it might have been otherwise.'[29] While Bell's priority in this discovery is clear, it was Magendie's more extended and widely circulated 1822 report of his independent discovery of the differing functions of the spinal nerve roots which effectively established the doctrine and must be credited as the more influential. For Psychology the significance of this is that it opened the way for new concepts of neurology and brain functioning, leading fairly directly to Hall's 'reflex action' model. Indeed the discovery was a necessary condition for the possibility of a physiological Psychology ever being realized.

The Anatomy and Philosophy of Expression (1806), the 1844 third edition of which greatly influenced Charles Darwin's *The Expression of the Emotions in Man and Animals* (1872), has been less discussed by disciplinary historians. It is an attempt – in some ways a rather curious one – to integrate aesthetics and neurology[30]. At one level Bell is striving to clarify the basis for our notions of human physical beauty by arguing that it involves an emphasis on – even an abstraction of – the most characteristically human, and a subordination or de-emphasis on that which is animal. But this engages us in the question of how our mental states (and especially our emotions) are visibly expressed via the body. In exploring involuntary emotional expression, particularly in Essay 3, he utilizes his notion of the unique qualities of the various components of the nervous system to produce an account which it is not too fanciful to read as adumbrating the James–Lange theory, although of course it goes less far in suggesting that experienced emotions are secondary to their physical manifestations. What he says is that just as externally directed sensory systems are possessed of unique qualities (vision, sound, etc.), so too are internal ones, and these may therefore be considered as producing emotions in the way the optic nerve produces perceptions. Accorded a central place in this are the nerves controlling the respiratory system, which is in turn determined by the heart. The dynamic is thus that the brain, on receiving some traumatic sensory information, affects the heart and thence, via that, the respiratory system through the motor nerves. Heart and respiratory systems together then bring in train all the involuntary aspects of emotional expression such as panting, blanching, blushing, gasping, shoulder-heaving, sobbing, and so forth. These are experienced via the internal sensory system as emotion. While the emotions as such remain located, like all psychological phenomena, in the brain, it is the body as a whole system which produces and responds to them.

A further aspect of Bell's account is that such outward manifestations of psychological state are not arbitrary but are clearly functional responses to the situation. This, of course, is Darwin's point of departure, but Bell remained committed to a pious Paleyite Natural Theology, to the extent that he provided illustrative notes for an edition of Paley's *Natural Theology* and contributed one of the Bridgewater Treaties: *The Hand: its mechanism and vital endowments, as evincing design* (1832). Given the success of *The Anatomy and Philosophy of Expression*, and its obvious cultural location in contemporary interest in physiognomy and phrenology (which he rejects), it is reasonable to infer that it was through this work as much as his specialized neurological writings, that his influence on Psychological thought was mediated[31]. At the very least the work demonstrated the potential value of a neurological and physiological approach to elucidating the nature of emotion from a functional viewpoint. But the 'Darwin connection' raises the further possibility that it made a vital contribution to the later extension of evolutionary theory into Psychological issues in *The Expression of the Emotions in Man and Animals*. That Bell would have been appalled at this we need not doubt.

Marshall Hall (1790–1857), while but sixteen years Bell's junior, seems to belong to a quite different intellectual era. One obvious difference between them is methodological: Bell had relied on dissection, while Hall, like his continental contemporaries Flourens, Müller and Weber, was pioneering genuinely experimental techniques. Without entering into the physiological minutiae of his findings regarding the structure of the spinal chord[32], the upshot of his extensive researches (published between 1837 and 1850) was a further recasting of the operation of the nervous system which had a greater long-term effect on Psychological theory than any other single neurological idea. This may be summed up in two phrases: 'reflex function' and 'reflex arc'.

His views, initially aired in two *Memoirs on the Nervous System* (1832, 1837), immediately embroiled him in a heated controversy regarding the originality of his ideas and the rejection of the second memoirs for publication by the Royal Society. The novelty in Hall's account was that it identified a class of behaviours in the explanation of which the brain played no part. To the efferent–afferent circuit, routed through the brain, which Bell had identified, Hall adds a subordinate 'diastaltic' nervous system centred on the spinal marrow, short-circuiting, as it were, the cerebrally controlled and monitored voluntary nervous sytem. Decerebrated lower animals could be experimentally shown to move and respond to stimuli. The 'reflex' concept had been introduced in the previous century, and used particularly by Prochaska (see above, p. 198), as had some of the phenomena of persistence of behaviour after decapitation, hence the controversy. But nobody before Hall had provided a full theoretical physiological account, and the term 'reflex' had remained rather loose and descriptive in meaning. First systematically expounded in *New Memoirs on the Nervous System* (1843) and receiving its final version in *Synopsis of the Diastaltic System* (1850), Hall's theory made rapid headway against the opposition with the backing of Müller in Germany and fellow British neurologist R.D. Grainger.

What Hall proposes is that part of the nervous system serves a general reflex *function*. This is comprised of a number of reflex 'arcs' which connect stimuli to motor responses with no conscious awareness and/or no exercise of voluntary control on the organism's part. This reflex function is, furthermore, implicated in the performance details of much voluntary behaviour. The model has serious consequences for Psychological theorizing, for a number of reasons. At the broadest level, it challenges the sufficiency of purely mentalistic approaches to the understanding of human behaviour. If the brain is the 'seat of the Soul', the source and recipient of all behaviour and sensation, then the physiological details of how these are engineered can be largely ignored for psychological purposes – Mind is in the driving seat and Psychology's concern is with its journeys, not the steering mechanism. But if behaviour is governed to a significant degree by a non-cerebral 'reflex function', then a more intimate involvement of Psychology with physiology becomes inevitable. As early as 1840

Thomas Laycock is writing:

> There are . . . numerous observations which, when compared, serve to extend the two great doctrines above alluded to [i.e. Bell's and Hall's] far beyond their original limits; placing on the one hand the sensorial fibres under the power of the will; on the other applying the laws of the excito-motory system to the phenomena, not of the spinal cord only and its prolongations, but to the brain also, and the diffused nervous system.[33]

Further exploration of this intimate mutual involvement is indeed what happens in the 1850s when figures such as Laycock, B. Brodie, H. Holland, W.B. Carpenter and R. Dunn produce their 'psychophysiological' works (though I am not suggesting that this development was due exclusively to Hall).

More specifically, the reflex action provides, for the first time, a kind of behavioural *unit* which can serve, in the analysis of behaviour, a role similar to that of simple ideas in Associationist philosophy. While this is not immediately apparent in Hall's work, and would have to await further elaboration of the reflex concept, it would prove central to behaviourally orientated US Psychologists in the run-up to Behaviorism, and also provided Dewey with the focus for one of the subtlest theoretical papers in nineteenth-century Psychology[34]. Finally, one implication of Hall's reflex concept was that a comprehensive Psychology would be unable to confine itself to conscious phenomena alone if it was to address behaviour adequately. Not that Hall himself ever discusses the question of the 'unconscious', his concerns were exclusively physiological, but the issue could not but surface in any attempted integration of his model into Psychology. The research tradition initiated by Hall continued unbroken through the latter half of the century, culminating in Sherrington's *The Integrative Action of the Nervous System* (1906), and from Bain onwards British and American Psychological writers usually sought to set their ideas within the context of current neurological understanding.

The work of Bell and Hall, taken in conjunction with the contemporary research and debates on brain function triggered by phrenology, was ineluctably rendering the division between the philosophically based 'Science of Mind' project and the increasingly experimental and materialist sciences of the body difficult to sustain. None the less, their fusion was a consummation which many, even of those centrally involved, devoutly did not wish. They saw the soul being driven from cover to cover, retreating from spinal column to brain and from cerebellum to cortex, while progressively being robbed of its functions by material physiological mechanisms. But as we shall now see, this alarm was not the result of neurology alone.

4 Proto-Anthropology

As philosophers strove to represent their accounts of the mind as being at least in some fundamental sense scientific (while undertaking no laboratory experiments and making no measurements) and phrenologists cultivated the image of themselves as practitioners of a true empirical science of human nature, two central questions of a broader kind remained to be tackled. The first may be termed the 'Man's Place in Nature' question, the second concerned the unity of the human race itself. While neither was a directly Psychological issue, the debates surrounding them, and the outcomes of these debates, were important factors in determining the character of British Psychology. With regard to the first: for as long as 'Mankind' remained partly superordinate to Nature – halfway between animals and angels on a Great Chain of Being, perhaps, or the being for whose benefit all other terrestrial life-forms were created, or the crowning end-product of a quasi-spiritual evolutionary process – major psychological barriers would remain against fully assimilating its study into the natural sciences; moral philosophical and religious matters would, under such circumstances, continue to underpin the agenda. With regard to the second question, doubts as to the unity of the human species were inextricably linked to basic ideological controversies (particularly about slavery)[35]. These in turn were one arena in which the rival psychologies or *mentalités* of the early to mid nineteenth century were visibly competing. However racist Psychology later proved, on occasion, to be, a different outcome to the unity-of-the-species debate would have made racism a central disciplinary dogma.

From the mid eighteenth century on, European thinkers had become more and more fascinated by the diversity of humankind which imperial expansion was bringing to their notice. This diversity took both cultural and physical forms. Cultural diversity, while raising disturbingly relativistic possibilities about morality (exploited most fully by the Marquis de Sade), was ultimately more intellectually manageable than physical diversity. By the time Blumenbach is collecting the skulls of savage head-hunters and Camper is pioneering cranial measurement at the turn of the century, the challenging hypothesis is being proposed in some quarters (e.g. by Blumenbach himself) that certain people, especially African black-hued ones, are actually members of a different species to Europeans. Their 'cranial line', it was claimed, disclosed a 'muzzle'-like form patently inferior aesthetically and physiognomically to that of whites. From then on the 'monogeny' versus 'polygeny' debate exercised ethnographers and anthropologists until late in the century (with spasmodic revivals since). Did the human race have a single origin? Or did it have more than one? Orthodox Christianity, of course, favoured the former, Adam and Eve, via Noah's sons, being the parents of us all – the first 'protoplast pair', as R.G. Latham would have put it[36]. This controversy was not settled before the end of the period being discussed here, but the monogenists were gaining the upper hand[37]. Their eventual victory was initially somewhat Pyrrhic, for the time-scale of human evolution had extended so much that while a single evolutionary origin for all *Homo sapiens sapiens* could be conceded, the divergences of racial groups could be placed so far back that erstwhile polygenists could salvage much of their message. This we cannot explore here.

In the rest of this section we shall be considering how the two questions were tackled by British anthropological writers in the first half of the nineteenth century. The most significant text during this period was William Lawrence's *Lectures on Physiology, Zoology, and the Natural History of Man* (1819). A second, highly successful and influential writer was Prichard, whose two major works in this field were *Researches into the Physical History of Mankind* (1813) and *The Natural History of Man* (1843)[38]. It was on these, rather than his psychiatric work, that his contemporary fame largely rested. Finally, by virtue of its cultural impact, Robert Chambers's notorious *Vestiges of the Natural History of Creation* (1844) must be taken into account, although its author was no scientist. All these can be read, naturally enough, as a run-up to Darwinian theory, but I am more concerned here with indicating how their several approaches involved a radical rethinking of human nature in a very general sense, which, along with Combe's *Constitution of*

Man, inevitably had psychological, and Psychological, *sequelae* of a far-reaching kind[39].

(i) William Lawrence (1783–1867)

The contumely heaped upon Hall by his medical-establishment opponents in 1837 somewhat pales beside that heaped upon Lawrence from much the same quarter eighteen years earlier. Lawrence eventually weathered the storm to become Sergeant-Surgeon to Queen Victoria herself, but kept mum for ever after on the issues he had raised. What he had done in his lectures was to place the study of 'Man' firmly within the framework of zoology and the biological sciences. Darlington (1959) summarizes his 'remarkable conclusions' as follows (I abbreviate them somewhat further):

> 1. Physical, mental and moral differences in man are hereditary.
> 2. Races of man have arisen by mutations such as are seen to distinguish different kittens or rabbits in a litter.
> 3. Sexual selection has improved the beauty of advanced races and governing classes.
> 4. Characters of races and nations are preserved by breeding barriers between them.
> 5. 'Selections and exclusions' are the means of change and adaptation. Differences, mental and physical, between races of men can never be related to differences in external conditions such as food, climate or government.
> 6. Men can thus be improved by selection in breeding, just as domesticated animals can. Conversely, they can be ruined by inbreeding . . .
> 7. Zoological study, the treatment of man as an animal . . . is the only proper foundation for teaching and research in medicine, in morals or even in politics. (pp. 19–20)

As Darlington notes, most of these had been mooted before (although he does not mention Gregory's advocacy of point 6 – see above, p. 229). What was new was the simultaneous, thorough and wholehearted fashion in which Lawrence expounded them. Lawrence, threatened with professional ruin, withdrew his support for the book's publication, but nine illicit editions were none the less published and it remained notorious for three decades. As far as the first question is concerned, then, Lawrence placed 'Man' firmly in zoological and biological context. The human race was to be studied just like any other species, and its character was governed by principles no different from those employed by stock-breeders. And yet, while treating the human species zoologically, he is anxious not to demote it too thoroughly:

> The peculiar characteristics of man appear to me so very strong, that I not only deem him a distinct species, but also put him in a separate order by himself. His physical and moral attributes place him a much greater distance from all other orders of mammalia, than those are from each other respectively. (p. 114)

This is elaborated later in a short chapter (VIII) on the faculties of the mind:

> Thrown on the surface of the globe, weak, naked, and defenceless, man appeared created for inevitable destruction. Evils assailed him on every side; the remedies remained hidden: but he received from his Creator the gift of inventive genius, which enabled him to discover them. (p. 198)

Tool-making and language elevate us high above the most intelligent of our fellow creatures.

On the second question Lawrence was a monogenist, departing in this from Blumenbach, to whom he dedicated the book. In adopting this position he is far from rejecting intrinsic differences in mental as well as physical qualities, urging us to compare, among other things:

> . . . the highly civilized nations of Europe, so conspicuous in arts, science, literature, in all that can strengthen and adorn society, or exalt and dignify human nature, to a troop of naked, shivering, and starved New Hollanders, a horde of filthy Hottentots, or the whole of the more or less barbarous tribes that cover nearly the entire continent of Africa. Are these all brethren? (p. 209)

First appearances, he deferentially concedes (having quoted Voltaire on the matter at length), naturally suggest a negative answer. It takes some time for Lawrence to explain why this is erroneous. His case is not, as one might expect, on the grounds of interfertility: this criterion is called into doubt by the evidence of cross-species hybridization yielding fertile offspring – and although this happens only as a result of human intervention, and generally among domesticated species, humans themselves are, if not domesticated, at any rate 'eminently domestic' (p. 232). It remains possible, therefore, that interracial fertility is of this kind. By what criteria, then, can we decide species identity? The answer is a little more convoluted, and derived from Blumenbach:

> If we see two races of animals resembling each other in general, and differing only in certain respects, according to what we have observed in other instances, we refer them without hesitation to the same species, although the difference should be so considerable as to affect the whole external appearance. (p. 231)

On this basis it transpires:

> There is no point of difference between the several races of mankind, which has not been found to arise, in at least an equal degree, among other animals, as a mere variety, from the usual causes of degeneration. Our instances are drawn chiefly from the domesticated kinds, which, by their association with man, lead an unnatural kind of life, are taken into new climates and situations, and exposed to various other circumstances, altogether different from their original destination. Hence they run into varieties of form, size, proportions, colour, disposition, faculties; which, when they are established as permanent breeds, would be considered, by a person uninformed on these subjects, to be originally different species. Wild animals, on the contrary, remaining constantly in the state for which they were originally framed, retain permanently their first character. (p. 232)

The variety of the human races is thus strictly analogous to that of domestic animals, 'mere varieties' becoming 'established as permanent breeds' in the various lands to which we have dispersed by breeding isolation. Lawrence's case is a purely zoological one, and in no way mitigates the view that present races are (as we now say) genetically different in qualities of all kinds, just as the dachshund and Border collie, the Great Dane and the Chihuahua, are among dogs.

Though he touches only briefly on strictly psychological matters, other than affirming the brain as the seat of mental phenomena and comparing the mental faculties of humans with other animals, and those of human races with one another, Lawrence firmly embeds human nature in Nature, and as far as its further investigation is concerned his message is clear.

(ii) James Cowles Prichard

Though Lawrence was silenced, his project was continued in part by his friend Prichard, who had encouraged him in producing the *Lectures* and whose own *Researches into the Physical History of Mankind* had appeared in 1813. Unlike Lawrence, Prichard devotedly expanded and revised his book (similarly dedicated to Blumenbach) over the ensuing decades. But while his position had earlier been almost the same as Lawrence's, the furore over the *Lectures* chastened him, and by the third edition (1836) he is backtracking on the kind of 'natural selection' model which both had adopted[40]. Even so, it remains significant for our purposes.

While Prichard is less inclined than Lawrence fervently to urge the necessity of treating 'Man' zoologically, his arguments for the monogenist case are couched primarily in zoological terms. He again expounds at length on the theoretical problem of identifying species and differentiating them from 'varieties', species being marked by possession of 'any peculiar character which has always been constant and undeviating' (vol. I, p. 105). On the hybridization issue he distinguishes between interspecies hybridization, which produces infertile offspring, and intervariety hybridization, the products of which are frequently even more reproductively vigorous than their parents. Where Prichard's case differs from Lawrence's is in the additional value he places on psychological criteria. Having cited evidence as to the high fertility of the offspring of parents from different races, he moves on to the 'psychic histories' of Bushmen or Hottentots, 'Esquimaux' and 'Negroes'. While accepting that

> No picture of human degradation and wretchedness can be drawn which exceeds the real abasement and misery of the Bushmen, as we find it displayed by the most accurate writers who describe this people. (p. 178)

he argues that nevertheless, on the account of a Mr Burchell, they possess 'traits of kind and social feelings, and all the essential attributes of humanity' (*ibid.*). Furthermore, their current miserable circumstances are due to their having been driven into the 'inaccessible rocks and deserts of the interior' by Europeans, and wars with other tribes. Their eager, positive responsiveness to Christianity is also cited in their favour. After similar reviews of the moral and religious ideas of Eskimos and 'Negroes', Prichard concludes:

> . . . it may be affirmed that the phenomena of the human mind and the moral and intellectual history of human races afford no proof of diversity of origin in the families of men; that on the contrary, in accordance with an extensive series of analogies above pointed out, we may perhaps say, that races so nearly allied and even identified in all the principal traits of their psychical character, as are the several races of mankind, must be considered as belonging to one species. (p. 216)

Not that he denies differences between them in mental capacity or 'the average degree of perfection in the developement [sic] of the brain', but:

> . . . it will be quite sufficient for my present argument, if it is allowed, that there are *some* Negroes whose mental faculties fully attain the standard of European intellect. (*ibid.*, original emphasis)

And this proposition 'can scarcely be disputed'. Only once he has settled the case for the 'psychic' unity of mankind does Prichard discuss skin colour and other physiological features. His general strategy here, in line with his earlier analysis of the nature of species, is to demonstrate that variations in such physiological traits can occur universally, and that a trait characteristic of one particular race may, even so, occasionally be found among members of others. Human races are thus 'varieties', not species. The main body of the work is a comprehensive survey of the physical and cultural variety of mankind, including some use of linguistic data for tracing their relationships.

Both Lawrence and Prichard are of relevance to Psychology as promoters of the idea of the essential psychological unity of the human race, and the adoption of natural historical and zoological methodologies in investigating human nature. Prichard in particular also recognizes the need to study functional and behavioural characteristics alongside anatomical ones.[41] While Prichard's approving references to missionary zeal and the civilizing effects of Christianity no doubt sounded reassuring, they cannot disguise the fact that he is continuing to further the project which he initiated with his friend Lawrence – notwithstanding his downplaying of evolutionary 'transmutation', except in the matter of 'varieties'. The later *Natural History of Man* adds little, so far as I can tell (except some very nice coloured plates), to the previous work, though the religious flights are perhaps more fervent:

> The Sacred Scriptures, whose testimony is received by all men of unclouded minds with implicit and reverential assent, declare that it pleased the Almighty Creator to make of one blood all the nations of the earth, and that all mankind are the offspring of common parents. (p. 5)

Large passages are lifted verbatim from the earlier work. In discussing the dramatic superficial differences between the races, Prichard invokes an extraterrestrial visitor being shown high-culture Europe, and then:

> . . . let the same person be carried into a hamlet in Negroland, in the hour when the sable race recreate themselves with dancing and barbarous music. (p. 487)

The argument for psychic unity continues to rest on a common belief in the afterlife and unseen agencies, on death rites, and on the universality of humane sentiments even amongst the most savage.

Some clue as to why Prichard is reluctant to search more deeply for psychological universals may be found in his afore-cited rejection of comparative Psychology (see above, p. 264). To apply too rigorously the criterion of common species behavioural and psychological traits, as well as physical ones, would be the thin end of an evolutionary wedge which Prichard – by now, at any rate – wishes to avoid.[42]

5 Other Areas

The four fields discussed cover the majority of proto-Psychological texts published before the 1850s, but one could obviously find numerous additional works reflecting the broad trends already outlined. Educational thought, and pressures for educational reform, continued. British writers on education were, however, of less importance than continental pioneers in the Rousseau tradition such as Herbart, Pestalozzi and Froebel, and do not appear to have introduced any significantly new psychological ideas. The same may be said in the closely related field of subnormality, in which Guggenbühl and Séguin were the principal pioneers. Natural-historical studies of animal behaviour began to make an appearance during this period (e.g. Kirby, 1834), but the methodology was anecdotal and undeveloped and the theoretical stance, such as it was, tended to be Natural Theological – the marvels of animal nest-building, migration, web-weaving and the like being evidence of Providential wisdom. The best examples of this are to be found in the Bridgewater Treatises (e.g. John Kidd, 1833). Although such work continued to appear until late in the century, occasionally in books of quite a substantial size[43], it is only among those written within the evolutionary Darwinian framework that we begin to find 'comparative Psychology' of a more modern kind. An increasing interest in trying to characterize more precisely the difference between animals and humans is, however, evident in the anthropological works already dealt with, which, in publishing terms, establish the genre to which Darwin's *Descent of Man* (1871) belongs. The analytical study of animal behaviour in its own right, with neither theological nor demarcational objectives, is rare before Darwin, notwithstanding the vast amount of exotic anecdote in travellers' and natural historians' works.

Linguistics was the virtual monopoly of the Germans throughout these years, although the Anglophone tradition would revive later in the century. This was, as explained above (pp. 114–5), in part due to Horne Tooke's baleful influence on the Associationist tradition and, in the Scottish school, Dugald Stewart's marginalization of linguistics as philosophically irrelevant.

One additional source, however, is staring us in the face: the novel. It is arguable that much of what we now consider to be research on personality and social psychology was being undertaken in this medium, above all in Britain, France and Russia. Again this is more evident – the Brontës and Charles Dickens excepted – in the latter half of the century (George Eliot being the prime example). Clear-cut cases of conceptual innovation among novelists would, however, be difficult to identify, central though they undoubtedly were in the cultural mediation and expression of psychological change. Finally, one might mention a lingering tradition of characterology persisting on the margins of physiognomy and phrenology, in which character sketches of typical classes of citizen are presented alongside an appropriate illustration. This eventually revived in Henry Mayhew's *London Labour and the London Poor* (1851–62), in which it metamorphosed into investigative sociological survey. During our period, Busby's modest *Costume of the Lower Orders of London* (1820) stands out for its honest empathy and the individuated nature of several of its character descriptions. Also Social Psychology in its fashion was C. Mackay's extraordinary *Popular Delusions and the Madness of Crowds* (1841, 1852; repr. 1956), which might be seen as descending from Thomas Browne's *Pseudodoxia Epidemica*. Much as such works are in need of renewed attention, they offer us little here in the way of conceptual novelty.

Conclusion

We are now in a position to understand more clearly the matrix of ideas in which the founding of British Psychology was embedded. The broad cultural reconceptualization of human nature, and the social background in which it originated, had reordered the priorities of reflexive discourse. A practical agenda was evolving for the 'Science of Mind' in which new questions and methodologies were rapidly replacing or transforming the metaphysical and epistemological concerns which had previously dominated philosophy and hamstrung physiology. Theologians, at bay, intensified their defence of religious orthodoxy after nearly a century of relative quiescence, and in 1840 Laycock was still able to lament:

> It is to be regretted that the physiology of the mind of man is made more difficult to study by speculations on the immortality of the soul. (1840, p. 89)

Such speculations had long been laid aside by his fellow physiologists and philosophers alike. In philosophy the once rival doctrines of Associationism and Reidian Common Sense had argued themselves more or less to a halt, and in some sense John Stuart Mill's assault on Sir William Hamilton in 1865 belonged to an era already past. Bain and Spencer – and even, as Daniel N. Robinson (1982) points out, John Stuart Mill himself – had absorbed much from the Scottish school. But Bain and Spencer, if not John Stuart Mill, also knew that a place for physiology has to be found in any account of human nature which is to carry conviction. How to accomplish this was perhaps unclear, and we might query whether it has yet been achieved, but there was no lack of people willing to try, particularly among the new breed of psychophysiologists such as Laycock, Noble and Carpenter.

With physiology another strand of ideas had to be addressed concerning 'Man's' status as an object of scientific enquiry. The likelihood that some kind of evolutionary account was required became inescapable in the years between Lawrence's *Lectures* and the appearance of the *Origin of Species* in 1859. This was reinforced by archaeological discoveries in Denmark and France implying the existence of a distant prehistoric 'Stone Age' phase. The authority of conventional wisdoms was being sapped across the board, as comprehensively, if not so dramatically, as it had been at the beginning of the seventeenth century. Meanwhile, society itself was demanding new kinds of wisdom: about how to manage education, crime, madness, deviancy, and socialization in an industrialized and increasingly urbanized culture for which history provided no precedent.

It was observed above that John Stuart Mill's proposed Ethology contained clear anticipations of the direction which British Psychology would take under Galton. Combean phrenology and Owenite utopian socialism provided competing reforming visions during the years we have been examining, and it is Roger Cooter's case that the former, locating the agency for change in the striving, competitive, self-examining and self-disciplined individual, won out, even if phrenology itself did not. John Stuart Mill, though an environmentalist in modern terms, implicitly endorses this by viewing social life as an aggregative product of individual actions with no emergent properties of its own. But the Owenite vision had an impact, none the less, in its stress on education and socialization – which John Stuart Mill would also have endorsed. Again, British Psychology might be located at the confluence of these two approaches, incorporating, after Darwin (in Galton especially), both a strong hereditarian and a managerial component.

Social historians now exhibit a fair degree of consensus that a net effect of all this was a change in mentality, characterized as the rise of an excessively individualistic consciousness, primarily relating to others as objects rather than subjects. And they would also see Psychology as being founded on this, amounting to nothing less than the creation of the realm of the psychological itself, as we now understand it. Only at this point can the operations of the individual mind become a delimitable target of investigation. While I am in broad sympathy with this position, I do not believe it was quite as sudden as this, happening over a few decades from about 1780 onwards. Norbert Elias (1978) locates its origins in the Renaissance, and I have argued that this emergence of the autonomous individual begins as early as the seventeenth century. Nor do I believe it adequately captures the shift in tone which we see in British writings from the first half of the nineteenth century, by contrast with Germany, where an older orientation is not only maintained but flourishes before a substantial collapse around mid century.

While it is somewhat nebulous to grasp, this change seems to involve abandoning an attitude, shared by both Romanticism and Enlightenment philosophy, in which the human race, and especially its present activities, were somehow of central cosmic importance. The human race was rationally or Romantically exalted, and glorified yet further in Germany after the turn of the century by writers such as Schelling, Fichte, Hegel and Oken for whom the human story is a triumphal spiritual progress heading towards fusion with the Absolute. This is not incompatible with science – indeed, the scientist is a hero in the very vanguard of this progressive advance. Human nature is governed by cosmic laws operating at successively higher and higher levels, driving matter into organism, organism into sensitivity, sensitivity into consciousness, consciousness into Reason, and Reason into Spirit. In France it is Comte who most clearly represents this orientation; in Britain, perhaps, Coleridge and Shelley – as well as Morell in his learned but sterile 1851 'odd' volume. In the British psychophysiologists, John Stuart Mill, Bain and even, strangely enough, Spencer (whose evolutionary philosophy was as cosmic as you could wish) this tone is absent. We are in a down-to-earth material world of physical causes and effects, a world the scale of which dwarfs rather than glorifies us in cosmic terms. The anthropocentric spiritual aspiration has finally evaporated, replaced by practical realities. Of course there remains a huge self-confidence in the superiority and competence of white educated males, especially if they are British. But this is a pale substitute for the intoxicating realms of Absolute Spirit and Man the supreme and culminating product of Nature, the product of aeons of labour by Mind aspiring to Realize itself. Or was the latter but a pale substitute for the joys of running an earthly Empire?

9
The French Route: Degenerating Dreams

In contrast to the previous century, the role of French thought in generating new psychological ideas and theories was now greatly reduced in significance, and few French writers (Ribot, Taine and Tarde being arguable exceptions) customarily figure among Psychology's founders. One distinct tradition of proto-Psychological thought is, even so, readily discernible: a preoccupation with the clinical and the abnormal. Not that this entirely monopolized the French Psychological agenda. There is a predictable philosophical reaction against the extreme materialism of late Enlightenment *idéologues* such as Cabanis and Bichat, but this tends to take the form (e.g. in Maine de Biran and Victor Cousin, the most eminent of those concerned) of variants on contemporary German Idealism. Central to the bizarre Theory of Universal Unity propounded by the cosmic utopian Charles Fourier[1] there is a theory (fantasy? delusion?) of human character which is quite *sui generis*, and known to Anglophone historians of Psychology primarily from Roback's account (Roback, 1928). It was the physiologists Magendie and Flourens, however, who made the most concrete contributions to the development of Psychology (as distinct from psychiatry). We shall consider in turn the psychiatric, philosophical and physiological aspects of French Psychological thought, and finish with a brief look at Fourier.

1 French Psychiatric Tradition[2]

Philippe Pinel (1745–1826) and his successor J.E.D. Esquirol (1772–1840) represent the triumph of the Enlightenment's optimistic, rational, humanitarian approach to madness and, in the view of medical historians, the beginning of modern psychiatry. They also, in the light of Foucault's now classic *Madness and Civilization* (1967), represent the paradigm example of the modern use of psychiatry as a managerial instrument of hegemonic social control in the interests of bourgeois norms and values[3]. Unlike Britain, France had already seen a period of increased incarceration of the insane in large official institutions, of which the Paris Bicêtre Asylum, scene of Pinel's famed casting off of inmates' chains in 1793, was one of the most important. Pinel's humane revolution in therapy and asylum organization had a rapid and international impact which similar efforts on a smaller scale (such as William Tuke's in York and Vincenzo Chiarugi's in Italy) had never achieved. Since he was the leading figure in French psychiatry, Pinel's adoption of 'moral treatment' had an authority which isolated provincial reformers and humanitarian pamphleteers lacked. Coupled with his two major works, the three-volume *Nosographie philosophique* (1798) and *Traité médico-philosophique sur la Manie* (1801), these practical reforms made Pinel the focal point of reference for subsequent psychiatric writers throughout Europe. Esquirol continued Pinel's work, producing a new nosology and introducing systematic record-keeping and statistical analyses of recovery rates and the incidence of different conditions. Reported recovery and improvement rates increased considerably under the Pinel–Esquirol regimes.

The conceptual innovations introduced by Pinel and Esquirol are more elusive than their therapeutic and managerial significance. At the most general level they succeeded in establishing the notion of madness as a *disease*, and thus the province of medicine. While, as we saw, this remained an issue in Britain and Germany for some time to come, the combination at the Bicêtre and Salpêtrière (where Pinel later moved and Esquirol practised) of an apparently 'moral' approach to treatment within a fully medicalized framework provided a crucial image, for psychiatry elsewhere, of the possibilities of reconciliation between the two. At a more specific level, Esquirol's nosology was also among the most influential over the coming decades (although it was an era as rich in such exercises as it was poor in deriving clear-cut therapies from them). This appeared in its most developed form in his two-volume *Des maladies mentales considérées sous les rapports médicals, hygiéniques et médico-legals* (1838). Some of this was new (differentiation of depressive states, *lypemanias*, from psychoses); some was clearer redefinition of existing concepts such as 'monomania'. Zilboorg (1941) also credits Esquirol with giving 'hallucination' its modern sense. His extensive listings of events implicated in precipitating madness may be read in two ways: traditionally, they were viewed by medical historians as heralding the acknowledgement of madness as – sometimes, at least – purely psychological in nature, but in Foucault they become a catalogue and medicalization of the deviancies found intolerable by contemporary bourgeois society, signifying psychiatry's role in defining the emerging social power relationships in post-Revolutionary French society.

In the background to all this lay a continued fascination with Mesmerism and 'Animal Magnetism' (see above, Chapter 6). As we saw, medical interest in this never entirely abated, and the major revival after 1860 led directly to Charcot's psychiatric usage of hypnosis at the end of the century. While clearly separate from psychiatry during the period we are are concerned with here, the indigenous Mesmeric tradition may be seen as evidence of a persistent French fascination with the psychologically abnormal.

Following Esquirol, French psychiatry, like psychiatry elsewhere, retreated from therapeutic optimism, and the management function increasingly dominated the therapeutic one. Although J.P. Falret, a pupil of Esquirol, continued to adopt a psychological level approach, advances in physiology began to shift psychiatric thinking back in the direction of physical aetiology. At this stage it is reasonable to see a correlation between physiological orientation and therapeutic pessimism, given the inability of medicine at that time to tackle neurological pathologies, even when they were identified – only the advent of modern pharmacology would change this. Psychological orientations, on the other hand, held out the possibility of cure by some form of behavioural re-education. This pessimism was bolstered by growing hereditarianism, particularly B.A. Morel's degenerationist model, expounded in his *Traité des dégénérescences physiques, intellectuelles et morales de l'espèce humaine* (1857). Morel's degenerationism reversed his earlier focus on the psychological nature of madness, probably as a result of his close friendship with the physiologist Claude Bernard. Of all European countries, France would later be the most culturally responsive to degenerationism, which eventually pulled together evolutionary theory, hypnotic suggestibility, madness and immorality into a comprehensively nightmarish vision of impending social and racial collapse. Further into this we cannot enter, but hints of things to come were already evident in the 1840s.

A further figure also concerned with the psychologically abnormal is Edouard Séguin, pioneer in the treatment of subnormality. Séguin devoted his life to devising practical methods for managing and improving the subnormal, and continued to do so in the USA after emigrating for political reasons following the 1848 Revolution. Among his lasting innovations was the humble 'form-board' – with variously shaped holes in which pegs of corresponding shapes are to be inserted. Apart from becoming a basic infant's toy, this device entered the Psychologist's battery of intelligence testing equipment and a vast number of variants were designed (especially between the two World Wars), some of considerable complexity[4]. Séguin worked in the Romantic educational tradition of Rousseau, Pestalozzi and Froebel; his methods involved a detailed empirical study of basic psychological processes and are an important, if neglected, link in the child-study lineage leading to modern Developmental Psychology[5].

2 French Philosophy

By the restoration of the Bourbon monarchy in 1815, the Materialist Sensationalist philosophy which had dominated French thought since Condillac had exhausted both its intellectual vigour and its social appeal, its utopian aspirations for social reform now seemed naive and obsolete. The last representatives of the school were the *idéologues*[6] such as Cabanis, Bichat, Broussais and Destutt de Tracy, with the University of Montpellier being the final bastion of materialism in French physiological thought. The inevitable reaction initially seems to have taken the form of an incorporation of the ideas of Reid, Stewart and Kant – first, in M. Laromiguière, in modifying the Condillac tradition, followed by Maine de Biran (1766–1824), and Royer-Collard (a translator of Reid and Stewart), who both opposed it. Maine de Biran's *Essai sur les fondements de la psychologie* (1813–1822)[7] was the first major French Idealist attack on the Condillac tradition, replacing it with a developmentally focused account of how the individual actively acquires an integrated sense of self. In this the will becomes the major explanatory factor. Notwithstanding his desire to integrate physiology and Psychology fully, his concept of Psychology remains as a science of consciousness. The work is basically a French version of the German genre of programmatic attempts philosophically to identify fundamental principles on which Psychology should be established, rather than actually to establish it. Its developmental character and emphasis on the will and attention are its most distinctive features, and according to D.B. Klein (1970) Piaget acknowledged the importance of Maine de Biran's account of the active interaction between child and environment.

In so far as French philosophy immediately made any further original moves, it was in the work of Victor Cousin (1791–1867), whose eventful career included being bailed out of prison by Hegel in Berlin in 1824 and being a Minister of Public Instruction under the Thiers government in 1840. Although he is now virtually forgotten outside France, Cousin's contemporary esteem was considerable, as a translator of classics, a historian of philosophy, and a thinker in his own right. His critique of Locke's *Essay* was especially influential in striking at the founding text of the materialist school. Part of this was translated into English and published in Hartford, Connecticut, in 1834 as *Elements of Psychology included in a critical examination of Locke's Essay on the Human Understanding*. The Introduction to this by the editor, C.S. Henry, seems to be the only extensive account of Cousin's system in English, although it came too early to deal with his most important book, *Du vrai, du beau, du bien* (1840), a transcript of lectures given in 1818. In retrospect, Cousin's philosophy appears to be yet another variant on contemporary German Idealism, although his nuances of difference seemed profound enough at the time. This is perhaps unfair; even if he is forgotten, there are some features which might strike us as prophetic.

For Cousin, human consciousness comprises – conventionally enough – three distinct levels: the sensible, the voluntary, the rational. Both the sensible and the rational are governed by necessity; the voluntary stands between them as the 'personal and imputable', the province of Will, and it is to this that the term 'Personality' applies. We find ourselves 'between these two orders of facts' (i.e. sensible and rational), from which we separate and distinguish ourselves:

> All light comes from the reason, and it is the reason that perceives both itself, and the sensibility which envelops it, and the will also upon which it imposes obligation, though without constraining it.[8]

Reason is in essence Divine and not, strictly speaking, ours. Psychology, the study of consciousness, envelops all of science in the way God envelops the world. The irreducible 'fundamental' Psychological 'fact' involves two ideas and their 'connexion or correlation'. First, there is the distinction between the 'me' and the 'not-me', but both of these pertain to what is finite, and together they contrast with what contains and explains them both: the infinite. This move has an obviously Hegelian dialectic character. Cousin also identifies four kinds of philosophical system, or expressions of the philosophical spirit: Sensualism, Idealism, Scepticism and Mysticism, each of which is useful; these exist and reappear 'in every great epoch'[9]. Cousin's own position must, we infer, be understood as transcending this quartet. The direct impact of the system just crudely sketched on Psychological thought appears to have been minimal, but obvious though the point is, we might see adumbrations of id, ego and superego in his sensible, voluntary, rational division. In this it resembles the German psychiatrist Heinroth's system (see above, pp. 313–4). For all these Idealist 'Eclectics', as they were known, the first generation of French Psychologists had nothing but disdain. Any direct influence of their work on the Psychology of Taine and Ribot would be hard to discover.

After Cousin, the next French philosopher of any international significance is Auguste Comte (1798–1857), himself reacting in his turn against the new Idealism. How far Comte influenced Psychology is a moot point. Although sympathetic to phrenology, he was basically hostile to the psychological level of analysis, favouring sociology (of which he was one of the founders). Boring (1950) gave him pretty short shrift, noting his rejection of introspection, his belief that all facts are social, and the fact that his concept of positivism as meaning 'based on observable facts' in some senses begs the question and differed from both Mach's positivism and that of the Logical Positivists. Murphy and Kovach (1972) deal even more briefly with him, noting only his evolutionism and the 'behaviourist' implications of his anti-introspectionism. D.B. Klein discusses Comte primarily as a harbinger of anti-introspective Behaviorism and Gilbert Ryle's philosophical attack on the feasibility of studying consciousness as if it were a parallel realm observable in the same sense in which the external world is (Ryle, 1949). More recently, Hearnshaw (1987) has conceded that 'he made no great impression on psychologists' (p. 183). John Stuart Mill's *Auguste Comte and Positivism* (1866, 2nd edn) early on provided English readers with a systematically diplomatic deconstruction of Comte's highest pretensions. On his rejection of Psychology, Mill impatiently comments: 'There is little need for an elaborate refutation of a fallacy respecting which the only wonder is that it should impose on any one' (p. 63). Later adding – more in sorrow than in anger, one feels:

> And what Organon for the study of 'the moral and intellectual functions' does M. Comte offer, in lieu of the direct mental observation which he repudiates? We are almost ashamed to say, that it is Phrenology! (p. 65)

For Psychologists, then, the mighty six volumes of Comte's *Cours de philosophie positive* (1830–42) have remained closed from the beginning – his rejection of introspection being repugnant to those of the nineteenth century and his version of Positivism being the opposite of that held by mainstream twentieth-century ones.

Only at the very end of the period we are concerned with are there signs of a move towards modern Psychology. Antoine Cournot (1807–77), in his *Essai sur les fondements de nos connaissances* (1851) seeks to embed Psychology within a vitalist biology, as part of a continuum in the ways the life-force manifests itself. He is anti-reductionist but also anti-metaphysical, and his system admits unconscious and instinctual levels. Brett (1953 edn) considers him comparable to Wundt and Bergson, but Herbert Spencer may be a closer contemporary figure, particularly with regard to the notion of instinct and reason being the lower and higher ends of a single continuum of increasingly complex synthesis. His position may be seen as a transitional one between the anti-mechanistic Idealism of the Eclectics and the more orthodox empiricism of Hippolyte Taine, whose *De l'intelligence* (1870, English transl. 1871) gave him a role in French Psychology analogous to that of Bain in Britain. Modern English language disciplinary histories are devoid of references to Cournot. A slightly earlier transitional figure who attempted to develop an introspective Psychology was Théodore Simon Jouffroy (1796–1842), another Reid and Stewart translator, whose *Mélanges philosophiques* (1833) has now been forgotten.

3 French Physiology

As they have been discussed previously, we need only note here the two major psychophysiological contributions during this period: (a) Magendie's confirmation, and clearer articulation, of Bell's discovery of the distinction between the afferent and efferent nerves (1822) and (b) Flourens's research on brain functioning which seemed to refute localization of function. These have been mentioned in the contexts of Bell's work and phrenology respectively. It was undoubtedly to Magendie's research that the widespread recognition of the difference in nerve functions was due[10]. His major psychophysiological book was *Leçons sur les fonctions et les maladies du système nerveux* (1839). Flourens's findings, first reported in 1824, effectively swung the physiological consensus of opinion against localization of cortical functioning until Broca's apparently authoritative announcement of the discovery of the speech area[11]. In addition, a good deal of sensory physiology and psychophysics was being conducted[12]. But unlike events in Germany, there was no obvious point at which this kind of research was co-opted from physiology into Psychology.

A second area in which physiology had long assumed significant proportions in France was in anthropology, the credit for founding which the French ascribed to Buffon. Among European imperial powers France was second to none in measuring the bodies, particularly the skulls, of its non-European subjects. Even if the localization of function question remained unsettled, the importance of brain-size as an index of intellectual power was apparently unquestioned (and Broca's, as it eventually turned out, was reassuringly huge). The French Natural History tradition of Buffon and Cuvier had already demonstrated the French penchant for classification, ordering and labelling, best expressed culturally, perhaps, in the Napoleonic Code. Esquirol's statistical analyses of his patients may be read in the same light, and French anthropology provided another arena. It is none the less somewhat anachronistic to talk of anthropology at this time as a distinct discipline, the Société d'Anthropologie being founded (by Broca) in Paris only in 1869. A Society of Ethnology had been founded in 1839, and the terms ethnology (referring to the theoretical side of the enterprise) and ethnography (referring to factual data-gathering) were the more commonly used. As in Britain, the monogenist–polygenist debate was a constant issue, with the latter position being more strongly represented in France than in Britain (Virey and A. Desmoulins being its main advocates against Cuvier). It was Cuvier's magisterial anti-'transformationist' attack on Lamarck, though, which created the climate in which the polygenist case could be effectively mounted, in contrast to Britain where, even if it was heretical, the evolutionary thinking introduced by Erasmus Darwin and William Lawrence continued to dominate discussions of the issue whenever it was allowed to surface[13]. In France, '*transformisme* was vanquished', P. Topinard tells us, in 1830, when Cuvier succeeded in defeating Lamarck's follower Geoffroy St Hilaire[14]. Topinard, while accepting *transformisme*, was still endorsing a variety of polygenism late in the century[15].

It was as ethnology or anthropology that the French saw the Science of Man as being realized, an aspiration which persisted via Durkheim and Lévy-Bruhl to Lévi-Strauss. In view of the close connections between physiology and ethnology, the possibilities of a Psychology appearing are not, in the early part of the century, that promising[16]. With French philosophy in creative decline, ethnology taking a role analogous to that of German *Völkerpsychologie*, and physiology ranging from what would now be termed 'physical anthropology' to psychophysics, there is little space for Psychology. This is exacerbated by the absence in France of any strictly articulated *Geisteswissenschaft–Naturwissenschaft* divide.

Physiology and natural history – along with ethnology, which in a sense bridged them – enjoyed an epoch of considerable success in early-nineteenth-century France. By contrast French philosophy, on which Psychological thought largely depended, could not compete with its German counterpart; nor, though to a lesser degree, could it match contemporary British philosophy either (in which James Mill, Dugald Stewart, Thomas Brown and Sir William Hamilton were all active). The researches of Flourens and Magendie would in time be seen as crucial steps in the history of physiological Psychology, and the less well-known psychophysical researches of their humbler contemporaries similarly fall into place retrospectively in the history of Psychological studies of the senses. At the time, however, their context was purely physiological (except for Flourens's role in combating phrenology). Before pulling the story of the French route to Psychology together, a look at Charles Fourier is in order, since his is the first – albeit fantastic – attempt at a 'modern' personality theory.

4 Charles Fourier (1772–1837)

If the case is being made that modern Psychology arose in large part as a response to social management pressures, then no better evidence might be found to support the hypothesis than Charles Fourier, would-be social manager *extraordinaire*. A reluctant but at times successful businessman, he sought respite from this apparently guilt-inducing vocation in constructing a vast cosmological system of 'Universal Unity' which involved a blueprint for a utopian planetary society, and at the heart of this lay a Psychological model of the nature of the diversity of the human race. We will, alas, have to leave aside here his beliefs that the elephant, oak and diamond were created by the Sun, and the cow, jonquil and topaz by Jupiter, as well as his Laws of Simple and Compound Immortality. Roback's fairly extended treatment of Fourier is charitably sympathetic and provides an adequate introduction to his Psychological system, although it omits some of its features (Roback, 1928).

The core metaphor on which Fourier's system is built is the musical scale, which provides him with a schema of cosmic harmony and much of his technical vocabulary, though all the sensory modes are analogically exploited[17]. The human life-cycle, like that of everything else in the universe from stars downwards, goes through a series of stages, punctuated by crises. Fully elaborated, there are 8 phases of 'ascending vibration' and 8 of slow decline comprising the 'descending vibration'. We begin with 'ascending limbo, or anterior subversion' – i.e. bodily formation in the womb – and end with 'descending limbo, or posterior subversion' – i.e. bodily decay in the grave (death itself being the 'Final crisis or posterior transition'). The intervening period comprises a fairly conventional succession through birth, childhood, adolescence, etc., to sterility and decline, but all translated into Fourier's curious terminology. There are twelve fundamental motivating 'passions', and these provide a basis for both individual personality and his plans for social harmony. At this point it should be noted that the human race as a whole is going through its own 32-stage career from 'Edenism' to an eventual decay and death, after which it will be removed to another more advanced 'globe'. Not to worry – we

Table 9.1 Frequency of Character Types in Charles Fourier's System

		Total per 810
1. Monogynes – 1 dominant, of whatever kind		576
A. *Dimixts*		80
2. Digynes – 2 dominant affectives, or one affective and one distributive		96
B. *Trimixts*		16
3. Trigunes		24
4. Tetragynes		8
C. *Tetramixts*		8
5. Pentagynes		2
	Total	810
. .		
D. *Pentamixts*	2 per	2432
6. Hexagynes	"	2434
E. *Heptamixts*	"	9728
7. Heptagynes	"	9740
8. Omnigynes	"	29222

adapted from C. Fourier (1851) Vol.2, pp.312–313

are as yet only at the relatively early (fifth) stage of 'Civilization', with 'Guaranteeism, Socialism and Harmonism' and the rest of the 24 ascending stages to follow.

The twelvefold classification of Passions is, as far as I can tell, at the 'Genera' level, because, like the branches of a tree, they can be subdivided into successively smaller types ('Classes, Orders, Genera, Species, Varieties, Diminutives, Tenuities and Minimities'). Individuals may be dominated by one or more of these twelve passions, the relative frequencies in the population being calculable by analogy with the musical scale (see Table 9.1). There are also mixed types in which no single passion is dominant, but which oscillate between two or more 'ralliant' passions. Out of 810 people 576 will be 'Monogynes', dominated by one passion; 96 'Digynes' dominated by two, 24 'Trigynes', 8 'Tetragynes' and 2 'Pentagynes'. Above this level, from 'Hexagynes' to 'Omnigynes', the frequencies become progressively smaller, until we reach 'Super-omnigynes' of the 'seventeenth' degree or power with a frequency of one in two-and-a-half to three billion[18]. There is also a similar increasing rarity of mixed types. These 'Dimixts', etc., are, at the Civilization stage, seen as contemptible, but will become very valuable in the Harmony stage.

Relationships between individuals are also mapped in an extraordinary table entitled 'Potential Gamut of the Accords of Friendship, and of the Accord of Love; with Analogies'[19]; this includes such delights as a variety of Love called 'Delphigamy', a variety of 'Visuism' possessed of the 'Ultra-ethereal eye', and a phase of 'Development' called 'Phanerophily'. The most important role of the personality type system, however, is as a basis on which to arrive at ideal forms of social organization. Fourier calculated that 1,600 people were necessary for a fully self-supporting 'social body'. Ideally, this would comprise 16 'tribes' of the different age groups, with roughly equal numbers of male and female, yielding 32 single-sex 'choirs'. Taken together, these constitute a 'Vortex' or 'Phalanx', a social or industrial self-supporting 'hive', headed by a 'Monarch'. These 'phalanges' in turn form national units (ruled by a 'duarch') and so on through successively higher scales of organization, including continents, ruled by 'Douzarchs' and 'Omniarchs' ruling the whole world – of whom there will be 32, each governing their own sphere of activity 'in the areopagus of the whole globe'. Thus will the 'spherical unity of mankind' be achieved. At every level harmony will be attained by ensuring the right ratios of the passionally defined personality types. I cannot leave Fourier without citing the English title of Volume 2, Part III, Section 1 of *The Passions of the Human Soul*: 'Of Parcours, Transits, Flitting Raptures, Passional Delights or Exhilirations, and of Unityism'.

This book, containing Fourier's Psychology, formed one volume of the nine-volume *La Théorie de l'unité universelle* (1822). In 1832, along with the socialist Saint-Simonians, Fourier founded a journal, *Le Phalanstère, ou La Réforme Industrielle*, for the promotion of his ideas, and the Fourier movement continued to play a part in the French radical political scene until the Revolutionary year 1848, which brought it to a halt. As well as other journals, two Fourierist publications, *La Phalange* and *Démocratie Pacifique* appeared as daily papers in the 1840s. The introduction to the English translation of *The Passions of the Human Soul* by Hugh Doherty (who knew Fourier) is probably the best contemporary account of his ideas in English, gaining by being largely uncritical, although even Doherty strains at a few gnats while swallowing most of the camel[20]. He proclaims: 'The Bible is the only book which treats of human destiny more deeply and more luminously than the writings of this man of genius' (p. xxxiii).

No psychologist since has attempted such an ambitious and all-encompassing project; their personality typologies seem rudimentary alongside Fourier's mathematico-musical system, and few, if any, have sought to find such rigorous order in the characterological ecology of the entire species. But none of his plethora of neologisms gained common acceptance, and although, as Roback observes, his system contains moments of genuine insight, it has become no more than a historical curiosity. The only comparable successor appears to have been someone called M. Edgeworth Lazarus, whose books, such as *Vegetable Portraits of Character* and *Passional Geometry*, Roback briefly mentions[21].

5 The French Route to Psychology

The canonical texts normally taken to mark the advent of a national Psychological discipline appeared in Britain and Germany in the decade 1855–1865[22], in France they are somewhat later: Taine (1870), Ribot (1870, 1876[23]) and G. Tarde (1884). While all these figures drew on the psychiatric tradition, and Tarde at least was influenced by Cournot and Comte[24], the main features of the new French Psychology were its anti-Idealist stance, its sympathetic orientation towards the British rather than the German approach, and its strong physiological orientation. The bias towards the abnormal became increasingly marked in the final years of the century as the synthesis of hypnosis, evolutionary theory and psychiatric thought – now bolstered by Tarde's Laws of Imitation – became consolidated, and with this its social managerial functions came increasingly to the fore (e.g. in Binet's work on education and intelligence testing and Le Bon's crowd psychology at the turn of the century[25]). The turbulent nature of French history during much of the nineteenth century undoubtedly disrupted the course of Psychology's development, particularly in periodic stiflings of radical thought and the consequent emigration of such potentially influential figures as Séguin. This disrupted history nevertheless helped to determine the focus on social control and management which marked the discipline from the 1880s onwards.

Having said this, we can, during the first half of the century, see a number of incipient ideas which later came to the fore; most significant among them is a preoccupation with the developmental process traceable back to Maine de Biran. A second is an increasing fascination with the unconscious and deviant conscious states with its twin sources in Mesmerism and the great psychiatric reforms at the beginning of the century. Conversely, the establishment of an evolutionary perspective was more fitfully accomplished than in Britain and Germany, owing to Cuvier's influence. Although the use of social statistics, pioneered by Quetelet, was extended rapidly for social management purposes, it failed to be assimilated into French Psychology's research methodology until the time of Binet, the psychiatric clinical tradition tending to dominate (Danziger, 1990). By then Galton and Pearson in Britain had already laid the basis for parametric statistical methods, particularly correlational techniques, in Psychology, and Spearman was working on a crude version of factor analysis.

Except possibly in the much later work of Henri Piéron, A. Michotte and Jean Piaget, Francophone Psychology never succeeded in becoming integrated with the mainstream of the discipline's development in Germany, Britain and North America. And even these exceptions occur during a relatively limited period: roughly from the 1920s to around 1960. On balance this apparent failure has been of enormous benefit to Western thought, since it eventually enabled France to sustain the autonomous and highly creative tradition which eventually produced such modern and post-modern luminaries as Sartre, Lévi-Strauss, Foucault, Derrida and Lacan. This tradition is hardly definable as 'Psychological', but it has had an enormous impact on the discipline – and it is precisely, in part, because matters psychological had not, in France, become the academic property of Psychology that it was able to flourish.

In summary, then, French thought from 1800–1850 played a major role in placing on Psychology's agenda the idea of unconscious and subconscious states, the relevance to Psychology of abnormal conditions in general, and the idea of developmental stages. More darkly, it saw the origins of degenerationism, which became the focal point of *fin-de-siècle* French Psychology (see Nye, 1975). Although the route to French Psychology never succeeded in becoming the sort of trunk road along which Anglo-American and German Psychology eventually managed to continue travelling, the alternative paths which French reflexive discourse took eventually carried it into regions both more scenic and more novel than those mapped by academic Psychology.

10
Conclusion: Making the Mind Up 1600–1850

We will now encircle the entire area.
(Crosby, Stills, Nash & Young)

The thesis underlying this book has been that novel psychological ideas have their source in changing exeriences of the world: discoveries and inventions continually enlarge the repertoire of concepts by which the inner world can be construed, social and economic changes likewise provide new images of order (or disorder) and new public social roles, as well as altering social relationships (especially power relationships) in such a way that the priorities of our self-scrutinies are modified. Those engaging in such scrutinies invariably do so in the context of ideological, political, economic or religious agendas (sometimes hidden, sometimes overt). There has been a modern illusion, which recent historiography has been striving to dispel, that such agendas can be ignored, and that a pure core of rationally evolving ideas can be identified and constitutes the proper target of historical enquiry. A sense that this approach was inadequate is not entirely new in the history of Psychology – Boring's invocation of the *Zeitgeist* signified a disquiet with it as early as 1929, while Joan Wynn Reeves (1958), almost incidentally, drops the remark:

> The current attitude of any period to questions of public health and to physical and social conditions is in itself interesting in relation to people's views on body and mind. (p. 172)

Since the late 1970s historians of Psychology have increasingly sought to align their labours with the contextualized and social constructionist approaches being adopted in other areas of post-Kuhnian history of science. Even so, the nettle has not been firmly grasped, since the very inclusion of Psychology within this enterprise begs the central question of the scientific status of the discipline. The questions of what the project of Psychology really *is*, what place it actually occupies in both the intellectual ecology and the social life of post-Renaissance Western culture, have remained largely unaddressed. At the same time, the conviction that Psychology has achieved membership of the natural sciences is itself a historical fact which requires explanation.

The present work has been written in the light of the meta-psychological problem of how 'psychological language' is possible in the first place, given that the phenomena to which it refers are ultimately subjective. The outlines of this are given in my previous book and the Introduction to this one and I will not discuss it again here. Its immediate relevance is that it requires that a historical treatment of the discipline of Psychology must be framed within a broader understanding of how psychological ideas of any kind are produced. If, as I hold, the process of physiomorphic assimilation of world-novelty into psychological novelty is a universal dynamic, mediated (most obviously, if not exclusively) by language, then Psychology as a discipline can be construed as a particular cultural form in which that process manifests itself. This move, the invention of Psychology, entailed, however, that its subject matter be constituted in a far more rigorous manner than previous modes of reflexive discourse had adopted. An autonomous, individualized realm of 'the psychological' had to be delimited as this discipline's natural object of inquiry. As late as the German and French Idealists of the early nineteenth century it was still being argued (e.g. by Heinroth and Cousin) that Reason, for example, was not individual, but transpersonal and Divine. If a consistent trend is perceivable in events during our period, it is the slow consolidation of the very idea of 'the psychological', of 'psychology', in this unitary subject-matter sense. And it is towards this that the multitude of more specific 'psychological ideas' being produced gravitate – usually, to pursue the metaphor, in more or less protracted spirals rather than headlong free fall (this metaphor, of course, comes easily only in an age of decaying satellites).

The historiographic programme seems, in this light, straightforward enough: to trace the world sources of psychological ideas, the stages by which they acquire psychological meanings, and the process by which they coalesced into proto-Psychological systems of ideas, finally becoming Psychology. In this way we would be able to track how the West made up its 'Mind'. We would also be able to identify the different impacts which these new ideas made at various levels, from popular modes of self-understanding to philosophy.

Unfortunately (or perhaps not), the past does not lend itself to quite such systematic decoding. Two difficulties immediately present themselves. First, the existence of an extensive body of History of Psychology literature providing the synoptic accounts of major figures, events and developments which are the indispensable point of embarkation for any author. These are both blessing and curse, since in trying to implement this programme one is constantly drawn into critiques of this literature in so far as the interpretations it offers appear to be flawed. Secondly, from the late seventeenth century onwards, the possibility of a unified story becomes increasingly artificial as distinct national traditions begin to crystallize out of what, through most of the seventeenth century, had been a genuinely international set of debates centring on the Scientific Revolution and philosophy. This had been possible because the number of *virtuosi* engaged in the debates was small, and the debates themselves were managed via personal correspondence networks extending across Europe, and even further[1]. During the eighteenth century a number of factors eroded this system, especially in areas of thought most relevant to us: increasing populations, the rise of the nation-state, the decline of Latin as a *lingua franca*, pursuit of different 'paradigms' (e.g. between Lockean in Britain and France versus Leibnizian in Germany) and diverging sociopolitical agendas (e.g. between proto-democratic Britain, the autocratic French *Ancien Régime*, and the feudal – if sometimes 'Enlightened' – despotism of the German States).

A third difficulty, previously mentioned, is that in seeking to redress the internalist bias of existing disciplinary histories and locate the more widespread origins of new ideas, the amount of potentially relevant territory demanding attention becomes intolerably vast. I can only hope that my peers look charitably upon the inevitably varied levels of expertise evident in my efforts to deal in some way adequately with this.

The upshot is that the implementation of the programme becomes beset with digressions which at times threaten to reduce it to the status of a hidden agenda. How is this confusion to be redeemed?

The remainder of this last chapter is an attempt to formulate a more coherent picture of the process by which psychological ideas originated in the modern period before Psychology's disciplinary debut.

1 The Sources of Psychological Ideas

How did external world sources amplify and change the body of psychological ideas during our period? This question can be answered by considering the following kinds of source: (i) 'scientific' discoveries; (ii) technological innovation; (iii) changes in forms of social life (in the broadest sense).

(i) 'Scientific' discoveries

During the seventeenth century the direct reflexive application of new scientific discoveries and ideas was, as we saw, limited. The reasons for this were twofold:

> (a) the Cartesian exclusion of the soul from the agenda of mechanistic Natural Philosophy, and the prevailing power of contemporary theological 'Pneumatology' to resist Natural Philosophical intrusion into its domain. High cultural level reflexive discourse on the psychological thus remained primarily theological and was conceptually conservative;
> (b) the Natural Philosophers' anti-rhetorical view of language, involving a hostility to metaphor, and the aspirations of Wilkins and others to reform language in such a way that it became a univalent codification of the world's contents, inhibited exercises in detailed psychological model-building in terms of newly discovered or invented 'scientific' phenomena or theories.

Nevertheless, these sources of resistance were overcome, either at the time or later, in the following ways:

> (a) via the usage of a variety of newly discovered 'mechanisms' and phenomena by physiologists trying to explain organic processes; as these usages changed the concept of the body, so in time reconstrual of bodily experience ensued and, via that, the terminology acquired PL meanings;
> (b) occasionally a Natural Philosopher might cautiously ignore theological boundary-policing and present a 'Psychological'

model – Hooke's theory of memory being the prime example[2]. This is very much a rule-proving exception;

(c) eventually some of the mechanistic explanations for behaviour offered by Descartes and Hobbes were retrospectively redefined as Psychological by the modern discipline (e.g. their adumbrations of the concept of the reflex);

(d) the Scientific Revolution raised the notion of a 'Science of Man' or 'Science of Mind' as part of the Natural Philosophy project's long-term goals. This is present in Bacon, and after Newton the quest is on among philosophers to be a 'Newton of the Mind'. This is first evidenced in a more detailed way in Frances Hutcheson's quasi-Newtonian moral calculus. Later, Hartley devised his physiological 'vibratiuncle' model explicitly in emulation of Newton, while Enlightenment French mechanists such as La Mettrie and Diderot constructed various hypothetical models of human nature using a *bricolage* of contemporary scientific and technological ideas.

In general, the seventeenth century did not immediately exploit contemporary scientific discoveries and ideas in the service of creating new psychological concepts in the way in which modern Psychology has systematically done. In the eighteenth century the inhibitions weaken and, as just noted, French mechanists are happy to introduce such concepts, but on the whole these are meant to be taken literally as physical models, not as models of the 'Mind'. The continued absence of innovation of this kind in Britain and France during the century requires further analysis. In Chapter 2 a survey of major contemporary linguistic positions showed that in all of them, for one reason or another, the direct generation of new psychological concepts was inhibited. Assumptions regarding the universally common and immutable character of the human mind also underlay contemporary philosophical schools of thought. In this climate existing psychological categories remained unchallenged as identifying objectively existing psychological realities. The task became either to analyse the mind reductively (in the case of the Lockeans) or to systematize and order the various 'Powers' of the mind as currently identified (in the case of Reidians). Only in Germany, after Leibniz, does the psychological vocabulary develop within a philosophical context, but even there this occurs in terms of elaborating on existing conceptual frameworks (such as the traditional 'faculties'), not by adopting scientific concepts.

Only at the end of the eighteenth century do we see a more dramatic physiomorphic assimilation of scientific phenomena beginning to occur in Mesmer and Puységur's conversion of 'Man' into 'Magnet', although physiologists had been pondering the role of the 'electrical fluid' for several decades. Fourier's bizarre doctrine of Universal Unity may also be seen as an exercise in introjecting contemporary mathematical and musical theory. By the first decades of the nineteenth century Romantic versions of evolution as a process of cosmic realization of the Spirit, with 'Man' at the forefront, mark the first wave of the psychological encounter with rapidly increasing time-scales and geological/ palaeontological data. The incorporation into Psychology of evolutionary ideas has continued, in many guises, ever since. Notions of degeneration and atavism, and of a 'beast within' (so different from the old concept of a wise primeval Adam), were beginning to stir, although their full efflorescence came after Charles Darwin's natural selection model. In a more general way the notion of 'Laws', comparable to scientific laws like Newton's and Boyle's, governing human life and the mind became widespread during the Enlightenment, but this was very much a metaphor returning, albeit transformed in meaning, to its source.

The most profound psychological impact of science before the mid nineteenth century is also the most elusive: a reconceptualization of 'Man's' place in Nature as part of a dynamic, rather than static, universe on a greatly expanded time-scale. The 'Great Chain of Being' was both temporalized and psychologized. Such a change is difficult to demonstrate at the simple lexical level, but is rather more pervasive, expressing itself in such things as an increasing concern with development and a sense, in Britain and France, of individual as well as social perfectibility (thereby raising the issue of psychological change). Thus education and child development became a focus of interest following Rousseau. The fixity and universality of human nature also begin to be challenged in the late eighteenth century under the impact of both this factor and the relativistic implications of the vast cultural differences in behaviour and customs which European imperial and economic expansion had brought to the attention of thinkers at home.

Even so, the central factors inhibiting direct Psychological utilization of scientific discoveries and theories diminished only slowly and then, ironically, because the essentially metaphorical nature of psychological concepts, a fact broadly recognized by linguists and philosophers, was lost sight of. The irony here from the present perspective is that those who understood this were unable to see its full psychological implications – namely, the constitutive function of psychological language and concepts. To have admitted this would have been to adopt a degree of radical relativism that was inconceivable within early-nineteenth-century-*Weltanschauungen*. Once the central linguistic insight had fallen from view, would-be Psychologists were in no danger of confronting this worrying thought, and happily began, from the mid nineteenth century onwards, building Psychologies out of contemporary scientific revelations and theories, believing that they were investigating objectively existing 'psychological' realities, and blind to the possibility that they themselves *were* 'the psychological', actively constituting itself in the course of these very investigations.

(ii) Technological innovation

While much that has been said in the previous section applies here also, there are some differences. It was to a large degree in terms of technological innovations, rather than scientific discoveries about the natural world, that much of the 'mechanistic' model building of how humans 'worked' in materialist terms was conducted – first by Descartes, and then more exuberantly by Condillac, Diderot, and La Mettrie. In these, musical instruments and vibratory phenomena played a large part. A second area in which technology stimulated an area now included in Psychology was perception; since Optics addressed the effects of lenses on light in general, the operation of the eye-as-lens was automatically included in its subject matter. In the era which saw the origins of modern optical scientific instruments, Natural Philosophers from Newton downwards were especially fascinated by the topic, and 'psychological' issues such as the nature of some visual illusions, binocularity and its involvement in depth perception, and perceptual learning thus start to receive attention during the seventeenth century and, more intensively, at the beginning of the eighteenth. Thereafter interest waned somewhat as the scientific study of light, and major innovations in optical instruments (bar John Dollond's invention of the achromatic lens) declined, to revive at the beginning of the nineteenth century in the wake of Thomas Young's wave theory of light, and in the context of new physiological theories.

After the mid eighteenth century such developments as the steam engine and other heavy industrial equipment began to influence psychology. Not only did they impress physiologists and anatomists by the evidence they provided of the capacities of 'mechanism', but they incorporated self-regulating devices such as the planetary valve. This, as we saw, provided physiologists with the possibility of modelling physiological processes in less hierarchical terms than hitherto: as incorporating unconscious, but purposive, regulatory mechanisms. This created a need to postulate unconscious levels of phenomena that still had to be thought of as in some sense mental. But the impact extended further, to the kind of factory production process in which these machines were used. This image of the factory, with its divisions of labour, specialized sections and adaptable character, provided, it was suggested, a complex metaphorical schema with which those living in such an environment would construe themselves, and this matched very neatly the formal structure and message of phrenology. The kind of mechanization of the body accomplished in the earlier part of the eighteenth century was now followed by a mechanization of the mind for which the new mechanical language of the body, and the increased (and more or less automatic) adoption of this language for referring to subjective experience, had paved the way. Now the brain itself was similarly analysed.

Popular PL often leads Psychology in adopting salient public technological innovations; terms relating to steam engines and railways (*go off the rails, full steam, blow a gasket*) and electricity (*electrifying* and *galvanized*) often entered PL quite rapidly. Without an exhaustive philological search, the full extent and rate of entry of such technologically rooted expressions cannot be gauged[3]. It is at least plausible to suggest, however, that what I have called the physiomorphic process operated at the cultural level with respect to such innovations throughout our period, partly transforming the nature of psychological language and introducing new psychological concepts, regardless of the philosophers' conceptual conservatism. Samuel Johnson's *Dictionary* included numerous terms of this kind derived from the physical sciences, few of which figured significantly in contemporary philosophical discourse as 'Psychological' innovations[4]. More seriously I would claim that it was at this level, by this kind of piecemeal shifting of PL in response to immediately public novelties, that the broader changes in *mentalité* which are now widely claimed for this period actually happened.

(iii) Changes in social life

This is at once the largest and most problematical source of changing ideas of the psychological – probably always, but especially throughout the period being covered here. New social roles, new kinds of social organization and institution, new economic relationships and practices, and new group interests (relating to social class, religion or region, for example) both entail psychological changes and provide ways of naming those changes. Public social roles, especially occupational ones, have always been endowed with psychological significance as engendering a particular Gestalt of traits and temperamental qualities in those occupying them. If we consider Britain alone, for generations down to the early seventeenth century these had remained essentially unchanged; few occupations in 1600 were unknown to Chaucer over two hundred years earlier, and they were long familiar to his audience. In urban life a few had been added – the alchemist, for example, and the playwright; while the Renaissance courtier had evolved into a far more cultured figure than the courtiers of Chaucer's day. In Britain some had disappeared – notably nuns, friars and pardoners. By and large, though, the occupational *dramatis personae* of everyday life was much the same as it had been for centuries. By 1800 the cast has altered almost beyond recognition: factory owners and their workers, engineers, canal-men, stockbrokers, chemists, novelists, newspaper columnists, literary critics and, indeed, scientists (in fact if not in name) are now on-stage, while alchemists, courtiers, and Puritan fanatics have gone. Jobs like doctor, soldier, teacher and painter have changed even while they have persisted. Farmers, blacksmiths, drapers, bakers and brewers continue too, but even here there are changes, albeit less far-reaching, as there are in the sex roles.

One new social role which has attracted the attention of historians of science is the role of scientist itself, a role which Steven Shapin has seen as deriving from the existing category of the Gentleman[5]. Renaissance Gentlemen do not call one another liars, they are honourable, and their word is to be trusted implicitly. (Well, of course they do and they aren't and it can't, but then they cease to be gentlemen; honourable gentlemen strive to take this code seriously.) One necessary condition of early science was that its practitioners believed what one another said about what had happened in the course of their researches. This mutual trust was already something on which the gentlemen who, for example, created the Royal Society and comprised most of the membership prided themselves. It was being self-consciously honourable gentlemen that enabled them to create the intellectual conditions in which new discoveries about the natural world could be communicated, interpreted and defined, and integrated with similar findings elsewhere. Now in every era there are a number of social roles which are used as symbols of the human condition itself, of the nature of the relationship between soul, or self, and the world of experience through which it lives. The culturally paramount male modes of these have included King, Farmer, Sailor (or ship's Captain), Pilgrim, Knight, Magus, and Shepherd. It was suggested in Chapter 1 that in the climate of the late seventeenth century a new role of this kind appeared – or at least, for those enacting it, it seemed to: namely, the Natural Philosopher himself, a *virtuoso*; reliant only on Reason and Observation, he seeks to read God's second book, the Book of Nature. It is a role combining the honour of the gentleman with the aspirations of the magus. Its central feature, though, is *seeking knowledge*, and I argued that the centrality of epistemology in Enlightenment philosophy constituted, in a sense, the adoption of this new social role as the key image of the individual's condition. In other words, the role of Natural Philosopher itself becomes reflexively assimilated as signifying a particular psychological condition or mentality of a highly valued kind (at least by those involved in science and philosophy). We must now pursue this line of thought further.

This new archetypal variety of magus is more Bacon than Faust; eventually he will become Frankenstein, Pasteur, Darwin, Einstein, Dr Strangelove . . . (and acquire one archetypal sister – Madame Curie). What I want to insist on here, though, is the entry on-stage at this time of a new archetypal social role identity, a new psychological model, which will henceforth underlie the ego-identities of all those scientists, philosophers, psychiatrists and would-be Psychologists of whom we have to speak. They are not Kings, Warriors, Pilgrims or Neo-Platonic Magi – they are Baconians, *Virtuosi*, Natural Philosophers, Scientists, Men of Reason; and Comte openly proclaims them the highest form of life on earth. I wish to stress this so much now because it is this very *mentalité*, in one or another of its various forms, which subsequently envelops and creates the subject matter of this book. In so far as we can talk, in a disciplinary history context, of a history of 'Psychological Ideas', it is within a predefined framework in which we (the Baconians, Natural Philosophers . . .) have already created an epistemological category of 'the Psychological' and, indeed, the epistemological category 'Idea'. Thus the idea of the Natural Philosopher as social role, fusion of magus (but more rational) and gentleman (but even more honourable), is in itself the source of a 'psychological idea' of more importance to our current task than any other – the idea of the psychological character of the *ideal* scientist-cum-philosopher in terms of which we (Baconians, etc.) define our own psychological parameters, psychological orientations, and – at the end of the day – the very nature of the psychological.

If the foregoing is correct, it locates one source of that 'individualization' and 'interiorization' which many now see as the hallmark of modern Western psychology in the very process whereby Western science was itself constituted. This is a conclusion at which others have arrived by different, perhaps less tortuous routes. But I believe my tortuosity has added something – it has rendered more visible the way in which this happened as a psychological process in its own right: by the reflexive interiorization of a novel social role as ego-identity, – differing only in the epochal nature of its content from the similar interiorisation which routinely, and necessarily, befalls new social roles as signifying new psychological states. Of course there are much wider collective social dimensions to all this, some of which we have discussed in the course of this book, and I must avoid being misunderstood as offering a simplistic individualist 'psychologistic' explanation of a social process. What I have described is a social process as much as it is a psychological one; it involves language, it involves the collective social construction of a new role and the collective endorsement of its reflex interiorization.

The psychological ideas which influenced Psychology necessarily either originated within, or were assimilated into, the terms of consciousness of that 'scientific psychology' just described. Their social origins are ubiquitous. For models of the psychological workings of the brain we move, in the course of the seventeenth century, from the castle of Holland's Pliny through Bacon's Renaissance bureaucracy and Willis's 'metropolis'. More technological models take over during the Enlightenment, but the social reappears in phrenology's cerebral factory (on the technology/social boundary) and its popular iconography of heads populated by a Dickensian δεμοσ of alimentive gourmands, venerable preachers and largely acquisitive misers. The revised nosologies of madness produced at the end of the eighteenth century are at one level catalogues of the deviant social behaviours abhorred by the newly middle class, pathologized into psychological conditions. At the same time, the growing fascination with the idea of childhood as a distinctive state of consciousness is inextricably bound up with a complex of demographic and economic developments which prioritize education and child-rearing. Even the first articulations in the early nineteenth century of some quasi-evolutionary hierarchy of the races, and the monogeny–polygeny debate, are set within the social contexts of the slavery controversy and power relations between white Europeans and the variously hued subjects of their empires.

Listing instances in this discrete fashion does not get to the heart of the matter. The entire Scottish Enlightenment project from Hutcheson and Reid onwards, through Hume, Home, Ferguson, Smith, Stewart and their associates, is motivated above all by a concern to identify and develop practical moral philosophical principles on which social life can rest in a secular age. In their various systems the passions and emotions are charted and coded increasingly in terms of social relations. The same is true south of the border, in Benthamite Utilitarianism.

The divergence of German philosophy from that of Britain and France during the Age of Reason is in part a reflection of the differing political-ideological agendas by which their philosophers were motivated. In Germany, working in state-owned universities under the eye of feudal rulers who enjoyed the monopoly of socio-economic power, philosophy inevitably turned inwards and tended to produce basically static and conservative (if cosmologically dynamic) metaphysical systems which offered no overtly subversive threat. Social problems are the prince's problem. Morality is defined in terms of *a prioristic* rational principles, not sought in the exigencies of social life. That these often rich and subtle systems, in adopting this very orientation, on occasion produced new Psychological concepts is not in dispute – indeed, the richness of the technical vocabulary of German philosophy regarding the psychological was a major factor in enabling a discipline of Psychology to emerge there earlier than anywhere else in the nineteenth century (and the term *Psychologie* was commonplace in Germany at a time when it was rare elsewhere). This is not to deny that German society underwent change during the Age of Reason, but to stress that this took the form of continued elaborations of the existing absolutist feudal structure rather than its restructuring and replacement. Large-scale industrialization begins in Germany only during the early nineteenth century, and only as it does do German psychiatric writers and philosophers begin to tackle madness, deviance, education and social order as *social management issues*, rather than philosophical ones.

A picture (blurred no doubt) emerges from all this regarding the relative weightings and roles of different kinds of source. The dynamic for conceptual change is ultimately provided by fundamental alterations in the forms of social life throughout the period and the content of such changes reflects the varied cultural locations of reflexive discourse within that process. It is factors of this kind which set the priorities for proto-Psychological enquiry, as well as actually producing psychological change – i.e. changes in the way life is experienced and responded to. The management of both these kinds of change is mediated via their articulation and analysis in reflexive discourse. It is within this social framework that the utilization of scientific and technological novelty as sources of new psychological ideas takes place.

Where reflexive discourse is culturally located within the Natural Philosophical subculture – as in England and France – the use of scientific and technological novelty as resources for reconstruing the psychological is more widespread than in situations where such discourse is located within a traditional university culture (as in Germany and Scotland). In England there are, even so, two inhibiting factors: (a) the broadly materialist and reductionist character of Natural Philosophy itself; and (b) linked with this, the linguistic character of Natural Philosophical discourse as anti-metaphorical. The former, in the lineage of Lockean philosophy, results in a conceptually spartan form of deconstruction of the mental into elementary epistemological processes, themselves foregrounded in such discourse just because Natural Philosophy is an epistemological enterprise. The latter induces a wariness in producing exercises in genuinely Psychological theory or model building in terms of new 'scientific' or technical concepts, the deployment of such ideas in writers like La Mettrie and his fellow Enlightenment *philosophes* is primarily literal in character, or as heuristic analogies for the physiological. As far as psychological language is concerned the received vocabulary is usually understood as a functionally non-figurative language which has evolved to name and classify a universal, pre-existing, objectively real set of mental phenomena and does not require change. The only 'Psychological' headway is made on the relatively restricted front of research into perception.

Where reflexive discourse is located in university subcultures, as in Scotland and Germany, less direct use is made of scientific and technical ideas. There are, though, differences in what happens in these two countries. In Scotland the isolation from Natural Philosophy was largely fortuitous – the Scots generally endorsed its aspirations – and far from total, especially in relation to medicine, in which Edinburgh was almost paramount, only Boerhaave's Leyden having a higher European reputation in the earlier part of the eighteenth century. The impact of social change is also far greater than in Germany. The strong French connection also brings French natural history into the Scottish purview as a paradigm of Natural Philosophical method. Here, then, there is a combination of anti-reductionism, social change and a classificatory concept of Natural Philosophy, which largely determines the character of the Scottish Enlightenment's version of the 'Science of Man' project. This takes the form of a cataloguing and ordering of the existing body of psychological concepts and a classificatory observational 'Social Psychology', again in terms of the existing conceptual corpus. The tension in this (as we saw clearly in the case of Thomas Brown) is between a continued tendency to accept the traditional view of human nature as fixed and universal, and the function of the project as in the service of social perfectibility or reform in a context of psychological change. In Germany, by contrast, reflexive discourse continued to be fundamentally metaphysical, struggling with the legacy of Leibniz, whose conceptual innovations it assimilates, and evolving new concepts from the traditional scholastic vocabulary. While addressing the mind more directly, sensitively and introspectively, it does so from the stance of the absolutist philosopher in the service of the absolute prince, providing rationales for the cultural status quo and couching its visions of social change in absolutist terms as a triumphal cosmological advance of Absolute Spirit. This stance, of course, pervades German science as a whole, enveloping it in metaphysics until the 1840s.

At the very heart of the situation lies the social creation of the new archetypal social role of the Natural Philosopher, introjected as signifying a new mode of consciousness, a 'scientific psychology'. It is with this that all those engaging in reflexive discourse in order to create some Science of Man or Science of the Mind identify, albeit with national variations. And, I argued, it is *within* this mode of consciousness or *mentalité* that all subsequent 'Psychological' discourse has occurred. The very idea of the 'psychological' as now understood, as well as the idea of a discipline of Psychology to study it, flowed from this move.

We may see those sharing this *mentalité* as forming, throughout the modern period, the social psychological centre where the psychological implications of novelty were most authoritatively processed. It was here that psychological ideas came home to roost; this was the point to which, as we said earlier, they eventually gravitated. It was from here that the new messages regarding human nature – sometimes optimistic, sometimes gloomy – were broadcast by philosophers, physiologists, anthropologists, and sometimes social utopians, Mesmerists and phrenologists. But all these are centrally identifying themselves with this new mode of consciousness; all see themselves (even if their peers disagree) as representing and embodying the spirit of Natural Philosophy or Scientific Reason. The new psychological ideas they are processing and from which they draw their conclusions do not, however, originate with them directly, but variously from the socioeconomic and cultural life around them, and from their own physical discoveries and inventions. Thus they are in no sense objectively outside the total historical process, detachedly surveying the mind and uncovering truths about it. On the contrary, they are carried along by continually varying contemporary political, economic, social and religious concerns. Their messages do indeed feed back into this overall process and are to some degree attempts at directing it, but as Dewey demonstrated of the reflex arc itself, attempts at differentiating between stimulus and response are misguided. And their guiding efforts fail because the mode of consciousness they have espoused is, after all, only one among many ever-present options. Their programme thereby acquires an expansionist imperative of its own – to universalize their own mode of consciousness as the only one adequate to the very task of psychological construal in which they are, from different disciplinary perspectives, engaged.

And is it not from this last imperative that Psychology the discipline ultimately derives? To reconstrue all other mentalities in terms of its own, and in so doing to prove itself finally at the top of the psychological pecking order – is this not scientific Psychology's deep ambition? One may observe, in mitigation, that Psychology has notoriously failed to gell, that its current practice remains as diverse as the sources from which we have seen it being constructed. One might also accuse the author of dodging the final reflexive twist of admitting that the present work remains part of the same enterprise. This observation and accusation, however, would miss the point. The conclusion is not by way of an arraignment or unmasking. The answer to the 'scientific consciousness' (which, remember, is in principle committed to the possibility of constant change and in the origin of which Locke's 'blank slate' played a significant role) is either to modify it with respect to those current facets of it which one finds offensive, redressing its remaining blindesses to certain kinds of 'data', or to find a mode of consciousness which can outflank it. The present work is more in the nature of the former than the latter – which would, though, I admit, be sweet to find.

The 'mechanization of the mind' and the 'discovery' of mental machinery has, in conclusion, been a more profound yet also more elusive process than has been hitherto described. We use the things we find in the outside world as schemata for understanding the things we find in the inner one, thereby shaping that inner one accordingly. What scientists have sought and found in the outer world are mechanisms, and when the 'scientific psychology' behind that quest turns its direction inwards, it will be no exception. The blind spot in this has been a failure to understand that this is how we *create* that inner realm, not how we discover pre-existing truths about it. In so far as the scientific world-view has become the touchstone of sanity, and succeeded in establishing the 'scientific psychology' which enabled it to create that world-view as the dominant mentality in our culture, so too have all our minds become 'mechanized'. Thus has emerged a psychology amenable to Psychology's exploration. And by the mid twentieth century George Kelly was explicitly universalizing the scientist as the core image of human nature, as if this was a Psychological discovery! Like the man in Magritte's painting, Psychology remains forever staring at the reflection of its own back. What I have been examining in this volume is why it never looks over its shoulder.

Notes

Introduction

1. Throughout this work I have adopted the orthographic practice of differentiating between discipline and subject-matter sense of the term 'psychology' and its derivatives by capitalizing the former as Psychology, Psychological, etc., and leaving the latter in lower case as psychology, psychological, etc. To demonstrate that the two are not always easily differentiable is perhaps part of my 'hidden agenda', but an attempt to do so is crucial. My efforts at establishing this as a convention within the discipline have so far failed to bear fruit; hence the persisting ambiguity of phrases like 'German psychology'. Remember, animal psychology is the subject matter of the study of their behaviour, etc.; animal Psychology, by contrast, would comprise experiments on perception performed by owls and treatises on learning written by rats. For various aspects of the current debate on the nature of Psychology, see Richards (1987a), R. Smith (1988), Danziger (1990), Leary (ed.) (1990), Rose (1987, 1990a, b), Romanyshyn (1982). An earlier, if orthodox, work on the language of Psychology is Mandler and Kessen (1959).
2. I am taking this Wittgensteinian point as read. See Richards (1989a), ch. 1, for its role in the present argument. The *locus classicus* for the 'Private Language' debate is Wittgenstein (1968), para. 259 ff.; see also Saul Kripke (1982), A.J. Ayer (1985), pp. 71–78; Budd (1989).
3. For this reason the possibility, now being canvassed by the Churchlands (1985, 1986), Stich (1983) and Braaten (1988), that the future will see a *replacement* of current PL by a new one couched in terms of neurophysiological understanding, must be considered very remote. After all, we can still be high-spirited, we still plough through books, and we can still experience melancholy, even though animal spirits, farming, and humoral typologies have ceased to figure in modern science or urban life. PL is basically cumulative, and innovations are never mere synonyms for existing terms; 'hold your horses' is not the same as 'stop running your current psychological programme', nor is it *quite* the same thing to say 'It's slipped my mind' as to say 'I can't access that for the

moment'. Their central error, perhaps, is their assumption that folk psychology constitutes a putative scientific theory. On the contrary, theorizing is one of the things it enables us to do (and 'to theorize' is now a folk-psychological category anyway). (See *On Psychological Language* for more on this issue.)

4. Many historians and philosophers of science do not, of course, accept that even what appear to be the natural objects of scientific enquiry are. The social constructionist case is that *all* objects of knowledge are ultimately artefacts of the intellectual and social community. But no one is denying that there are rocks; what they deny is that the 'scientific' account of rocks (Jurassic, sedimentary, fossiliferous, etc.) is a neutral depiction of 'facts'. This geological vocabulary and theoretical corpus is a collective invention endowing the phenomena with a particular range of meanings ultimately rooted in the assumptions, values and motives of the geological community which coined them (see Rudwick, 1972 on fossils, for example). The problem for Psychology is that there is *no* ostensible object of enquiry at all in this sense. Psychology is about the meanings of reflexive discourse while itself being reflexive discourse. Geology is the creation of a meaningful discourse about rocks, but it isn't itself rock. The issue is not simply one of 'visibility'; particle physics creates the phenomena it studies in a far more thoroughgoing way than geology, via the mediating processes it uses to render them 'visible'. The 'reality' is as invisible for particle physics as it is for Psychology; even so, the discourse of particle physics is not itself particle physics (except in the most reductive sense). Psychological discourse *is* 'psychology'. There is no phenomenal 'middle term' in the equation. It could be said that *all* discourse is psychological, because it is all in one way or another about or expressive of conscious experience. But this merely brackets the question without solving it (like saying everybody is selfish); in our linguistic life we have to choose (even if routinely the appropriate choice is obvious) between construing utterances as 'about' the speaker's 'psychological' state or 'about' the public world – and the choice we make may creatively constitute the reality (see Richards, 1989a, ch. 2). The social constructionist discovery of a 'psychological' dimension to geological discourse is an unmasking not of its 'true' meaning but of the fact that those who believed it to be univalent, possessed of only a single 'objective' referential meaning, were mistaken. To deny that Lyell was writing about rocks would be silly. To affirm that he was also unwittingly writing about something else, to identify what that something else was, and to discern the interactions between the two, is profound scholarship.

5. A late additional note: D.A. Leary's volume of papers *Metaphors in the History of Psychology* (1990) appeared too late to be taken into account in writing the present book. His introductory essay, 'Psyche's Muse', will become an essential reference point for future work; among the other papers the most relevant to us appear to be James Averill's (on metaphors of emotion), Kenneth Gergen's and Kurt Danziger's. None of the contributors has, however, been prepared to reach similar theoretical conclusions to my own, even though these implications seem obvious enough.

PART ONE: THE SEVENTEENTH CENTURY

Chapter 1 Vast Confusions and New Paradoxes

1. From the Shilleto edn of 1896.
2. The most important of these being N. Coeffeteau (1621), E. Reynoldes (1640), J.F. Senault (1649), T. Wright (1601).
3. e.g. John Earle (1628), Sir T. Overbury (1614).
4. e.g. Thomas Hill (1556, 1613).
5. e.g. Timothy Bright (1586).
6. e.g. R.T. Ascham (1570), J.A. Comenius (1657, 1658, 1896), W. Kempe (1588), R. Mulcaster (1581).
7. See M.T. Hodgen (1964).
8. See R. Mulcaster, *op.cit.*; T. Phayre (1545).
9. e.g. E. Brerewood (1614).
10. See Appendix.
11. The standard edition of Francis Bacon is Spedding, Ellis and Heath (1851–1874).
12. G. Richards (1989 a,b).
13. See C. Fox (1987).
14. T. Phayre (1545, A.ii.iv). On 'terrible dreames and feare in the slepe' of children he is quite unmystical: '. . . which effecte commeth of the arysyng of stynking vapours out of the stomake into the fantasye, and sences of the brayne'.
15. See J.W. Saunders (1983) and M. Spufford (1981). Spufford's estimates seem to be somewhat lower. her book is a valuable source of information regarding the lower end of the publishing market and seventeenth-century popular reading habits.
16. This relative paucity of sixteenth- and seventeenth-century material cited in current general textbooks can be indicated by listing the figures cited in five of them:

    Hearnshaw (1987): Descartes, Hobbes, Leibniz, Locke, Spinoza;
    Kantor (1963) Boyle, Descartes, Hobbes, Leibniz, Locke, Newton;

Leahey (1987): (Bacon, More *passim* in Introduction), Descartes, Hobbes, Leibniz, Locke, Pascal, Spinoza;
Murphy and Kovach (1972): Descartes, Hobbes, Leibniz, Locke, Spinoza;
Schultz (1975): Locke.

Even E.G. Boring (1950) has only Descartes, Harvey, Hobbes, Leibniz and Locke (plus four lines on Willis). Baldwin (n.d.), however, adds Gassendi and Malebranche, but one has to go to Brett (1912–21) to find Comenius, Cudworth, Geulincx, More, and Overbury (and R.S. Peters's 1953 abridgement cuts out some of these).

17. Descartes's primacy in creating the reflex concept is not beyond dispute. Canguilhem (1955) argues that only in the following century was the *concept* of the reflex clearly formulated.
18. Patrides (1980), p. 4.
19. The paradigm text here is Robert Boyle's *Christian Virtuoso.*
20. Only in recent years has the influence of the Cambridge Platonists on the major English figures of the Scientific Revolution (especially Newton) become fully appreciated.
21. See E. and F.S. Michael (1989) and J.W. Yolton (1984).
22. e.g. J.W. Yolton (1956, 1984), G.M. Ross (1988), E. and F.S. Michael, *op.cit.*
23. M. Jacob (1976).
24. S. Schaffer (1987), p. 57.
25. 'The Mechanization of Mind' story still explicitly structures Leahey's account: ch. 4, 'The Mechanization of the World Picture'.
26. S. Schaffer, *op. cit.*, p. 57.
27. Also G.B. della Porta (1658).
28. See K. Thomas (1971), F. Yates (1964, 1966, 1972), B. Vickers (ed.) (1984).
29. The impact of the microscope was not, however, without its ambiguities: see C. Wilson (1988).
30. See note 2.
31. This section draws heavily on J. Morgan (1986).
32. See also J.T. Cliffe (1988).
33. See especially Christopher Hill (1971, 1974, 1981, 1984): see also N. Smith (ed.) (1983). Space considerations preclude any discussion here of Gerrard Winstanley the Leveller, whose *Law of Freedom* (1652, repr. 1973) must be seen as a counter-text to Hobbes's *Leviathan*, with which it is almost exactly synchronous; on Winstanley, in addition to Hill (*passim*), see T. Wilson Hayes (1979).
34. Z. Barbu (1960).

35. This section draws heavily on D. Morse (1989)
36. *TLS* ref. My knowledge of this is not due to any scouring of archives, the cutting happened to be slipped into my copy when I purchased it; in fact it is by John Middleton Murry and reprinted in Murry (1922).
37. see Basil Willey (1934, repr. 1977) on Browne. For a sympathetic account of Browne, see also R.D. Stock (1982).
38. She figures frequently in Antonia Fraser's *The Weaker Vessel*, a mine of information on all aspects of the position of women during this period. We must hope that Kathleen Jones's recent biography of her (1988) has opened the way for more detailed research into Margaret Cavendish's writings.
39. For a general survey of theories of Melancholy, see S.W. Jackson (1986).
40. I have used the Molesworth standard edition, but referenced chapters rather than pages here as being more useful to the general reader, given the number of editions of *Leviathan* circulating.
41. See also S. Goyard-Fabre (1979); T. Lott (1979); H.R. Bernstein (1980); M.M. Slaughter (1982).
42. But see S. Claus (1982), pp. 546–53), who discerns in Wilkins something ancestral to Foucault.
43. See V. Salmon (1974); his aspirations continued to be endorsed (e.g. by Joseph Priestley [1762]).
44. Much of the work is structured as a commentary on a report by Sir Kenelm Digby of the treatment in Spain of the younger brother of the 'Constable of Castile' by the priest J.P. Bonet, who published the first work on the topic in 1620. Digby's report is printed in full, but Bonet is not mentioned by name. Curiously, E.B. Tylor (1878, chs 1–6) does not notice Bulwer in spite of an extensive overlap in their concerns; while Bonet, the French eighteenth-century work of Sicard (1800) and many others are cited.
45. D.H. Tuke (1884), *Influence of the Mind upon the Body* (2nd edn) vol. 1, p. 232, to be precise.
46. See A. Debus (1965, 1977).
47. Much of this section first appeared in the *Newsletter* of the History and Philosophy Section of the British Psychological Society.
48. Huarte's work was first published in English as *Examen de Ingenios. The Examination of Men's Wits* by John Juarte, translated by M. Camillo Camillo and 'Englished from the Italian by R.C. Esquire', London: Adam Islip for Richard Watkins, 1594. This was a partial translation of a translation only; although often reprinted it was not replaced until 1698, when it reappeared in full as *Examen de Ingenios or the Tryal of Wits*, Juan Huartes, transl. 'Mr Bellamy' (London:

Richard Sale). The former is better as literature but harder to understand! An additional significant work which should by noted here is the anonymous *Anthropologie abstracted; or, the idea of Humane nature reflected in briefe Philosophicall and anatomical collections* (1655), the first 'volume' of which is entitled 'Psychologie' and deals with 'the nature of the rational soule' (see G.A.J. Rogers, *in press*).

Another forgotten anticipatory text which has been rediscovered is Marius D'Assigny's *The Art of Memory: A Treatise Useful for Such as are to Speak in Publick*, discussed by A.B. Laver (1973). It was in part derivative from Guglielmo Grataroli's *De memoria reparanda, augenda, sevandaque* of 1553 which had appeared in English translation (by William Fulwood) in 1562 as *The Castel of Memorie*. This in turn derived from Johannes Michael Albertus de Carrara's *De omnibus ingeniis augende memorie* of 1491. D'Assigny was a Protestant citizen of Jersey. The *locus classicus* for Renaissance theories of memory is, of course, Frances Yates (1966).

49. See M.T. Hodgen (1964), p. 334.

PART TWO: PSYCHOLOGICAL IDEAS IN THE EIGHTEENTH CENTURY

Introduction

1. J.R. Milton (1981), p. 182 – which provides a thorough review of the history of the concept.
2. *ibid.*, p. 195.
3. See especially his *Physico-Theology*, containing the 1711 and 1712 Boyle Lectures (Derham, 1720). This also contains the following warning about flying, which

   > might prove of dangerous and fatal Consequence: as for Instance, by putting it in Man's Power to discover the Secrets of Nations and Families, more than is consistent with the Peace of the World, for Man to know. (p. 268)

4. See J.T. Boulton's Introduction to Edmund Burke (1958). The Reverend Archibald Alison's 1790 *Essays on the Nature and Principles of Taste* more closely follows the Associationist party line; 'Emotions of Sublimity' involve the exercise of imagination, 'which consists in the indulgence of a train of thought'; the distinctive features of the chain of thought characteristic of Sublimity are that each idea in the chain is associated with a simple 'Idea of Emotion', and that the chain as a whole is connected by a common emotional principle (pp. 42–7).

Chapter 2 The Vehicle of Conjecture

1. That only males engaged in such debates at this time is important; the literary genres espoused by women tended to be quasi-oral, such as letters and devotional books of prayer (Davies, 1987), in contrast to the new priority of written over spoken represented by Wilkins.
2. *Essay*, Book III, chs 10: 'Of the Abuse of Words' and 11: 'Of the Remedies of the Foregoing Imperfection and Abuses'.
3. See S.K. Land (1986) for a full analysis of the complexities regarding Locke's treatment of language within the context of this wider philosophical position.
4. The most prominent modern advocate of a similar position is G.W. Hewes (1973, 1976).
5. See Aarsleff (1983), esp. pp. 102–8.
6. See Max Müller (1887), in which the 121 Sanskrit 'roots' are enumerated.
7. These, incredibly, were: *ag, bag, dwag, gwag, lag, mag, nag, rag, swag.*
8. Some of the most impressive, yet neglected, 'Psychological' views on language published in Britain in the wake of Tooke appear in the psychiatrist John Haslam's two works *Sound Mind* (1819) and *On the Nature of Thought, or the Act of Thinking & its connexion with a Perspicuous Sentence* (1835). As a sample: attacking the view that Ideas as such constitute the instruments of thought, he writes:

   > Thought does not result from this rapid and tumultuous rush of Ideas; but is a very deliberate, and in many cases painful elaboration: and must, when committed to writing, be subjected to subsequent revisals and repeated corrections, and which must be applied to the *words* constituting the sentence in which the thought is contained. (1835, p. 24)

   While obviously strongly influenced by Tooke, Haslam's observations are often remarkably insightful and original, as well as being pithily expressed. His neglect may well have been due to his loss of public reputation following his resignation from Bethlem in 1815 as a result of the Norris affair.
9. This reflects the influence on the Scottish Enlightenment philosophers of French Buffonian natural history.
10. D. Stewart (1818), ch. 2, p. 212.
11. *Ibid.*, ch. 3, p. 234.
12. For an account of the runners-up, see Paul B. Salmon (1989).
13. I am indebted to Simon Schaffer for drawing my attention to Coleridge's significance in this context.

14. This ambivalence over whether his job was to describe or reform is also noted in S.I. Landau (1984), p. 53.
15. The classic analysis of this is W.K. Wimsatt's *Philosophic Words* (1948). I intend to consider this in an appendix to the second part of the present work.
16. See R. Holmes (1982) for a clear, brief, overview of Coleridge.
17. Not with the German psychiatrist Heinroth, as F.G. Alexander and S.T. Selesnick claim (1966, p. 141), unless he was Coleridge's source, which is quite possible.
18. 1956 edn, p. 92. Contemporaneously, William Whewell at Cambridge was also attending to the issue of authoritative linguistic innovation in the sciences (himself coining the word 'scientist') and stressing the role of the classical languages as resources in creating terms which had a clear scientific meaning but lacked the irrelevant connotations, etc, of everyday words.
19. Even he implies that Alexander Bain was hardly aware of Coleridge – unlikely in view of the J.S. Mill quote (which he himself gives on p. 6) and the fact that Mill was Bain's philosophical mentor.
20. See Elias (1978), especially the new Preface.

Chapter 3 Sensible Reasoning

1. Such as Henry Dodwell (1708), for whom the issue seems to have boiled down to how one should interpret St Justin Martyr's Dialogue with Tryphon.
2. See Basil Willey (1940, repr. 1986), ch. iv, for a summary of Ashley Cooper's ideas and an evocation of his character.
3. Peter Browne's absence from the secondary literature (except in Yolton's works) is quite remarkable. He is absent not only from Ernst Cassirer (1932), Harald Höffding (1955) and Bertrand Russell (1962), but also from Mary W. Calkins's edition of Berkeley (1929) and both Mary Warnock's and George Pitcher's books on Berkeley (1953, 1977 respectively) – contexts in which his appearance would be most expected.
4. See Gladys Bryson (1945), esp. ch. 5.
5. See G.P. Brooks and S.K. Aalto (1981) for a full account of this.
6. *Ibid*; note Archibald Campbell, *An Enquiry into the Original of Moral Virtue* (1728, 1733); Anonymous, *An Introduction towards an Essay on the Origins of the Passions* (1741); Anonymous, *An Enquiry into the Origin of the Human Appetites and Affections, Shewing how each arises from Association* (1747; an extension of the previous title); and a parody of moral algebra by Richard Griffith, masquerading as by Lawrence Sterne, in *The Posthumous Works of a Late Celebrated*

Genius (1770).

7. What follows is geared to elucidating Berkeley's significance for Psychological thought, rather than expounding his doctrines in detail. George Pitcher (1977) is the fullest of more recent accounts, while Mary Warnock's Penguin (1953) provides a concise introduction to his thought. There is a vast literature on Berkeley (see Pitcher).
8. That the light travels through a greater thickness of intervening atmosphere when the Moon is on the horizon, thereby appearing hazier and fainter, one of the distance cues he has identified; his explanation is thus a variant of the 'it looks bigger because it looks further away' theory. (See pp. 76–79 above.)
9. Richards (1989a), ch. 2.
10. See her Introduction (Berkeley, 1962 edn), pp. 26–30.
11. Richards (1989a) ch. 2, n. 9.
12. See Kurt Danziger (1990) on the difference between experimental introspection and traditional philosophical reflection.
13. Jonathan Swift's 'Meditation upon a Broomstick' (1711) parodies Boyle's moral philosophizing, and Bernard de Mandeville's *Treatise of the Hypochondriacal and Hysterical Diseases* (also 1711) held up 'the speculative' Willis's 'brain as an alembick' model, which he quotes *in extenso*, as a prime example of futile analogizing (1730 edn, pp. 95–8).
14. This 'dissertation' appeared as a preliminary to E. Law's translation of Archbishop William King's *An Essay on the Origin of Evil* (see Bibliography under Gay).
15. See M.E. Webb (1988) for a fully documented account.
16. For some odd reason, Huguelet says that the latter is twice the length of the former, when it appears to me to be 57 pages shorter.
17. See C.U.M. Smith (1987) for an account of Hartley's Newtonianism.
18. A position explored further by Henry Home, Lord Kames (1751). More rigorously thought through, this solution might have come close to Kant's (see below, pp. 295–298).
19. Again, the literature on Hume is vast. Two papers exploring his 'Psychology' are E.F. Miller (1971) and J. Bricke (1974). As in the case of Berkeley, my treatment of Hume is directed specifically to his role in the history of Psychology, and necessarily leaves much of the detail of his philosophical doctrines untouched.
20. R.D. Stock (1982) is less impressed with the soundness of Hume's refutation than I am.
21. It is worth noting that he uses a sort of printing metaphor for this, and a little later uses a painting metaphor in differentiating Memory from Imagination: 'the former faculty paints its objects in more distinct colours' (p. 9).

22. Ernst Mach (1883) and W. K. Clifford (1885) being the key texts.
23. Such as the Reverend Vince, Plumeian Professor of Astronomy at Cambridge.
24. See T.H. Huxley (1887), esp. pp. 52–3.
25. The same string is still being plucked by Henry Home (1779 edn; see pp. 23–5).
26. This particular delusion seems to have been a common one during the eighteenth century. Thomas Arnold (1806) cites a number of cases, and casual references to it like Thomas Reid's frequently crop up.
27. See Aaron Ben-Zeev (1986, 1990), who compares Reid's position with J.J. Gibson's.
28. As noted elsewhere, P.B. Wood (1990) links this to the influence of French natural history.
29. Such as Captain Cook's account of life on Tahiti.
30. See, for example, G.D.H. Cole's introduction to the 1913 edition of Rousseau's *Social Contract.*
31. E.E. Evans-Pritchard (1981) identifies Montesquieu's *Esprit des Lois* (1748) and Condorcet's *Esquisse d'un tableau historique des progrès de l'esprit humain* (1795) as constituting, along with John Millar's *The Origin of the Distinction of Ranks* (17171) and Henry Home, Lord Kames's *Sketches of the History of Man* (1774), the founding texts of modern anthropology.
32. The *locus classicus* for this topic remains A.O. Lovejoy's *The Great Chain of Being* (1933).
33. See F. Rigotti (1986) for the French situation in particular.
34. See P. Harth's introduction to the 1970 edition for a full discussion of the background of the work and contemporary responses.
35. J.B. Bossuet (1627–1704), *Discours sur l'histoire universelle* (1681).
36. See E.J. Hundert (1986) for an account of this aspect of Mandeville's thought.
37. And it is no coincidence that the monetarist economist Hayek is eloquent in praise of Mandeville (Hayek, 1978).
38. See above, Note 30.
39. See Bryson, *op. cit.*, ch. 2 for a manageable synopsis of Adam Ferguson's philosophical thought, which she takes as representative of Scottish Enlightenment moral philosophy in general.
40. Though not, as I discovered, at a conference at nine o'clock in the morning.
41. It should be emphasized that the social philosophies of Adam Ferguson and Adam Smith belong in a fairly extensive genre of texts produced in Scotland during this period. Others include Kames's *Sketches of the History of Man*, and Monboddo's *Dissertation*

on the Origin and Progress of Language (1773–92) (touched on in Chapter 4) as well as lesser-known works such as James Dunbar's *Essays on the History of Mankind in Rude and Cultivated Ages* (1780). Although they were frequently in disagreement (e.g. over whether humans were one species [Dunbar] or several [Kames]), and although Monboddo's views often appeared bizarre even to his contemporaries, there remains an underlying homogeneity of aims, feeling, values and method which justifies us in viewing them as a distinct 'school'.

42. This was commoner on the Continent – e.g. Marchese di Cesare Beccaria's work on punishment, which appeared in English in 1767 and went through many editions.
43. Jeremy Bentham's other principal work of relevance here is *Deontology; or the Science of Morality* (1834).
44. cf. Haslam's position: above, ch. 2, Note 7.

Chapter 4 Practical Pressures

1. Cited in Roy Porter (1983).
2. See above, pp. 47–48.
3. Two secondary sources of paramount importance for this topic are Edwin Clarke's 1981 translation of Max Neuberger (1897) *The Historical Development of Experimental Brain and Spinal Cord Physiology before Flourens*, which carries exhaustive additional annotation of subsequent work and comments on Neuberger's text; and Franklin Fearing (1930) *Reflex Action. A Study in the History of Physiological Psychology*, which, while an orthodox internalist work, is an invaluable data source. Also of general use is E.G.R. Liddell (1960), although this concentrates on the neuroanatomical rather than theoretical side of the story. I cannot claim to have done justice to any of these here.
4. e.g. J.F. Unzer (1771; transl. Laycock, 1851).
5. See the Discussion of Mesmerism in Chapter 6 below for more on this point.
6. Haller's *Elementa physiologiae* (1757) remained the canonical textbook almost down to the time of Johannes Müller's *Handbuch der Physiologie des Menschen* (1834–40).
7. 'Stimulus' is derived from a Latin word, *stig-mulus*, meaning a prod for mules (see Diamond [1973] for more on this).
8. See R.K. French (1969) from a detailed account of Whytt's work and differences with von Haller.
9. See K. Danziger (1983); also D.J. Murray (1983), ch. 4.
10. Less than half, in fact; see Colin Gordon (1990) and the responses

to this in the same volume; Chapter 4 of the original edition has now been translated and published in the *History of the Human Sciences* (1991), vol. 4 (1), pp. 1–26.

11. Some of these works will be referenced in due course. Leigh's second volume never seems to have materialized.
12. See, for example, P.-G. Boucé (ed.) (1982) G.S. Rousseau and R. Porter (eds) (1987), as well as journals such as *Signs, International Journal of Women's Studies*, and *Journal of Homosexuality*.
13. See Belinda Meteyard (1980) for a full account of this, and critiques of the interpretations of Lawrence Stone and Edward Shorter (1975).
14. On the growth of 'rational domesticity' and mutual emotional interdependence among family members (including siblings) from the mid-sixteenth century onwards, see Irene Q. Brown (1982).
15. See papers by R. Trumbach, P.-G. Rousseau, T. Castle and L. Friedli in G.S. Rousseau and Roy Porter (eds), *op. cit.*, for various facets of this; also Louis Crompton (1980–81) for a broad review of the legal position of lesbianism in European culture from 1270 to 1791.
16. For this and the sex war generally, see especially Felicity Nüssbaum (1983); also M.S. Kimmel (1990) and Randolph Trumbach (1990).
17. See W.A.C. Stewart (1972). See H.C. Barnard (1961, chs 1–3) for a handy outline of eighteenth-century educational options; also Lawrence Stone (1977) *passim*.
18. One at Rugby in 1797, where pupils blew up the door of the headmaster's study with gunpowder, having to be suppressed by the army.
19. J.A. Axtell (1968) lists 21 editions before 1800, excluding those in complete editions of Locke's works, plus 16 French, 6 Italian, 3 German, 2 Dutch translations and one Swedish.
20. The most famous and successful of these being Henry Peacham's *The Compleat Gentlemen*, of which the 1661 3rd edn is considered the best by the antiquarian trade.
21. Apart from those to be discussed here there are Joseph Priestley's *Essay on a Course of Liberal Education* (1765) and *Miscellaneous Observations relating to Education* (1778), J. Ash, *Sentiments on Education* (1777), Henry Home (Lord Kames), *Loose Hints upon Education* (1781), J. Whitchurch, *Essay upon Education* (1772), D. Williams, *A Treatise on Education* (1774) and *Lectures on Education* (1789), and Clara Reeves, *Plans of Education* (1792) (see C.W.J. Higson [ed.] 1967, 1976 for bibliographical details).
22. Given the variety of different editions, references are to the paragraph numbers of Locke's final, 5th, edn (which all later editions

preserve), rather than page numbers.

23. Her view of Rousseau may be gauged from the following:

> He does not paint an innocent woman ruined, repenting, and restored; but with a far more mischievous refinement, he annihilates the value of chastity, and with pernicious subtlety attempts to make his heroine appear almost more amiable without it. . . . With a metaphysical sophistry most plausible, he debauches the heart of woman . . . (*Strictures on . . . Female Education*, (1818, 12th edn, vol. I, p. 34)

Her approach to Lockean curriculum design would not seem promising either:

> But who suspects the destruction which lurks under the harmless or instructive names of *General History, Natural History, Travels, Voyages, Lives, Encyclopedias, Criticism*, and *Romance*? Who will deny that many of these works contain much admirable matter . . . ? But while 'the dead fly lies at the bottom', the whole will exhale a corrupt and pestilential stench. (*ibid.*, p. 33).

24. 'Rhime, as well as fiefs and duels, owes its origin to the barbarousness of our ancestors' (p. 273) and is 'the legitimate offspring of barbarism and necessity, nursed by ignorance' (p. 274). There is more – much more.
25. He went on to edit Swift's complete works, while Swift's *A Proposal for Correcting, Improving and Ascertaining the English Tongue* (1712) is frequently his point of departure.
26. See Stone (*op. cit.*) pp. 380–86 on 'spinsters'. Regarding female education, C.W.J. Higson (*op. cit.*) includes the following works explicitly on female education, apart from those mentioned in the text (the topic was also usually touched on in general works): J. Bennet, *Strictures on Female Eduction* (1788); J. Burton, *Lectures on Female Education* (1793, 2nd edn); Erasmus Darwin, *A Plan for the Conduct of Female Education* (1797); Mary Wollstonecraft, *Thoughts on the Education of Daughters* (1787) (see Higson (*ibid.*, n. 21) for bibliographic details).
27. Nikolas Rose (1987) sees this episode as a crucial signification of the appearance of the 'moral subject', the crystallization of the individual's total character – behavioural, motivational, ethical, etc. – as a target for scientific scrutiny, and thus the possibility of a third 'Science of Man' separate from philosophy and physiology. I am not entirely clear how far he means to ascribe subsequent events directly to Itard's influence, and how far he has selected it as symbolizing the change in *mentalité* in question. The latter would, in any case, seem the more defensible position.

Chapter 5 Rethinking Eighteenth-Century Psychology

1. cf. Freudian neologisms which came with a whole set of instructions, as it were, regarding how the user could experience their referents.
2. There may be a covert input; I have not had time to explore the time of entry of such expressions as *highly strung, off key, to trumpet, crotchety, quavering*, and (possibly) *on the fiddle*. None of these, bar the first, in any case quite refers to the *topos* being discussed here.
3. As long ago as 1966 a short paper by Marcello Truzzi appeared in the *Journal of the History of the Behavioral Sciences* relating Smith to modern Social Psychology, but the topic has received little further exploration.
4. Though 'moral' and 'mental' were often synonymous during this period, so the label may not be that significant. (see below, Chapter 8, Note 23.)
5. The Scottish school was also the more influential in determining 'Mental and Moral Science' curricula of universities and seminaries in the United States, an influence which persisted until the rise of Psychology in the 1880s. This dimension will be explored in Part Two of this work.
6. See Robert M. Young (1972).
7. K. Danziger's (1982) title reference to it as 'a neglected Chapter in the History of Psychology' reinforces my point, of course.
8. Norbert Elias (1978) locates the turning point with the rise of a heliocentric cosmology at the end of the Renaissance.
9. See C.B. Macpherson (1962), quoted in Shotter (1990), p. 166.
10. See P.-G. Boucé (1982).
11. e.g. *evolution*, used by A. von Haller and Charles Bonnet but referring to their preformationist theory of embryological development

Chapter 6 Reading the Body and Ruling the Mind

1. See also Giustino (1975); Shortland (1987).
2. The Andersonian University of Glasgow, for example, inaugurated a Chair of Phrenology in 1846, though – understandably, by that date – with very limited success.
3. On education: George Combe, *Lectures on Popular Education* (1833); Andrew Combe (1840); on insanity: Andrew Combe, *Observations on Mental Derangement* (1830); on ethnology: J.W. Jackson, *Phrenology and Ethnology* (1863); W.E. Marshall, *A Phrenologist among the Todas* (1873); on statistics: H.C. Watson, *Statistics of Phrenology; being a Sketch of the Progress and Present State of that Science in the British Isles* (1836).

4. Phrenology's last major advocates were the Brighton-based phrenologist Millot Severn and the doctor Bernard Hollander.
5. J.C. Lavater met and travelled with Goethe (then twenty-five) in 1774, and apparently even corresponded with Goethe's mother.
6. See Paolo Mantegazza (n.d.); G. Tytler (1982 ch. I).
7. See Roy Porter (1985a) for more on this point.
8. Parsons's lectures are primarily anatomical and foreshadow Charles Bell (1806) rather than Lavater. He opposes any analogy between human physiognomy and that of 'brutes' and confesses himself to have learned of John Bulwer's *Pathomyotomia* (see above, p. 72) only 'when my intire Treatise, except the List of Authors, and this Preface, was printed off' (p. ii). In the event, he dismisses it as of little importance. Publication dates of the 44 works cited in his bibliography are distributed as follows: pre-1550= 11; 1550–74= 4; 1575–99= 4; 1600–24= 11; 1625–49= 10; 1650–74= 0; 1675–99= 2; 1700+ = 2. This seems to support the notion of a collapse in interest after the mid seventeenth century.
9. See G. Tytler, *op. cit.*, pp. 48–50 for an extensive list of nineteenth-century physiognomical titles.
10. Indeed, at least one plate (XII, 'the Impure') enters the standard iconographic repertoire – reappearing, for example, reversed and in cruder form, as Figure 4, 'Coarse-grained, gross, and carnal', of R.B.D. Wells (n.d.) *New Illustrated Hand-Book of Phrenology, Physiology and Physiognomy*, published about fifty years later.
11. Alfred David, in a paper entitled 'An Iconography of Noses: Directions in the History of a Physical Stereotype', is harsher on Lavater than Tytler (whom he criticizes), doubting that he 'ever exerted any truly profound influence' (p. 91) and seeing in such influence as he did exert a more 'sinister' aspect: promoting a climate sympathetic to stereotyping and racism (of which Lavater himself was not guilty) by adhering to a notion of 'ideal beauty'. In the light of Tytler's evidence, such a view would need to be established on a much broader basis than David provides in his short paper, and the charge he lays against Lavater is, even so, fundamentally anachronistic. Unfortunately, my copy copy of this paper, published in the mid 1980s, lacks both date and source (other than being Chapter 4 of something). For an apposite nineteenth-century physiognomical satire, see Eden Warwick (1848) *Nasology; or Hints towards a classification of noses.*
12. Although it must be said that the rather sensitive and individualized portrait drawings by the young Scots artist Alexander Johnson seem to subvert the very assumption on which the whole book rests.
13. See Sander Gilman (ed.) *The Face of Madness* (1976), in which two

works by Hugh W. Diamond (1856) and John Connolly (1858) are reprinted.

14. See Max Neuberger, 1981, pp. 267 ff. for a summary of these.
15. Camper, incidentally, also published an attack on Tyson (1699) in a work called *An Account of the Organs of Speech of the Orang-Outang* in 1779, although I have been unable to ferret out the bibliographical details.
16. Howard Spoerl (1936, p. 223) observes, though, that Gall's concept of the 'general attributes' and 'determinate faculties' operating as rectangular co-ordinates is fundamentally different from the Scottish approach of simply enumerating the Intellectual Powers and Active Powers as 'side-by-side' lists.
17. G. Lanteri-Laura (1970) notes that Spurzheim's neologisms, while just about – *à peine* – acceptable in English, were ridiculous in French.
18. See *ibid.*, esp. ch. 3.
19. See Ramón Carnicer, (1969); Luis S. Granjel (1973). I am unaware of any English work on Cubi i Solar. My thanks to Denis Gahagan for making these, and other European material, available.
20. Michael Herwig's *The Art of Curing Sympathetically or Magnetically, Proved to be the Most True by its Theory and Practice* (1700) proves not to be among these, in spite of its title. It is a rather grim, degenerate little Paracelsian tract, using the term 'magnetism' analogically – synonymously, even – with 'sympathy'. It makes no reference to therapeutic usage of magnets. Herwig does, however, believe that smearing a 'loadstone' with garlic stops it attracting iron. His one mention of electricity is to point out that it differs from magnetism principally in that it does not 'communicate some of its own virtue' to objects. There may be a tenuous link between Mesmer and Paracelsian thought, but Herwig's work forms no part of it.
21. See Geoffrey Sutton (1981) for a fuller account of this episode.
22. See Roy Porter (1984).
23. On Perkinism, see E.T. Carlson and M.M. Simpson (1970); Roy Porter (1985b).
24. See Stanley W. Jackson (1986), p. 123.
25. *OED*, 2nd edn; the 1st edn gives Franklin only.
26. 'Galvanic', referring to Galvani's work, dates from 1797, and is recorded figuratively in a PL sense in 1807, but the first *OED* entry for 'galvanize' with a PL sense is Charlotte Brontë in *Villette* (1853).
27. Other widely read mid-century English texts include C.H. Townshend (1839, rev. 1844) *Facts in Mesmerism*, and J.B. Dodds (1876) *The Philosophy of Mesmerism and Electrical Psychology.*

28. As a stronger synonym for 'attractive', 'magnetic' is older – Ben Jonson's title *The Magnetic Lady* of 1632 being the first *OED* entry.
29. Simon Schaffer, personal communication. I gather that Godwin's authorship of this has only recently come to light.
30. One current view seems to be that English Mesmerism at this time is something of a myth, and that all the practitioners were primarily followers of Puységur and Mainauduc. It is also possible that, following the French Royal Society of Medicine's rejection of Mesmer in 1784, they were avoiding being identified with his name for public-relations reasons.
31. See Adam Crabtree (1988) for a comprehensive bibliography of 'Animal Magnetism' and Mesmerism.
32. Martin ascribes to Cue the 16-page pamphlet *A true and genuine Discovery of Animal Electricity and Magnetism* (1790), but Stearns confusingly suggests that it was by a John Parsons, who was also publisher of his own response to it. There is clearly a bibliographical muddle here; time precludes any resolution of this in the present work. Not having Crabtree, *op. cit.* to hand, I am assuming that it was by Pearson.
33. This won the Fothergillian Medal of the Medical Society in 1784, and a 2nd edn appeared in 1791: a medical study of the power of mental over physical processes, noting, for example, how the mental state of a patient can affect their recovery.
34. This passage is very similar to one by Puységur quoted in Richard Harte (1902, pp. 85–6).
35. See Roy Porter (1985b).
36. I have used a bound volume, in my own possession, of seven of ten numbers published between 1846 and 1848. A study of the full run is badly needed.
37. O. Hashnu Hara (n.d.; *c.* 1910).
38. George Prochaska (1851 edn), pp. 434–5.
39. He numbers 66, but there are two additional cases, 10a and 27a.
40. James Braid (1846), repr. as Appendix III of Waite's 1899 edn, which also contains an annotated bibliography of Braid's writings.
41. See James Cowles Prichard (1835, pp. 420–21), who provides a good near-contemporary forty-odd-page survey of French and German views of Mesmerism; also Albert Moll (1890), ch. 1.
42. Prichard, *op. cit.*, pp. 422–39.

PART THREE: 1800–50: THREE ROUTES TO PSYCHOLOGY

Chapter 7 The German Route

1. One particularly useful recent paper on this is F. Gregory (1989).
2. I gleaned the data on universities here from my old B. Vincent (1910) *Haydn's Dictionary of Dates*, an indispensable database!
3. M. Norton Wise (1990).
4. cf. phrenology's 'factory' model of the mind in Britain: above, Chapter 6.
5. In this they were adumbrating Gestalt Psychology's mid-twentieth-century anti-reductionist rhetoric.
6. See D.B. Klein (1970), pp. 71–2.
7. cf. William James's 'Transcendental Ego' concept (1890, ch. X).
8. e.g. by Ernst Haeckel; see Hans Schwarz (1981).
9. Leary (1982a) goes so far as to trace modern concerns with 'individuation' (Jung), 'self-actualization' (Maslow) and kindred concepts back to Hegel.
10. The best English summary of Herbart's doctrine remains E.G. Boring's (1950), though D.B. Klein's (1970) discussion and H.B. Dunkel (1970, ch. 8) are a valuable supplement.
11. See E.B. Boring, *op. cit.*, pp. 255–6.
12. See D.B. Klein, *op. cit.*, p. 770.
13. H.B. Dunkel, *op. cit.*, p. 141.
14. *General Thoughts for a Pedagogical Plan of Instruction for the Higher Studies* (1801); *Pestalozzi's Idea of an ABC of Sense Perception*; and *On Pestalozzi's Latest Writing: "How Gertrude Teaches Her Children"* (both 1802); *General Pedagogy* (1806). His two other works on the subject postdate his philosophy: *Letters on the Application of Psychology to Education* (1831) and *Outlines of Pedagogical Lectures* (1835). The original German texts were published as a collected edition; see J.F. Herbart (1873–5).
15. See H.B. Dunkel, *op. cit.*, for a full account of this.
16. Lotze was medically trained and author of *Medicinische Psychologie* (1852), which was his main explicitly Psychological text.
17. This, while deriving ultimately from the astronomer Bessel's reappraisal of the significance of the discrepancies in timing of stellar transits between Maskelyne and Kinnebrook, had rapidly become a topic of physiological interest, taken up by Johannes Müller in the 1830s.
18. See G. Murphy and J.K. Kovach (1972), ch. 6.
19. A later discussion, E.G. Boring (1961), reprinted in E.G. Boring (1963), should also be noted.

20. This might be an exaggeration; E.G. Boring (1942) mentions some French work on hearing from this period of which the same might be said (see Chapter 9 below).
21. I know nothing about E.R. Murray, and come across the book in the British Library catalogue. On a purely subjective level, I got the impression that Murray was a woman. I note that Robert Quick (1890) observes in awe: 'For the full attainment of Froebel's standpoint perhaps a few additional centuries may be necessary' (p. 385); he also has an informative footnote on p. 413 on current proponents of Froebel. Quick's book, I discover – somewhat late in the day – has essays on pre-Locke English educational writers, Locke, Basedow, Rousseau, Pestalozzi, Jacotot and Herbert Spencer, but not Herbart.
22. G. Stanley Hall's references to either in *Adolescence* are mostly negative or in passing: 'the cult of Herbart and Froebel flourishes as a finality instead of a prologue to a great drama now well on in its first act' (1905, II, p. 496).
23. *ibid.*, p. 81.
24. Doerner (1981), p. 240.
25. Forty-eight according to Gregory Zilboorg (1941).
26. Doerner, *op. cit.*, p. 241.
27. *ibid*, p. 244.
28. Cited in Hannah S. Decker (1977).
29. Doerner, *op. cit.*, p. 272.
30. Griesinger, 1867, p. 207.
31. *ibid.*, original emphasis.
32. *ibid.*, p. 278.
33. *ibid.*, p. vi.
34. It should be added that Griesinger's text is 'profoundly Herbartian' (R. Smith, personal communication), although considerations of space prevent further exploration of the point.
35. For the influence of this on US Social Psychology, see Fay Berger Karpf (1932, repr. 1972).
36. E.G. Boring (1942, 1950) does discuss many of these, but later Anglophone historians have left them aside.

Chapter 8 The British Route

1. See Christopher Turk (1988).
2. Translated into English in 1849. It was this which brought to wider notice the Stone Age – Bronze Age – Iron Age sequence.
3. In Ruskin's famous lines, from a letter to Henry Acland in May 1851: 'If only the Geologists would let me alone, I could do very well, but those dreadful Hammers! I hear the clink of them at the end of every

cadence of the Bible verses . . .' (Ruskin [1909], p. 115).

4. See Seymour Drescher (1990) for a recent discussion of the contextual dimensions of this in relation to the slave trade.
5. See G.N. Cantor (1991).
6. The French philosopher Destutt de Tracy was also, apparently, an influence.
7. See John A. Mills (1987) for Brown's account of perception.
8. e.g. James Mark Baldwin (n.d.).
9. D.B. Klein (1970), pp. 706–7.
10. By Bacon, who '"purified" the temple of the mind' (*Lectures*, p. 21).
11. 1953 edn, p. 432.
12. Meaning reconstruction, restoration and even apparently, in Bacon, 'resuscitation', according to William Fleming (1876).
13. See K. Danziger (1982).
14. All references are to the 1967 reprint of the 1875 9th edn. Book VI remained unchanged from the 1st edn.
15. The term 'Ethology' seems to have been stillborn in Mill's sense, reviving in its modern usage, as the naturalistic study of animal behaviour, only in the mid 1950s. The *OED* notes its use in French in 1859, and English instances in 1897 and 1910, but H.C. Warren (1933) includes only the Millean sense (plus a third – the study of ethics). A 1956 quote in the *OED* is from O.L. Zangwill, writing of the new discipline being 'christened', so it was clearly being perceived as a neologism at this point.
16. An argument by which Daniel N. Robinson (1982) is unimpressed.
17. In Alexander Shand (1910) and an 1896 *Encyclopaedia Britannica* article.
18. The Foucault interpretation of the French situation.
19. 1979, pp. 70–71.
20. *ibid.*, p. 70. As mentioned in Chapter 1 with reference to alchemical imagery, psychological change had been explored at the end of the Elizabethan period. This period also saw utopian schemes for social reform (obviously in Thomas More himself earlier, and later in Bacon and Campanella). It had diminished with the rise of the Natural Philosophical law-governed universe and Rational Religion, which stressed the immutability of the physical and social universes.
21. Scull, *op. cit.*, p. 71.
22. Notably by Sir Alexander Morison (1825).
23. Vieda Skultans (1975), pp. 10–11; Nikolas Rose (1987), pp. 23 ff.
24. Pinel's figures being 464:219 and Esquirol's a 4:1 ratio: Prichard (1835), pp. 176–7.
25. William Falconer (1791) is an important earlier exception, although he does not much address psychopathology.

26. I omit W.B. Carpenter, since his greatest impact was post-1850. Other 'Psychophysiologists' of this period include Sir Benjamin Brodie (1783–1862), Sir Henry Holland (1788–1873), R. Dunn (1799–1877) and D. Noble (1810–1885); see L.S. Hearnshaw (1964), pp. 19–20.
27. For the priority dispute with F. Magendie, etc., in addition to E.G. Boring (1950, pp. 45–46), see Franklin Fearing (1930) and especially Max Neuberger (1981 edn p. 253, n. 20).
28. Quoted in E.G. Boring, *op. cit.*, p. 84.
29. Sir Charles Bell (1844), p. 85.
30. The work's first appearance coincided with a growing interest in anatomy among artists tired of the traditional obsession with classical Greek ideal forms; this led to a radical change in the role of the life-drawing class.
31. His combination of aesthetics and physiology reappeared later in Francis Warner's *Physical Expression: Its Modes and Principles* (1885), published in Kegan Paul, Trench & co.'s prestigious International Scientific Series.
32. See E.G.T. Liddell (1960), Neuberger, *op. cit.*, and especially Fearing, *op. cit.*, ch. IX.
33. Laycock, (1840) pp. 85–6.
34. John Dewey (1896). Dewey's paper on the reflex arc concept did not, of course, endorse the stimulus–response account but attacked it on the grounds that the two were objectively indistinguishable. The distinction is a purely functional one in a given behavioural situation. They always exist 'inside a coordination and have their significance purely from the part played in maintaining or reconstituting the coordination' (Dennis edn, 1948, p. 357). 'It is the coordination which unifies that which the reflex arc concept gives us only in disjointed fragments. It its the circuit within which fall distinctions of stimulus and response as functional phases of its own mediation or completion' (*ibid.*, p. 365). This 'top–down' model was all too subtle for J.B. Watson, who claimed that he could never understand what Dewey was talking about.
35. See Note 4.
36. I notice that Mrs Noah is never mentioned; Latham's expression is from R.G. Latham (1850).
37. The leading polygenist of the ensuing period was James Hunt, whose 1863 paper 'The Negro's Place in Nature' was the fullest 'scientific' statement of the position, and briefly revived the polygenist camp's fortunes. He concludes: 'there is as good reason for classifying the Negro as a distinct species from the European, as there is for making the ass a distinct species from

the zebra' (p. 51). It is, I must say, an extraordinary document, and must be understood in the context of Hunt's pro-Confederacy campaigning, the American Civil War then being at its height. For nineteenth-century attitudes to race, see M.D. Biddiss (ed.) (1979) and on polygeny, G.W. Stocking Jr (1968).

38. The editions of Lawrence (1819) and Prichard (1813) used here are the 3rd (1823), and 3rd (1836) respectively. The contents of Lawrence remained unchanged; Prichard's altered and expanded considerably, and the later editions are historically the more important.
39. On Lawrence and Prichard see especially C.D. Darlington (1959), and for a stab at a synoptic review of the topic in general, see G.D. Richards (1987), ch. 2. Surveys of the 'races of Mankind' constitute an identifiable Victorian publishing genre; other examples include C. Hamilton Smith (1852), C. Pickering (1854), Oscar Peschel (1876) and A.H. Keane (1899).
40. Leigh (1961) has a useful biographical sketch of Prichard, who was born into a Quaker family and converted to Anglicanism, which enabled him to enter Cambridge University.
41. He also, in this chapter, praises Gall and Spurzheim for 'rescuing us from the trammels of doctrines and authorities, and directing our attention to nature' (p. 204), though he remains noncommittal on their phrenological doctrines as such.
42. Darlington, *op. cit.*: '. . . Prichard loses his nerve. He begins to admit the possibility of a direct action of the environment (guided by our Maker) and as he does so natural selection fades from his picture' (p. 18).
43. e.g. W. Lauder Lindsay (1880) *Mind in the Lower Animals* in two volumes of over 500 pages each, with chapters on such topics as stupidity, suicide, and crime among animals.

Chapter 9 The French Route

1. Not to be confused with his contemporary, the mathematician J.B.J. Fourier.
2. The extensive accounts and analyses of the work of Pinel and Esquirol in Gregory Zilboorg (1941), F.G. Alexander and S.T. Selesnick (1966), Michel Foucault (1967) and Klaus Koerner (1981), via which changes in historiographical interpretation may be tracked, render a detailed treatment of the background and character of Pinel and Esquirol's psychiatries unnecessary here. This section is restricted to their conceptual innovations.
3. More recent works on this include R. Castel (1988) and J. Goldstein (1987), which have modified the now classic Foucauldian picture.

4. The British Psychological Society's equipment collection housed at Royal Holloway and Bedford New College Psychology Department has a considerable number of these.
5. Edouard Séguin's major work was Séguin (1846). Nikolas Rose (1987) places great importance on the fascination for French Enlightenment philosophers of sensory handicaps such as blindness and deafness as a factor in the creation of the 'moral subject'. Séguin may be seen as continuing this tradition.
6. The adoption of this name was at first puzzling to English-speakers: '. . . by a strange fortune, the word Ideology became in France the distinctive appelation of the doctrine of exclusive sensualism'. (C.S. Henry, p.x. of Introduction to Cousin, 1834). Another French Kantian philosopher of this period was the mathematician Sophie Germain (1776–1831). For accounts of preceding Enlightenment French proto-Psychology from La Mettrie to the *idéologues*, see S. Moravia (1978, 1983) and Charles E. Goshen (1966) for Jean Louis Alibert's work on the 'passions'.
7. E.G. Boring (1950), p. 218 (not p. 277 as indexed) erroneously has 1812.
8. Henry, Intro to Cousin (1834), p. xvii.
9. *ibid.*, p. xxxi.
10. See Max Neuberger (1981) p. 253, n. 20.
11. See Robert M. Young (1970) for extensive discussion of this.
12. E.G. Boring (1942) mentions Cloquet's studies of the sense of smell, which appeared first in 1815 and then, in an enlarged edition, in 1821 (according to him, the most cited source on the topic for over seventy years [p. 439]); C.E.J. Delezenne's researches on pitch discrimination ([1827], *ibid.*, pp. 339–41); and F. Savart on the limits of hearing (*ibid.*, pp. 333–4).
13. The palaeontologist Richard Owen's anti-evolutionism came to the fore only in the 1850s.
14. See P. Topinard (1890), p. 520.
15. See also M.D. Biddiss, (ed.) (1979), Introduction.
16. This is notwithstanding the early emergence in France of the distinct 'moral realm' signified, for Nikolas Rose, by Itard's study of the Victor 'Wild Boy of Aveyron'; see above, Chapter 4, Note 27.
17. Roback (1928) comments that 'he seems to have been possessed of an extraordinary degree of synaesthesia': p. 168.
18. *ibid.*, p. 179.
19. Fourier (1851), vol I, p. 18.
20. For a modern account, see J. Beecher (1986).
21. Roback could discover nothing about this author, whose works seem to have been published in the USA in the 1850s (Roback, p. 180).

22. Taking these to be, in the British case, Bain (1855, 1859) and Spencer (1855), and in Germany Fechner (1860) and Wundt (1863).
23. Ribot's founding of the *Revue Philosophique de la France et de l'Etranger*, which corresponded in character to *Mind* (founded by Bain in the same year).
24. For Gabriel Tarde, see Fay Berger Karpf (1932, repr. 1972, pp. 93–107).
25. For Gustav Le Bon, see R.A. Nye (1975) and Karpf, *ibid.*, pp. 134–44.

Chapter 10 Making the Mind Up

1. See R. Mandrou (1978) on the correspondence networks of Pierre Gassendi and N. Peiresc; Henry Oldenberg, secretary of the Royal Society, represented the major British hub of this communication system.
2. This is the only extended instance I have come across; the 'occasionally' here is really to hold the door open to the possibility of others being unearthed.
3. But 'gauge' was in use in this sense before 1600!
4. See W.K. Wimsatt (1968).
5. See, for example, Steven Shapin (1991).

Appendix

PUBLICATIONS IN ENGLAND OR IN ENGLISH ABROAD BEFORE 1641

In the early phase of preparing this work, I felt that a survey of the kinds of books published in Britain before 1641 would help to provide a picture of prevalent cultural concerns (although censorship existed throughout virtually the whole period). In addition, such data may provide a way of checking the impressionistic generalizations to which anyone attempting to write about whole historical epochs is necessarily prone; for example, if Zevedei Barbu (1960) was correct in talking of increased secularization during the sixteenth century, we would expect this to be reflected in the proportion of total publications which were religious in character. In order to shed light on this, I undertook a survey of the entries in the second edition of Pollard and Redgrave's *A Short-Title Catalogue of Books Printed in England, Scotland & Ireland and of English Books printed abroad, 1475–1640* (STC for short). A full report of this would be out of place in the present work, but the overall picture may be of some help or interest.

In brief, I sampled every entry ending in a zero – which, since the entry numbers were sometimes decimalized, amounted to a sample of around 8 per cent (2,647). (Details of procedure, etc., will, it is hoped, be published in due course.) The two issues of interest here are (a) the relative frequencies of different genres of books; and (b) variations in the proportion of religious books over time. These are presented below in Tables Appendix 1 and Appendix 2 respectively.

Table Appendix 1. % of publications by subject

SUBJECT	NO.	%	
Religion	1,096	41.	1,139: 43% including Church Admin.
Law & Civ.Adm.	328	12.4	
Verse	240	9.1	Includes non-Classical Latin
Sciences	106	4.0	Includes maths, medicine (49), navigation, geography, astronomy.
Politics	85	3.2	
History	79	3.0	
News	70	2.6	Inc. 29 Newsbooks. Excluding ballads.
Drama	67	2.5	
Education	67	2.5	
Language	57	2.2	Including dictionaries, occasional arbitrariness *vis-à-vis* Education.
Philosophy	51	2.0	
Husbandry etc.	48	1.8	Includes all practical instruction excepting navigation.
Popular	44	1.7	Books of wit, scandals, etc.
Classics	41	1.5	Livy, Euclid, Galen, under History, maths & medicine respectively[a].
Church of Eng.	38	1.4	Admin. documents.
Crime	22	0.8	inc. pre-execution confessions.
Occult	22	0.8	Astrology, witchcraft, ghosts.
Biography	20	0.8	Exc. hagiographies properly belonging under religion.
Fiction	17	0.6	A difficult category; anything apparently in prose of a fictional nature.
Travel	16	0.6	
Military	14	0.5	
Scottish Adm.	13	0.5	
Music	12	0.45	
Orations, etc.	10	0.4	Formal orations, prose elegies, obituaries (other than sermons)
Scot. Univ. Theses	6	0.23	
Scot. Church Adm.	5	0.2	
Genealogies	5	0.2	a block by Speed
Emblems/Heraldry	5	0.2	
Psychology	5	0.2	Burton, Earle, Overbury, Wright
Epigrams/Satires	2	0.08	
Economics	2	0.08	
Complaints	2	0.08	One about the roads, one about the destruction of woods.

Other	35	1.3	Varying from chess to a book on the Frankfurt Book Fair and a Bill of Mortality.
Unclassified	32	1.2	Cases where, either from ignorance or insufficient information, I was unable to identify the subject matter of a work.
Total	2,647	100.52	(due to rounding-up)

Note

a. The Classics market was being supplied primarily by the Italian publishers (such as Aldine) or the Dutch (Elsevier) throughout this period. This figure is thus a considerable underestimate of their relative popularity. It is nevertheless still remarkable that none of Plato's works had been published in English translation before 1640 (although one erroneously ascribed to him had been); the first to appear was a 1672 translation of the Phaedo by Bentley.

Comment

The sheer domination of religious and Church-related publications is the most obvious feature, these amounting to nearly 43%. Science, philosophy and 'psychology' amount to a bare 6.2%, of which nearly a third are on medicine. Language and Education alone, however, make up about nearly 5%, which, if combined, would put them in fourth place after Religion, Civil Administration and Verse.

Table Appendix 2 Changes in Proportion of Religious Books

Period	%
pre-1550	40.6
1511–1555	47.5
1556–1560	39.0
1561–1565	37.1
1566–1570	33.4
1571–1575	38.4
1576–1580	46.6
1581–1585	43.9
1586–1590	40.2
1591–1595	42.2
1596–1600	34.8
1601–1605	35.5
1606–1610	46.7
1611–1615	49.4
1616–1620	46.8
1621–1625	53.7
1626–1630	46.3
1631–1635	44.7
1636–1640	45.1

These data suggest an oscillation for the post-1550 period, with three peaks and three troughs: peaks in the early 1550s, late 1570s and early 1580s, and 1611 to the mid 1620s (though remaining high thereafter); troughs in the late 1560s, 1595–1605 and, if only relatively, the early 1630s. On these figures, 'secularization' appears to be more of a late-sixteenth- than early-seventeenth-century phenomenon.

Bibliography

Abbreviations

JHBS	*Journal of the History of the Behavioral Sciences*
PR	Pennington, D and Thomas, K. (1978)

Square brackets denote works published anonymously.

Aarsleff, Hans (1976) 'John Wilkins', in C.C. Gillespie (ed.), *Dictionary of Scientific Biography*, vol. XIV, New York: Scribner's.

Aarsleff, Hans (1983, 2nd edn) *The Study of Language in England 1780–1860*, Minneapolis: University of Minnesota Press / London: The Athlone Press.

Abercrombie, John (1840, 1st edn 1830) *Inquiries Concerning the Intellectual Powers and the Investigation of Truth*, London: John Murray.

Alexander, F.G. and Selesnick, S.T. (1966) *The History of Psychiatry*, New York: Harper & Row.

Alison, Archibald (1790) *Essays on the Nature and Principles of Taste*, Dublin: P. Byrne, J. Moore, Grueber and M'Allister, W. Jones, & R. White.

Allport, Gordon W. (1937) *Personality: A Psychological Investigation*, New York: Henry Holt.

[Anon.] (1655) *Anthropologie abstracted; or, the idea of Humane nature reflected in briefe Philosophicall and anatomical collections*, London.

[Anon.] (1741) *An Introduction towards an Essay on the Origins of the Passions in which it is . . . shown how they are acquired and that they are all no other than associations of ideas of our own making, or what we learn of others*, London: R. Dodsley.

[Anon.] (1747) *An Enquiry into the Origin of the Human Appetites and Affections, Shewing how each arises from Association*, London: R. Dodsley.

[Anon.] (1800) *Lavater's Looking Glass or Essays on the Face of Animated Nature from Man to Plants*, London: Millar Ritchie.

[Anon.] (1849) *The Life of John Kaspar Lavater, Minister of St. Peter's Church, Zurich*, London: Religious Tract Society.

Apel, Karl Otto (1977) 'Types of Social Science in the Light of Human Interests of Knowledge', *Social Research*, vol. 44 (3), pp. 425–70.

'Aristotle' (pseud.) (n.d.) *The Works of Aristotle the Famous Philosopher. Containing his complete masterpiece and family physician; his experienced midwife, his book of problems and his remarks on physiognomy*, London: Clifton, Chambers (usually known as '*Aristotle's Masterpiece*').

Arnold, Thomas (1806, 2nd edn; 1st edn 1782, 1786) *Observations on the Nature, Kinds, Causes, and Prevention of Insanity*, (2 vols), London: Richard Phillips.

Ascham, Roger (1570) *The scholemaster or plaine and perfite way of teachyng children, the Latin tong*, London: J. Daye.

Ash, M.G. and Woodward, W.R. (eds) (1987) *Psychology in Twentieth-Century Thought and Society*, Cambridge: Cambridge University Press.

Axtell, J.A. (1968) *The Educational Writings of John Locke*, Cambridge: Cambridge University Press.

Ayer, A.J. (1985, repr. 1986) *Ludwig Wittgenstein*, Harmondsworth: Penguin.

Aylmer, G.E. (1978) 'Unbelief in Seventeenth Century England' in PR, pp. 22–48.

Bacon, Francis (1857–74) *The Works of Francis Bacon*, vols IV–V, ed. James Spedding, Robert Leslie Ellis and Douglas Denton Heath, London: Longman.

Bain, Alexander (1855) *The Senses and the Intellect*, London: Longmans Green.

Bain, Alexander (1859) *The Emotions and the Will*, London: Longmans Green.

Bain, Alexander (1861) *On the Study of Character, including an Estimate of Phrenology*, London: Parker, Son & Bourn.

Bakan, David (1966) 'The Influence of Phrenology on American Psychology', *JHBS*, vol. 2 pp. 200–20.

Bakan, David (1975) *Sigmund Freud and the Jewish Mystical Tradition*, New York: Beacon.

Baldwin, James Mark (n.d.; Preface date 1913) *History of Psychology: A Sketch and an Interpretation*, London: Watts.

Bamborough, J.B. (1952) *The Little World of Man*, London: Longmans Green.

Barbu, Zevedei (1960) *Problems in Historical Psychology*, London: Routledge & Kegan Paul.

Barfield, O. (1974) 'Coleridge's Enjoyment of Words', in John Beer (ed.), pp. 204–18.

Barnard, H.C. (1961) *A History of English Education from 1760*, London: University of London Press.

Battie, William (1758) *A Treatise on Madness*, London: J. Whiston & B. White, (repr. ed. R. Hunter & I. Macalpine, 1962, London: Dawsons of Pall Mall).

Baugh, A.C. (1959) *A History of the English Language* (2nd edn), London: Routledge & Kegan Paul.

Beattie, James (1770) *Essay on the Nature and Immutability of Truth*, Edinburgh: William Creech.

Beccaria, Marchese di Cesare (1767) *Del delitti e delle pene. An Essay on Crimes and Punishments*, London: J. Almon.

Beck, Cave (1657) *The Universal Character*, London: Thomas Maxey for William Weekley.

Beecher, J. (1986, repr. 1990) *Charles Fourier: The Visionary and his World*, Berkeley, CA: University of California Press.

Beer, J. (ed.) (1974) *Coleridge's Variety: Bicentenary Studies*, London: Macmillan.

Bell, Sir Charles (1811) *Idea of a New Anatomy of the Brain: Submitted for the Observations of his Friends*, London: Strahan & Preston.

Bell, Sir Charles (1844, 3rd edn; 1st edn 1806) *The Anatomy and Philosophy of Expression as connected with the Fine Arts*, London: John Murray.

Bell, Sir Charles (1865, 7th edn; 1st edn 1832) *The Hand: its mechanism and vital endowments, as evincing design*, London: Bell & Daldy.

Bell, John (1788) *An essay on Somnambulism or Sleep-walking, produced by Animal Electricity and Magnetism As well as by Sympathy etc.*, Dublin: 'for the author'.

Bell, John (1792) *The General and Particular Principles of Animal Electricity and Magnetism &c, in which are found Dr Bell's Secrets and Practice as delivered to his pupils*, Dublin: 'the author'.

Beneke, F.E. (1832) *Lehrbuch der Psychologie als Naturwissenschaft*, Berlin: Mittler.

Beneke, F.E. (1845) *Die neue Psychologie*, Berlin: Mittler.

Benjamin, A.E., Cantor, G.N. and Christie, J.R.R. (1987) *The Figural and the Literal: Problems of Language in the History of Science and Philosophy, 1630–1800*, Manchester: Manchester University Press.

Bennington, G.	(1987) 'The Perfect Cheat: Locke and Empiricism's Rhetoric', in A.E. Benjamin *et al.* (eds), pp. 103–23.
Bentham, Jeremy	(1789) *An Introduction to the Principles of Morals and Legislation*, London: T. Payne & Sons.
Bentham, Jeremy	(1834) *Deontology; or the Science of Morality* (2 vols), London: Longman & Co.
Ben-Zeev, Aaron	(1986) 'Reid's Direct Approach to Perception', *Studies in the History and Philosophy of Science*, vol. 17 (1), pp. 99–114.
Ben-Zeev, Aaron	(1990) 'Reid's Opposition to the Theory of Ideas', in M. Dalgarno and E. Matthews (eds) *The Philosophy of Thomas Reid*, Dordrecht: Kluwer, pp. 91–101.
Berkeley, George (ed. G.J. Warnock)	(1710 repr. 1962) *The Principles of Human Knowledge*, London: Collins Fontana Library.
Berkeley, George	(1901) *The Works of George Berkeley* (4 vols), Oxford:
(ed. A.C. Fraser)	Clarendon Press.
Berkeley, George (ed. Mary Whiton Calkins)	(1929 repr. 1957) *Essay, Principles, Dialogues with Selections from other writings*, New York: Scribner's
Bernstein, H.R.	(1980) '*Conatus*, Hobbes, and the young Leibniz', *Studies in the History and Philosophy of Science*, vol. 11(1), pp. 25–37.
Biddiss, M.D. (ed.)	(1979) *Images of Race*, Leicester: Leiceester University Press.
Boas, F.S.	(1950) *An Introduction to Tudor Drama*, Oxford: Clarendon Press.
Bonelli, M.L.R. and Shea, W.R.	(1975) *Reason, Experiment, and Mysticism in the Scientific Revolution*, London: Macmillan.
Bonet, J.P.	(1620) *Reduction de las Letras, y Arte para enseñar à ablar los Mudos*, Madrid: F. Abarca de Angulo.
Bonnet, C.	(1779–1783) *Œuvres d'Histoire naturelle et de Philosophie* (18 vols), Neuchâtel: Samuel Fauche Libraire du Roi. (vols 13–14, *Essai analytique sur les facultés de l'âme* [1760]; vol. 17, *Essai de Psychologie* [1754]).
Boring, E.G.	(1942) *Sensation and Perception in the History of Experimental Psychology*, New York: Appleton- Century- Crofts.
Boring, E.G.	(1950, 2nd edn, repr. 1957) *A History of Experimental Psychology* New York: Appleton-Century-Crofts.
Boring, E.G.	(1963) *History, Psychology & Science, Selected papers*

(ed. R.I. Watson and D.T. Campbell), New York: Wiley.

Bossuet, J.B. (1681) *Discours sur l'Histoire universelle à Monseigneur le Dauphin*, Paris: S. Mabre-Cramoisy.

Boucé, P.-G. (ed.) (1982) *Sexuality in Eighteenth-Century Britain*, Manchester: Manchester University Press.

Braaten, J. (1988) 'Elimination, Enlightenment and the Normative Content of Folk Psychology', *Journal for the Theory of Social Behavior*, vol. 18 (3), pp. 251–68.

Braid, J. (ed. A.E. Waite) (1899) *Braid on Hypnotism*, London: George Redway.

Brerewood, E. (1614) *Enquiries concerning the diversity of languages, and religions through the cheefe part of the world*, London: John Bill.

Brett, G.S. (1912–1921) *A History of Psychology* (3 vols), London: Allen & Unwin.

Bright, T. (1586) *A Treatise of Melancholie*, London: Vautrollier.

Bricke, J. (1974) 'Hume's Associationist Psychology', *JHBS*, vol. 10, pp. 397–409.

Bronowski, J. (1954) *William Blake 1757–1827: A Man without a Mask*, Harmondsworth: Penguin.

Brooks, G.P. (1976) 'The Faculty Psychology of Thomas Reid', *JHBS*, vol. 12, pp. 65–77.

Brooks-Davies, D. (1982) 'The Mythology of Love: Venerean (and Related) Iconography in Poe, Fielding, Cleland and Sterne', in P.-G. Boucé (ed.), pp. 176–97.

Broughton, John (1703) *Psychologia or, an Account of the Nature of the Rational Soul*, London: W.D. for T. Bennet and A. Bosville.

Brown, Irene Q. (1982) 'Domesticity, Feminism, and Friendship: Female Aristocratic Culture and Marriage in England, 1660–1760', *Journal of Family History*, Winter pp. 406–24.

Brown, Thomas (1836; 1st edn 1820) *Lectures on the Philosophy of the Human Mind* (2 vols), Hallowell: Glazier, Masters & Smith.

[Browne, Peter] (1728) *The Procedure, Extent, and Limits of Human Understanding*, London: William Innys.

[Browne, Peter] (1733) *Things Divine and Supernatural Conceived by Analogy with Things Natural and Human*, London: William Innys and Richard Manby.

Browne, Sir Thomas (1915; 1st, unauthorized, edn 1642) (ed. W.A. Greenhill) *Religio Medici*, London: Macmillan, 1915.

Browne, Sir Thomas (1890; 1st edn 1646) *Pseudodoxia Epidemica* (*Vulgar Errors*), in Simon Wilkin (ed.) *The Works of Sir Thomas Browne*, London: George Bell & Sons.

Bryson, Gladys (1968; 1st edn 1945) *Man and Society: The Scottish Inquiry of the Eighteenth Century*, Princeton, NJ: Princeton University Press (repr. New York: Augustus M. Kelley).

Budd, Malcolm (1989) *Wittgenstein's Philosophy of Psychology*, London: Routledge.

Buffon, G.L.C. (1749) *L'Histoire naturelle de l'homme*, in vol. II of *Histoire naturelle, générale et particulière . . .* , Paris: L'Imprimerie Royale.

Buikerood, J.G. 1985 'The Natural History of the Understanding: Locke and the Rise of Facultative Logic in the Eighteenth Century', *History and Philosophy of Logic*, vol. 6, pp. 157–90.

[Bulwer, John] ('J.B.') (1644) *Chirologia, or the Naturall Language of the Hand*, London: Thos. Harper.

[Bulwer, John] ('J.B.') (1648) *Philocophus, or the Deafe and dumbe man's friend*, London: Humphrey Moseley.

[Bulwer, John] ('J.B. The Chirosopher') (1649) *Pathomyotomia or a Dissertation on the Significative Muscles of the Affections of the Minde*, London: W.W. for Humphrey Moseley.

Bulwer, John (1653) *Anthropometamorphosis: Man Transformed: or, The Artificiall Changeling*, London: William Hunt.

Burgess, T.H. (1828) *The Physiology or Mechanism of Blushing*, London: John Churchill.

Burke, Edmund (1958; 1st edn 1757) *A Philosophical Enquiry into the Origin of our Ideas of the Sublime and Beautiful*, ed. J.T. Boulton, London: Routledge & Kegan Paul.

Burton, Robert (ed. A.R. Shilleto) (1896) *The Anatomy of Melancholy* (3 vols), London: George Bell & Sons, 1896 (1st edn published 1621; went through 6 revised edns, the last, quoted here, in 1651–2).

Busby, T.L. (1820) *Costume of the Lower Orders of London*, London: Baldwin, Craddock & Joy.

Campbell, Archibald (1728) *Απετη – λογια or An Enquiry into the Original of Moral Virtue*, London: B. Creake.

Canguilhem, G. (1955) *La Formation du concept de réflex aux XVIIe et XVIIIe siècles*, Paris: Presses Universitaires de France.

Cantor, G.N. (1991) 'Between Rationalism and Romanticism:

Whewell's Historiography of the Inductive Sciences', in M. Fisch and S. Schaffer (eds) *William Whewell: A Composite Portrait*, Oxford: Clarendon Press, pp. 67–86.

Carlson, E.T. and Simpson, M.M. (1970) 'Perkinism vs Mesmerism', *JHBS*, vol. 6, pp. 16–24.

Carnicer, Ramón (1969) *Entre la ciencia y la magia: Mariano Cubi*, Barcelona: Seix Barral.

Cassirer, Ernst (1934, repr. 1955; 1st German edn 1932) *The Philosophy of the Enlightenment*, Boston, MA: Beacon.

Castel, R. (1988) *The Regulation of madness: the origins of incarceration in France*, Berkeley, CA: University of California Press.

[Chambers, R.] (1845, 4th edn; 1st edn 1844) *Vestiges of the Natural History of Creation*, London: John Churchill.

Chambre, Marin C. de la (1648–62) *Les Caractères des Passions* (5 vols), Paris

Cheyne, G. (1733, 1742) *The English Malady: or, a Treatise of Nervous Diseases of all Kinds . . . with the Author's Own Case at Large*, London: G. Strahan & J. Leake.

Christie, J.R.R. (1987) 'Adam Smith's Metaphysics of Language', in A.E. Benjamin *et al.* (eds), pp. 202–29.

Churchland, P.M. (1985) 'Reduction, Qualia, and the Direct Introspection of Brain States', *The Journal of Philosophy*, vol. 82 (1), pp. 8–28.

Churchland, P.S. (1986) *Neurophilosophy: Towards a Unified Science of the Mind/Brain*, Cambridge, MA: MIT Press, 1986.

Claus, Sidonie (1982) 'John Wilkins'Essay Toward a Real Character: Its Place in the Seventeenth-Century Episteme', *Journal of the History of Ideas*, vol. 43 (4), pp. 531–53.

Cleland, John (1749, repr. 1977) *Memoirs of a Woman of Pleasure*, London: Mayflower Books.

Cliffe, J.T. (1988) *Puritans in Conflict: The Puritan Gentry during and after the Civil Wars*, London: Routledge.

Clifford, W.K. (1885) *The Common Sense of the Exact Sciences*, London: Kegan Paul, Trench & Co.

Coeffeteau, F.N. (1621) *A Table of Humane Passions with their Causes and Effects*, London: Nicholas Okes.

Coleridge, S.T. (1956; 1st edn 1817) *Biographia Literaria*, London: Dent (Everyman edn).

Combe, Andrew (1830) *Observations on Mental Derangement: being an application of Phrenology to the elucidation . . . of insanity*, Edinburgh: John Anderson Junior/London: Longman, Rees, Orme, Brown & Green.

Combe, Andrew (1840) *A Treatise on the Physiological and Moral Management of Infancy*, Edinburgh: McLachlan & Stewart.

Combe, George (1833) *Lectures on Popular Education*, Edinburgh: John Anderson Jr.

Combe, George (1836, 4th edn) *Elements of Phrenology*, Edinburgh: Maclachlan & Stewart & John Anderson/London: Longman & Co. & Simpkin, Marshall & Co.

Combe, George (1860, 9th edn; 1st edn 1828) *The Constitution of Man and its Relations to External Objects*, Edinburgh: Maclachlan & Stewart/London: Longman & Simpkin, Marshall (1st edn, Edinburgh: Neill).

Comenius, John Amos (1657) *Opera Didacticae Omnia*, Amsterdam: D. Laurentii de Geer.

Comenius*, John Amos (1658) *Orbis sensualium pictus*, Nuremberg.

Comenius, John Amos (ed. M.W. Keatinge) (1896) *The Great Didactic of John Amos Comenius*, London: Adam and Charles Black.

Comte, A. (1830–42) *Cours de philosophie positive* (6 vols), Paris: Rouen Frères (Bachelier).

Condillac, E.B. de (An VI, 1798) *Œuvres de Condillac* (23 vols), Paris: Ch. Houel (vol. 1, *Essai sur l'origine des connaissances Humaines*; vol. 3, *Traité des Sensations & Traité des Animaux*; vol. 6, *L'Art de penser*).

Condorcet, M.J.A.N. Caritat, Marquis de (1795) *Esquisse d'un tableau historique des progrès de l'esprit humaine*, n.p. 1795 (English transl. *Outlines of an Historical View of the Progress of the Human Mind*, London: J. Johnson, 1795).

Cooper, Anthony Ashley (Lord Shaftesbury) (ed. & intro. David Walford) (1977; 1st edn 1711) *An Inquiry Concerning Virtue, or Merit*, Manchester: Manchester University Press, 1977.

Cooter, Roger (1984) *The Cultural Meaning of Popular Science: Phrenology and the Organization of Consent in Nineteenth-Century Britain*, Cambridge: Cambridge University Press.

Cournot, A.A. (1851) *Essai sur les fondements de nos connaissances et sur les caractères de la critique philosophique*, Paris.

Cousin, Victor (1834) *Elements of Psychology included in a criti-*

* catalogued in the British Library as Kominsky.

cal examination of Locke's Essay on the Human Understanding, transl. C.S. Henry, Hartford, CT: Cooke & Co.

Cousin, Victor (1840) *Cours de philosophie . . . sur le fondement des idées absolue du vrai, du beau, du bien*, Brussels.

[Coward, William] (Estibius Psychalethes) (1702) *Second Thoughts Concerning Human Soul*, London: R. Basset.

Cowling, Mary (1989) *The Artist as Anthropologist in Victorian England: the Depiction of Type and Character in Victorian Art*, Cambridge: Cambridge University Press.

Crabtree, Adam (1988) *Animal Magnetism, Early Hypnotism, and Psychical Research, 1766–1925. An Annotated Bibliography*, New York: Kraus International Publications.

Crichton, Sir A. (1798) *An Inquiry into the Nature and Origin of Mental Derangement*, London.

Crombie, A.C. (1864) 'Early Concepts of the Senses and the Mind', *Scientific American*, vol. 210 (5), pp. 108–16.

Crompton, Louis (1980/81) 'The Myth of Lesbian Impunity: Capital Laws from 1270 to 1791', *Journal of Homosexuality*, vol. 6 (1/2), pp. 11–25.

Cudworth, R. (1678) *The True Intellectual System of the Universe*, London: Richard Royston.

Dalgarno, G. (1661) *Ars Signorum*, London: J. Hayes.

Danziger, Kurt (1982) 'Mid-Nineteenth-Century British Psycho-Physiology: A Neglected Chapter in the History of Psychology', ch. 5 in William R. Woodward and Mitchell G. Ash (eds) *The Problematic Science: Psychology in Nineteenth-Century Thought*, New York: Praeger.

Danziger, Kurt (1983) 'Origins of the Schema of Stimulated Motion: Towards a Pre-history of Modern Psychology', *History of Science*, vol. xxi, pp. 183–210.

Danziger, Kurt (1990) *Constructing the Subject: Historical Origins of Psychological Research*, Cambridge: Cambridge University Press.

Darlington, C.D. (1959) *Darwin's Place in History*, Oxford: Basil Blackwell.

Darwin, Charles (1859) *The Origin of Species*, London: John Murray.

Darwin, Charles (1871) *The Descent of Man*, London: John Murray.

Darwin, Charles (1872) *The Expression of the Emotions in Man and Animals*, London: John Murray.

d'Assigny, Marius (1697) *The Art of Memory. A treatise useful for such as are to speak in public*, London: J.D. for Andr. Ball.

Davidson, John (1906) *A New Interpretation of Herbart's Psychology and Educational Theory through the Philosophy of Leibniz*, Edinburgh and London: William Blackwood & Sons.

Davies, Tony (1987) 'The Ark in Flames: Science, Language and Education in Seventeenth-century England', in A.E. Benjamin, *et al.* (eds), pp. 83–102.

Dawkins, R. (1976) *The Selfish Gene*, London: Oxford University Press.

Day, Thomas (1783–9) *Sandford and Merton*, London: A. Millar/ Edinburgh: G. Hamilton & J. Balfour.

Debus, Allen G. (1965) *The English Paracelsians*, London: Oldbourne Press.

Debus, Allen G. (1977) *The Chemical Philosophy: Paracelsian Science and Medicine in the Sixteenth and Seventeenth Centuries* (2 vols), New York: Watson Academic Publications.

Decker, Hannah S. (1977) 'Freud in Germany: Revolution and Reaction in Science, 1893–1907', *Psychological Issues*, vol. XI (1), Monograph 41, New York: International Universities Press.

Defert, Daniel (1982) 'The Collection of the World: Accounts of Voyages from the Sixteenth to the Eighteenth Centuries', *Dialectical Anthropology*, vol. 7, pp. 11–20.

Degerando, Jh.M. (An VIII, 1800) *Des signes et de l'art de penser considérés dans leurs rapports mutuels*, vol. III. Paris: Goujon, Fuchs, Henrichs.

Dennis, W. (ed) (1948) *Readings in the History of Psychology*, New York: Appleton-Century-Crofts.

Derham, W. (1720, 5th edn; 1st edn 1711, 1712) *Physico-Theology: or a Demonstration of the Being And Attributes of God from his Works of Creation. Being the Substance of Sixteen Sermons*, London: W. & J. Innys.

Derrida, J. (1982, 1986) *On the Margins of Philosophy*, Sussex: Harvester Press.

Descartes, René (1650) *The Passions of the Soule in three Bookes*, London: A.C.

Descartes, René (1680) *Six Metaphysical Meditations; wherein it is proved that there is a God*, with a life by W. Molyneux, London: B.G. for Benj. Tooke.

Descartes, René (1967; 1st edn 1911) *The Philosophical Works of Descartes Vol. 1*, transl. E.S. Haldane and G.R.T.

Ross, Cambridge: Cambridge University Press.

Dewey, John (1896) 'The Reflex Arc Concept in Psychology', *Psychlogical Review*, vol. III, pp. 357–70. reprinted in W. Dennis (ed.) (1948) *Readings in the History of Psychology*, New York: Appleton-Century-Crofts, pp. 355–65.

Diamond, Solomon (1968) 'Marin Cureau de la Chambre (1594–1669)', *JHBS*, vol, 4, pp. 40–54.

Diamond, Solomon (1973) 'Gestation of the Instinct Concept' in Mary Henle *et al.* (eds), pp. 150–65.

Dobbs, B.J.T. (1975) *The Foundations of Newton's Alchemy, or, 'the Hunting of the greene lyon'*, Cambridge: Cambridge University Press.

Dodds, J.B. (ed J. Burns) (1876) *The Philosophy of Mesmerism and Electrical Psychology*, London: James Burns, Progressive Library.

Dodwell, Henry (1708) *The Natural Mortality of Humane Souls clearly Demonstrated from the Holy Scriptures*, London: for E. Curll & E. Sanger.

Doerner, Klaus (1981; 1st German edn 1969) *Madmen and the Bourgeoisie: A Social History of Insanity and Psychiatry*, Oxford: Blackwell.

Drescher, Seymour (1990) 'The Ending of the Slave Trade and the Evolution of European Scientific Racism', *Social Science History*, vol. 14 (3), pp. 415–50.

Drever, James (1966) 'The Historical Background for National Trends in Psychology: On the Non-existence of English Associationism', *JHBS*, vol. 1, pp. 123–30.

Dunbar, James (1780) *Essays on the History of Mankind in Rude and Cultivated Ages*, Edinburgh and London: W. Strahan & T. Cadell and J. Balfour.

Dunkel, H.B. (1970) *Herbart and Herbartianism: An Educational Ghost Story*, Chicago and London: Chicago University Press.

[Earle, John] (1628, repr. 1904) *Micro-cosmographie or a peece of the World Discovered; in essays and characters*, London: William Stansby for Robert Allott (repr. Westminster: A. Constable).

Edgeworth, Maria and Richard Lovell (1798) *Practical Education* (2 vols), London: J. Johnson.

Elias, Norbert (1939, repr. 1978) *The Civilizing Process: The History of Manners*, transl. Edmund Jephcott, Oxford: Basil Blackwell.

Emmet, Dorothy (1974) 'Coleridge on Powers in Mind and Nature', in John Beer (ed.), pp. 166–82).

Esquirol, J.E.D. (1838) *Des maladies mentales considérées sous les rapports médicals, hygiéniques et médico-légals* (2 vols), Paris.

Evans-Pritchard, E.E. (1981) *A History of Anthropological Thought*, London: Faber & Faber.

Evelyn, J. (1667) *Publick Employment and an Active Life prefer'd to Solitude, and all its Appanages*, London: J.M. for H. Heringman.

Everett, C.W. (1966) *Jeremy Bentham*, London: Weidenfeld & Nicolson.

Falconer, William (1791) *A Dissertation on the Influence of the Passions upon Disorders of the Body*, London: C. Dilly.

Fearing, Franklin (1930) *Reflex Action. A Study in the History of Physiological Psychology*, London: Baillière, Tindall & Cox.

Fechner, Gustav (1860) *Elemente der Psychophysik* (2 vols), Leipzig: Breitkopf & Härtel.

Ferguson, Adam (1768, 3rd edn; 1st edn 1767) *An Essay on the History of Civil Society*, London: Miller & Cadell/Edinburgh: Kincaid & Bell.

Ferguson, Adam (1769, 1773) *Institutes of Moral Philosophy. For the use of Students in the College of Edinburgh*, Edinburgh: Kincaid & Creech, and J. Bell.

Ferguson, Adam (1792) *Principles of Moral and Political Science*, Edinburgh: Strahan & Cadell.

Fleming, William (1876) *The Vocabulary of Philosophy*, London: Charles Griffin.

Flourens, M.J.P. (1824) *Recherches expérimentales sur les propriétés et les fonctions du système nerveux, dans les animaux vertébrés*, Paris: Crevot.

Flourens, M.J.P. (1842) *Examen de la Phrénologie*, Paris: Paulin.

Flugel, J.C. (rev. D.J. West) (1964; 1st edn 1933) *A Hundred Years of Psychology*, London: Methuen.

Foucault, Michel (1967) *Madness and Civilization: A History of Insanity in the Age of Reason*, transl. Richard Howard, London: Tavistock.

Foucault, Michel (1976, transl. 1979) *The History of Sexuality, vol. 1*, transl. Robert Hurley, London: Allen Lane.

Foucault, Michel (1919) 'Experiences of Madness', transl. Ania Chevallier, *History of the Human Sciences*, vol. 4 (1), pp. 1–25.

Fourier, Charles (transl. J.R. Morell) (1851) *The Passions of the Human Soul* (2 vols), London: Hippolyte Baillière.

Fox, Christopher (ed) (1987) *Psychology and Literature in the Eighteenth Century*, New York: AMS.

Fox, Christopher (1987) 'Defining Eighteenth-Century Psychology: Some Problems and Perspectives', in Fox, ed., pp. 1–22.

Fraser, Antonia (1984) *The Weaker Vessel: Woman's Lot in Seventeenth-Century England*, London: Weidenfeld & Nicolson.

French, R.K. (1969) *Robert Whytt, the Soul, and Medicine*, London: Wellcome Institute for the History of Medicine.

Froebel, Friedrich (1826, transl. 1887) *The Education of Man*, New York and London: D. Appleton.

Froebel, F. (1843) *Mutter- und Kose- Lieden (Mother Songs)*, Blankenburg.

Froebel, F. (1862–83) *F.F.'s gesammelte pädagogische Schriften* (3 vols), Berlin (vols 1 & 2) and Vienna (vol. 3).

Gall, Franz Joseph (1809) *Recherches sur le système nerveux en général, et sur celui du cerveau en particulier*, Paris: Schoell.

Gay, Rev. Mr (1731) *Dissertation Concerning the Fundamental Principle of Virtue or Morality*, Prefixed to W. King, *An Essay on the Origin of Evil* transl. E. Law, Cambridge: W. Thurlbourn.

Gilman, Sander L. (1976) *The Face of Madness: Hugh W. Diamond and the Origin of Psychiatric Photography*, New York: Brunner/Mazel.

Giustino, David de (1975) *The Conquest of Mind: Phrenology and Victorian Social Thought*, London: Croom Helm.

Glanville, Joseph (1661) *The Vanity of Dogmatizing*, London: E.C. for Henry Eversham.

Glanville, Joseph (1681) *Sadducismus Triumphatus or full and plain evidence concerning witches and apparitions*, London: J. Collins & S. Lownds.

Goldstein, J. (1987) *Console and Classify: The French Psychiatric Profession in the Nineteenth Century*, Cambridge: Cambridge University Press.

Gordon, Colin (1990) '*Histoire de la folie:* An Unknown Book by Michel Foucault', *History of the Human Sciences*, vol. 3 (1), p. 3–26.

Goshen, Charles E. (1966) 'The Psychology of Jean Louis Alibert, 1768–1837', *JHBS*, vol. 2, pp. 357–70.

Goyard-Fabre, Simone (1979) 'Right and Anthropology in Hobbes's Philosophy', in J.G. van der Bend (ed.) *Thomas Hobbes: His View of Man*, Amsterdam: Ridopi.

Graham, H.G. (1908) *Scottish Men of Letters in the Eighteenth Century*, London: Adam & Charles Black.

Granjel, Luis S. (1973) *La frenologia en España (vida y obra de Mariano Cubi)*, Salamanca: Universidad de Salamanca Ediciones del Instituto de Historia de la Medicina Española.

Grave, S.A. (1965) 'Thomas Reid', *Encyclopedia of Philosophy*, vol. 7, New York: Collier Macmillan.

Gregory, F. (1989) 'Kant, Schelling, and the Administration of Science in the Romantic Era', *Osiris*, 2nd ser. vol. 5, pp. 17–35.

Gregory, John (1798 'new edn'; 1st edn 1765) *A Comparative View of the State and Faculties of Man with those of the Animal World*, London: T. Cadell Jr & W. Davies.

Griesinger, Wilhelm (1867; 1st German edn 1845, 2nd German edn 1861) *Mental Pathology and Therapeutics*, transl. of 2nd edn C. Lockhart Parkinson and James Rutherford, London: New Sydenham Society.

Griffith, R. (1770) *The Posthumous Works of a Late Celebrated Genius*, London: W. & J. Richardson.

Hall, G. Stanley (1905; 1st US edn 1904) *Adolescence: Its Psychology and its Relation to Physiology, Anthropology, Sociology, Sex, Crime, Religion and Education* (2 vols), London: Sydney Appleton.

Hall, Marshall (1832, repr. 1833) *On the reflex functions of the medulla oblongata and medulla spinalis*, London: J. Mallett.

Hall, Marshall (1832, 1837) *Memoirs on the Nervous System*, London: Sherwood, Gilbert & Piper.

Hall, Marshall (1843) *New Memoirs on the Nervous System*, London: Hippolyte Baillière.

Hall, Marshall (1850) *Synopsis of the Diastaltic System*, London.

Haller, Alberto von (1757) *Elementa Physiologiae corporis humani*, Lausanne: Marci-Michael Bousquet.

Hamilton, Elizabeth (1803, 3rd edn; 1st edn 1801) *Letters on the Elementary Principles of Education*, Bath: R. Cruttwell for G.J. Robinson.

Hamilton, Elizabeth (1815) *Hints addressed to patrons and directors of schools, principally intended to shew that the benefits derived from the new modes of teaching may be increased by a partial adoption of the plan of Pestalozzi*, London.

Hamilton, Sir William — (ed. H.L. Mansell and J. Veitch) (1859) *Lectures on Metaphysics and Logic* (4 vols), Edinburgh and London: William Blackwood.

Harris, James — (1765, 2nd edn; 1s edn 1751) *Hermes or a Philosophical Enquiry concerning Language and Universal Grammar*, London: John Nourse & Paul Vaillam.

Harte, Richard — (1902) *Hypnotism and the Doctors I. Mesmer, De Puységur*, London: L.N. Fowler.

Hartley, David — (1749, repr. 1966) *Observations on Man, His Frame, His Duty, and His Expectations*, London: S. Richardson; repr. with Introduction by Theodore L. Huguelet, Gainsville, FL: Scholar's Reprints.

Harvey, E. Ruth — (1975) *The Inward Wits: Psychological Theory in the Middle Ages and the Renaissance*, London: Warburg Institute Surveys VI.

Hashnu Hara, O. — (n.d.; *c.* 1910, 3rd edn) *Practical Hypnotism*, London: Apocalyptic Press.

Haslam, John — (1810) *Illustrations of Madness: exhibiting a singular case of Insanity and a no less remarkable difference of Medical opinion developing the Nature of Assailment, and the manner of Working Events: with a description of the tortures experienced by Bomb-Bursting, Lobster-Cracking and Lengthening the Brain*, London: G. Hayden.

Haslam, John — (1819) *Sound Mind; or, Contributions to the Natural History & Physiology of the Human Intellect*, London: Longman, Hurst, Rees, Orme & Brown.

Haslam, John — (1835) *On the Nature of Thought, or the act of Thinking & its connexion with a Perspicuous Sentence*, London: Longman, Rees, Orme, Brown, Green & Longman.

Hatfield, G.C. and Epstein, W. — (1979) 'The Sensory Core and the Medieval Foundations of Early Modern Perceptual Theory', *Isis*, vol. 70, pp. 363–84.

Hayek, F.A. — (1978) *New Studies in Philosophy, Politics, Economics and the History of Ideas*, London: Routledge & Kegan Paul.

Hearnshaw, L.S. — (1964) *A Short History of British Psychology 1840–1940*, London: Methuen.

Hearnshaw, L.S. — (1987) *The Shaping of Modern Psychology*, London: Routledge & Kegan Paul.

Hebb, D.O. (1949) *Organization of Behavior*, New York: John Wiley.

Heinroth, J.C.A. (1818) *Lehrbuch der Störungen des Seelenlebens vom rationalen Standpunkt aus entworfen*, Leipzig: Vogel.

Henle, M, Jaynes, J. and Sullivan, J. (eds) (1973) *Historical Conceptions of Psychology*, New York: Springer.

Henry, John (1989) 'Robert Hooke: The Incongruous Mechanist', in M. Hunter and S. Schaffer (eds) *Robert Hooke: New Studies*, Woodbridge: Boydell.

Herbart, J.F. (1816) *Lehrbuch zur Psychologie*, Königsberg and Leipzig: A.W. Unzer.

Herbart, J.F. (1824–5) *Psychologie als Wissenschaft*, Königsberg: A.W. Unzer.

Herbart, J.F. (1839–40) *Psychologische Untersuchungen*, Göttingen.

Herbart, J.F. (1873–5) *Johann Friedrich Herbart's pädagogische Schriften* . . . (2 vols), Leipzig.

Herwig, H.M. (700) *The Art of Curing Sympathetically or Magnetically, Proved to be the Most True by its Theory and Practice*, London: n.p.

Hewes, G.W. (1973) 'An Explicit Formulation of the Relationship between Tool-using, Tool-making, and the Emergence of Language', *Visible Language*, vol. 7 (2), pp. 101–27.

Hewes, G.W. (1976) 'The Current Status of the Gestural Theory of Language Origin', in S.R. Harnad, H.D. Steklis and J. Lancaster (eds) *Origins and Evolution of Language*, New York: New York Academy of Sciences.

Higson, C.W.J. (ed.) (1967; Supplement, 1976) *Sources for the History of Education*, London: Library Association.

Hill, Christopher (1971) *Antichrist in Seventeenth-Century England*, London: Oxford University Press and University of Newcastle upon Tyne Publications.

Hill, Christopher (1974) *Change and Continuity in Seveteenth-Century England*, London: Weidenfeld & Nicolson.

Hill, Christopher (1981) *The World Turned Upside Down: Radical Ideas during the English Revolution*, Harmondsworth: Penguin.

Hill, Christopher (1984) *The Experience of Defeat*, New York: Viking.

Hill, T. (1556) '*A brief and most pleasaũt Epitomye of the whole Art of Phisiognomie* . . .' London: John Waylande.

Hill, T. (1613) *A Pleasant History: declaring the whole Art of Phisiognomy* . . .' London: W. Jaggard.

Hobbes, Thomas (1839–45) *The English Works of Thomas Hobbes* (11 vols), ed. Sir William Molesworth, London: Bohn.

Hodgen, M.T. (1964) *Early Anthropology in the Sixteenth and Seventeenth Centuries*, Philadelphia: University of Philadelphia Press.

Höffding, Harald (n.d.; 1st Eng. transl. 1955) *A History of Modern Philosophy: A Sketch of the History of Philosophy from the close of the Renaissance to our own day* (2 vols), New York: Dover.

Holmes, Richard (1982) *Coleridge*, Oxford: Oxford University Press.

Home, Henry (Lord Kames) (1779 'corrected and improved'; 1st edn 1751) *Essays on the Principles of Morality and Natural Religion*, Edinburgh: Bells/London: Murray.

Home, Henry (Lord Kames) (1774) *Sketches of the History of Man*, Edinburgh: W. Creech/London: W. Strahan and T. Cadell.

Hooke, Robert (1705) *An Hypothetical Explication of Memory; how the Organs made use of by the Mind in its Operation may be mechanically understood*, in R. Waller (ed.) *The Posthumous works of Robert Hooke, M.D., S.R.S., . . . containing his Cutlerian lectures, and other discourses, read at the meetings of the illustrious Royal Society*, London: Smith & Walford (Printers to the Royal Society).

Howell, Francis (1824) *The Characters of Theophrastus; translated from the Greek, and illustrated by Physiognomical Sketches. To which are subjoined the Greek text, with notes and Hints on the Individual Varieties of Human nature*, London: Josiah Taylor, Architectural Library.

Huarte, John (Eng. transl. 1594, 1698*) *Examen de Ingenios. The Examination of Mens Wits*, London: Adam Islip for Richard Watkins; *Examen de Ingenios, or The Tryal of Wits*, London: Richard Sale.

Hume, David (1964 repr. of 1888 edn; 1st edn 1739–40) *A Treatise of Human Nature*, London: John Noon; repr. ed. L.A. Selby-Bigge, Oxford: Clarendon Press.

Hume, David (1748, rev. 1777) *Enquiry Concerning the Human Understanding*, repr. ed. L.A. Selby-Bigge† (1902, repr. 1963), Oxford: Clarendon Press.

* Author as Juan Huartes.

† This includes D. Hume (1751) also as *Enquiries concerning the Human Understanding and concerning the Principles of Morals*.

Hume, David (1751) *Enquiry Concerning the Principles of Morals*, repr. ed. L.A. Selby-Bigge (1902, repr. 1963), Oxford: Clarendon Press.

Hume, David (1779, repr. 1947) *Dialogues Concerning Natural Religion*, repr. ed. N. Kemp Smith, Indianapolis, IN: Bobbs-Merrill.

Hundert, E.J. (1986) 'Bernard Mandeville and the Rhetoric of Social Science', *JHBS*, vol. 22, pp. 311–20.

Hunt, James (1865) 'The Negro's Place in Nature', *Memoirs read before the Anthropological Society of London*, vol. 1, 1863–4, pp. 1–64, London: Trübner.

Hunter, Ian (1991) 'George Combe, 1788–1858: Why did he champion Phrenology?', Paper delivered at the British Psychological Society History and Philosophy Section Annual Conference, Lincoln, 25–27 March.

Hunter, Michael (1981) *Science and Society in Restoration England*, Cambridge: Cambridge University Press.

Hunter, Michael (1985) 'The Problem of "Atheism" in Early Modern England', *Transactions of the Royal Historical Society*, 135–57.

[Hutcheson, Frances] (1725) *An Inquiry into the Original of our Ideas of Beauty and Virtue: in Two Treatises*, London: J. Darby for Will and John Smith.

[Hutcheson, Frances] (1728) *An Essay on the Nature and Conduct of the Passions and Affections with Illustrations on the Moral Sense*, London: John Smith, William Brice.

Huxley, T.H. (1887) *Hume*, London: Macmillan.

Jackson, J.W. (1863) *Phrenology and Ethnology as an aid to the historian*, London: Trübner/Edinburgh: Maclachlan & Stewart.

Jackson, Stanley W. (1986) *Melancholia & Depression from Hippocratic Times to Modern Times*, New Haven, CT and London: Yale University Press.

Jacob, J.R. (1977) *Robert Boyle and the English Revolution*, New York: Burt Franklin.

Jacob, Margaret C. (1976) *The Newtonians and the English Revolution 1689–1720*, Sussex: Harvester Press.

James, William (1890) *Principles of Psychology*, New York: Henry Holt.

Jaynes, Julian (1973) 'Introduction: The Study of the History of Psychology', in M. Henle *et al.* (eds), pp. ix–xii.

Jaynes, Julian (1973) 'The Problem of Animate Motion in the Seventeenth Century', in M. Henle *et al.* (eds), pp.

166–79.

Johnson, Samuel (1818; 1st edn 1755) 'Plan of an English Dictionary', 'Preface to the English Dictionary' in *Works of Samuel Johnson* (10 vols), London: F. Offor *et al.*, vol. I.

Jones, Kathleen (1988) *A Glorious Fame: The Life of Margaret Cavendish, Duchess of Newcastle, 1623–73*, London: Bloomsbury.

Jouffroy, T.S. (1833) *Mélanges philosophiques*, Paris.

Kant, Immanuel (1963; 1st German edn 1781, 1787) *The Critique of Pure Reason*, transl. N. Kemp Smith, London: Macmillan.

Kant, Immanuel (1788) *Kritik der praktischen Vernunft (The Critique of Practical Reason)*, Leipzig: Reclam.

Kant, Immanuel (1969; 1st German edn 1790) *The Critique of Judgement*, transl. J. Creed Meredith, Oxford: Clarendon Press.

Kantor, J.R. (1963) *The Scientific Evolution of Psychology, Vol. 1*, Chicago and Granville, OH: Principia Press.

Karpf, Fay Berger (1972; 1st edn 1932) *American Social Psychology: Its Origins, Development, and European Background*, New York: Russell & Russell.

Kassler, Jamie C. (1984) 'Man a Musical Instrument: Models of the Brain and Mental Functioning before the Computer', *History of Science*, vol. xxii, pp. 59–62.

Keane, A.H. (1899) *Man Past and Present*, Cambridge: Cambridge University Press

Kempe, William (1588) *The Education of Children in learning; declared by the Dignitie, Utilities, and Method thereof. Meete to be knowne, and practised as well of parents as schoolemasters*, London: Thomas Orwin for John Potter & Thomas Gubbin.

Kidd, John (1833) *On the Adaptaton of External Nature to the Physical Condition of Man*, Second Bridgewater Treatise, London: William Pickering.

Kimmel, M.S. (1990) '"Greedy Kisses" and "Melting Extasy": Notes on the Homosexual World of Early 18th Century England as found in *Love Letters between a certain late Nobleman and the famous Mr Wilson*', New York: Harrington Park Press.

Kirby, Rev. W. (1834) *On the History, Habits and Instincts of Animals*, London: Pickering.

Klein, D.B. (1970) *A History of Scientific Psychology: Its Origins and Philosophical Background*, London: Routledge & Kegan Paul.

Koffka, Kurt (1935) *Principles of Gestalt Psychology*, New York: Harcourt & Brace.

Kripke, Saul (1982) *Wittgenstein on Rules and Private Language, an elementary exposition*, Oxford: Basil Blackwell.

La Mettrie, Offray de (1750, 2nd edn; [1st Eng. edn 1749, Dublin]; 1st French edn 1748) *Man a Machine*, London: G. Smith.

Land, Stephen K. (1986) *The Philosophy of Language in Britain: Major Theories from Hobbes to Thomas Reid*, New York: AMS.

Landau, S.I. (1984, repr. 1989) *Dictionaries and the Art of Lexicography*, Cambridge: Cambridge University Press.

Lange, Karl (1907) *Apperception: A Monograph on Psychology and Pedagogy*, Boston, MA: D.C. Heath.

Lanteri-Laura, G. (1970) *Histoire de la Phrénologie*, Paris: Presses Universitaires de France.

Latham, R.G. (1850) *The Natural History of the Varieties of Man*, London: John van Voorst.

Lauder Linday, W. (1880) *Mind in the Lower Animals* (2 vols), London: Kegan Paul, Trench & Co.

Lavater, Johann Kaspar (or Caspar) (1775–8, 1783–7) *Physiognomische Fragmente zur Beförderung des Menschenkenntniss und Menschenliebe* (4 vols), Leipzig & Winterthur. Major English eds: Transl. H. Hunter under T. Holloway's supervision, London, 1789–98 (3 vols); transl. T. Holcroft, London: G.G.J. & J. Robinson, 1789 (3 vols); transl. Rev. C. Moore, London: H.D. Symonds, 1797 (3 vols).

Lavater, Johann Kaspar (or Caspar) (1788; 1789, 2nd edn) *Aphorisms on Man*, London: J. Johnson.

Lavater, Johann Kaspar (or Caspar) (1795) *Secret Journal of a Self-Observer, or Confessions and Familiar Letters* (2 vols), London: R. Cadell Jr & W. Davies.

Laver, A.B. (1973) 'D'Assigny and the Art of Memory', *JHBS*, vol. 9, pp. 240–50.

Lawrence, William (1823, 3rd edn; 1st edn 1819) *Lectures on Physiology, Zoology, and the Natural History of Man*, London: James Smith.

Layard, A.H. (1849) *Nineveh and its Remains* (2 vols), London:

John Murray.

Laycock, Thomas (1840) *A Treatise on the Nervous Diseases of Women; comprising an inquiry into the nature, causes, and treatment of Spinal and Hysterical Disorders*, London: Longman, Orme, Brown, Green, & Longmans.

Leahey, Thomas Hardy (1987, 2nd edn) *A History of Psychology: Main Currents in Psychological Thought*, Englewood Cliffs, NJ: Prentice Hall.

Leary, David E. (1978) 'The Philosophical Development of the Conception of Psychology in Germany, 1780–1850', *JHBS*, vol. 14, pp. 113–121.

Leary, David E. (1982a) 'Immanuel Kant and the Development of Modern Psychology' in W.R. Woodward and M.G. Ash (eds), *The Problematic Science: Psychology in Nineteenth-Century Thought*, New York: Praeger.

Leary, David E. (1982b) 'The Fate and Influence of John Stuart Mill's Proposed Science of Ethology', *Journal of the History of Ideas*, vol. 43, pp. 153–62.

Leary, David E. (ed) (1900) *Metaphors in the History of Psychology*, Cambridge: Cambridge University Press.

Leibniz, Gottfried W. (ed. G.H.R. Parkinson) (1973) *Philosophical Writings*, London: J.M. Dent.

Leigh, Denis (1961) *The Historical Development of British Psychiatry, Vol. 1 18th and 19th Century*, Oxford: Pergamon Press.

Lelut, M. (1858) *La Phrénologie, son histoire, ses systèmes et sa condemnation*, Paris: Adolphe Delahaye.

Lewis, C.S. (1960) *Studies in Words*, Cambridge: Cambridge University Press.

Liddell, E.G.T. (1960) *The Discovery of the Reflexes*, Oxford: Oxford University Press.

Locke, John (ed. A.C. Fraser) (1894; 1st edn 1690) *Essay Concerning Human Understanding* (2 vols), Oxford: Oxford University Press.

Locke, John (1705, repr. 1710; 1st edn 1693) *Some Thoughts Concerning Education*, London: n.p.

Locke, John (ed. James L. Axtell) (1968) *The Educational Writings of John Locke*, Cambridge: Cambridge University Press.

Lott, Tommy L. (1979) 'Hobbes's Mechanistic Psychology' in J.G. van der Bend (ed.) *Thomas Hobbes: His View of Man*, Amsterdam: Ridopi, pp. 63–76.

Lotze, Hermann (1852) *Medicinische Psychologie oder Physiologies der Seele*, Leipzig.

Lotze, Hermann (1885; 1st German edn 1856–64) *Microcosmus: An Essay Concerning Man and his Relation to the World*, transl. E. Hamilton and E.E. Constance Jones, (2 vols), Edinburgh: T. & T. Clark.

Lovejoy, A.O. (1933) *The Great Chain of Being: A Study in the History of an Idea*, Cambridge, MA: Harvard University Press.

Lowthorp, John (1705) *Philosophical Transactions and Collections to the end of the Year 1700 Abridg'd and Dispos'd under General Heads*, London: Thomas Bennet, Robert Knaplock, Richard Wilkin.

MacDonald, Michael (1981) *Mystical Bedlam: Madness, Anxiety, and Healing in Seventeenth-Century England*, Cambridge: Cambridge University Press.

Mach, Ernst (1883) *Die Mechanik und ihre Entwicklung, historisch-kritisch dargestellt*, Internationale wissenschaftliche Bibliothiek, Bd. 59.

Mack, Mary P. (1962) *Jeremy Bentham: An Odyssey of Ideas 1748–1792*, London: Heinemann.

Mackay, C. (1841, 1852; repr. 1956) *Memoirs of Extraordinary Popular Delusions and the Madness of Crowds*, London: G.G. Harrap.

[Mackenzie, George] (1665) *A Moral Essay Preferring Solitude to Publick Employment, and all it's Appanages . . .*, Edinburgh: Robert Brown.

Mackenzie, Henry (1771) *The Man of Feeling*, London: T. Cadell.

Macpherson, C.B. (1962) *The Political Theory of Posssessive Individualism: Hobbes to Locke*, Oxford: Oxford University Press.

McKusick, James C. (1986) *Coleridge's Philosophy of Language*, New Haven, CT and London: Yale University Press.

McNish, Robert (1836, 3rd edn) *The Philosophy of Sleep*, Glasgow: W.R. M'Phunn.

Magendie, F. (1839) *Leçons sur les fonctions et les maladies du système nerveux*, Paris.

Maine de Biran, P. (1813–20, repr. 1920) *Essai sur les fondements de la psychologie*, in Paul Tisserand (ed.) *Œuvres de Maine de Biran accompagnés de notes et d'appendices*, Paris: Alcan.

Mandeville, B. de (1970; 1st edn 1723) *The Fable of the Bees: or, Private Vices, Publick Benefits*, ed. Phillip Harth, Harmondsworth: Penguin.

Mandeville, B. de (1730, 2nd edn; 1st edn 1711) *A Treatise of the*

Hypocholdriacal and Hysterical Diseases, London: J. Tonson.

Mandler, G. and Kessen, W. (1959) *The Language of Psychology*, New York: John Wiley/London: Chapman & Hall.

Mandrou, R. (1978; 1st French edn 1973) *From Humanism to Science 1490–1700*, Harmondsworth: Penguin.

Mantegazza, Paolo (n.d.) *Physiognomy and Expression*, London: Walter Scott.

Marshall, W.E. (1873) *A Phrenologist amongst the Todas*, London.

Martin, John (1790) *Animal Magnetism Examined: in a Letter to a Country Gentleman*, London: 'for the author'.

Mayhew, Henry (1851, repr. 1861–2) *London Labour and the London Poor* (3 vols), London: Griffin, Bohm & Co.

[Mayne, Zachary] (1728) *Two Dissertations Concerning Sense and the Imagination with an Essay on Consciousness*, London: J. Tonson.

Meteyard, Belinda (1980) 'Illegitimacy and Marriage in Eighteenth-Century England', *Journal of Interdisciplinary History*, vol. x (3), pp. 479–89.

Micale, M.S. (1989) 'Hysteria and its Historiography: A Review of Past and Present Writings I', *History of Science*, vol. xxviii, pp. 223–51.

Micale, M.S. (1990) 'Hysteria and its Historiography: The Future Perspective', *History of Psychiatry*, vol. i, (1), pp. 33–124.

Michael, E. and F.S. (1989) 'Corporeal Ideas in Seventeenth-Century Psychology', *Journal of the History of Ideas*, vol. 50, pp. 31–48.

Midgley, Mary (1979) *Beast and Man: The Roots of Human Nature*, London: Methuen.

Mill, James (1869; 1st edn 1929) *Analysis of the Phenomena of the Human Mind* ed. J.S. Mill, A. Bain, G. Grote and A. Findlater, London: Longmans, Green, Reader & Dyer.

Mill, John Stuart (1967; 1st edn 1843, 8th edn 1875) *A System of Logic – Ratiocinative and Inductive – Being a Connected View of the Principles of Evidence and the Method of Scientific Investigation*, London: Longmans, Green.

Mill, John Stuart (1865) *An Examination of Sir William Hamilton's Philosophy and of the principal philosophical questions discussed in his writings*, London: Longmans.

Mill, John Stuart (1866, 2nd edn) *Auguste Comte and Positivism*, London: Trübner.

Millar, John (1806, 4th edn; 1st edn 1771) *The Origin of the Distinction of Ranks or an Inquiry into the Circumstances which gave rise to Influence and Authority in the different Members of Society*, Edinburgh: John Craig.

Miller, E.F. (1971) 'Hume's Contribution to Behavioral Science', *JHBS*, vol. 7, pp. 154–68.

Miller, Jonathan (1973) 'Mesmerism', *The Listener*, 22 November.

Mills, J.A. (1987) 'Thomas Brown on the Philosophy and Psychology of Perception', *JHBS*, vol. 22, pp. 37–49.

Milton, John R. (1981) 'The Origin and Development of the Concept of the "Laws of Nature"', *Archives of European Sociology*, vol. XXII, pp. 173–95.

Moll, Albert (1890) *Hypnotism*, London: Walter Scott.

Monboddo, Lord (James Burnett) (1773–92) *Dissertation on the Origin and Progress of Language* (6 vols), Edinburgh.

Montesquieu, C.L. de Secondat, Baron de (1750; 1st French edn 1748) *The Spirit of the Laws*, London (10 English edns by 1773).

Moravia, S. (1978) 'From *Homme Machine* to *Homme Sensible*: Changing Eighteenth-Century Models', *Journal of the History of Ideas*, vo. 39 (1), pp. pp. 45–60.

Moravia, S. (1983) 'The Capture of the Invisible: For a (pre)history of Psychology in Eighteenth-Century France', *JHBS*, vol. 19, pp. 370–78.

More, Hannah (1818, 12th edn; 1st edn 1799) *Strictures on the Modern System of Female Education with a view of the principles and conduct prevalent among women of rank and fortune*, London: T. Cadell.

Morel, B.A. (1857) *Traité des dégénérescences physiques, intellectuelles et morales de l'espèce humaine* . . . Paris: J.B. Baillière.

Morell, J.D. (1853) *Elements of Psychology. Part 1*, London: William Pickering.

Morgan, John (1986) *Godly Learning: Puritan Attitudes towards Reason, Learning, and Education, 1560–1640*, Cambridge: Cambridge University Press.

Morgan, Michael J. (1977) *Molyneux's Question: Vision, Touch and the Philosophy of Perception*, Cambridge: Cambridge University Press.

Moriarty, Michael (1987) 'Figures of the Unthinkable: Diderot's materialist Metaphors', in A.E. Benjamin *et al.* (eds), pp. 147–75.

Morison, (1825) *Outlines of Lectures on Mental Disease*, Lon-

Sir Alexander — don: Longman, Rees, Orme, Brown & Green, and Highley.

Morison, Sir Alexander — (1838) *The Physiognomy of Mental Disease*, London.

Morse, David — (1989) *England's Time of Crisis: from Shakespeare to Milton. A Cultural History*, London: Macmillan.

Mudie, Robert — (1838) *Mental Philosophy: Popular View of the nature, immortality, phenomena, and conduct of the Human Mind*, London: Wm S. Orr.

Mulcaster, Richard — (1581) *Positions wherein those primitive circumstances by examined, necessarie for the training up of children*, London: T. Vautrollier.

Müller, Johannes — (1834*–40) *Handbuch der Physiologie des Menschen*, Coblenz.

Müller, F. Max — (1887) *The Science of Thought*, London: Longmans Green.

Müller, F. Max — (1888) *Three Introductory Lectures on the Science of Thought*, London: Longmans.

Murphy, Gardner and Kovach, J.K. — (1972) *Historical Introduction to Modern Psychology*, London: Routledge & Kegan Paul.

Murray, D.J. — (1983) *A History of Western Psychology*, Englewood Cliffs, NJ: Prentice Hall.

Murray, E.R. — (1914) *Froebel as a Pioneer in Modern Psychology*, London: George Philip & Son.

Murry, J. Middleton — (1922) *Countries of the Mind: Essays in Literary Criticism*, London: Collins.

Nadelhaft, Jerome — (1982) 'The Englishwoman's Sexual Civil War: Feminist Attitudes towards Men, Women, and Marriage 1650–1740', *Journal of the History of Ideas*, vol. 43, pp. 555–79.

Neuberger, Max — (1981; 1st German edn 1897) *The Historical Development of Experimental Brain and Spinal Cord Physiology before Flourens*, transl. and ed. Edwin Clarke, Baltimore, MD and London: Johns Hopkins University Press.

Newton, Isaac — (1704) *Opticks: or a treatise on the reflections, refractions, inflections and colours of light*, London: Sam Smith & Benj. Walford.

Nicholl, Charles — (1980) *The Chemical Theatre*, London: Routledge & Kegan Paul.

* E.G. Boring (1950) gives 1833.

Nichols, T.L. (1873) *Esoteric Anthropology (The Mysteries of Man): A Comprehensive and confidential treatise . . .*, Malvern: T.L. Nichols.

Norton, D.F. (1981) 'The Myth of British Empiricism', *History of European Ideas*, vol. 1 (4), pp. 331–44.

Nüssbaum, Felicity (1983) *The Brink of All We Hate: English Satires on Women 1660–1750*, Lexington, KY: University Press of Kentucky.

Nye, R.A. (1975) *The Origins of Crowd Psychology: Gustav Le Bon and the Crisis of Mass Democracy in the Third Republic*, London and Beverly Hills, CA: Sage.

Overbury, Sir Thomas (1614) *A wife now the widdow of Sir T. Overburye. Whereunto are added many witty characters*, London: L. Lisle.

Owen, Robert (1813–14) *A New View of Society: or, Essays on the Principle of the Formation of the Human Character, and the Application of the Principle to Practice*, London: Cadell & Davies (Essay First), Richard & Arthur Taylor.

Owen, Robert (1849) *The Revolution in the Mind and Practice of the Human Race: or, the coming change from irrationality to rationality*, London: Effingham Wilson.

Paine, Tom (Part 1 1791; Part 2 1792) *The Rights of Man*, London: J. Johnson (1791); J. Parsons (1792).

Parker, Ian and Shotter, John (eds) (1990) *Deconstructing Social Psychology*, London: Routledge.

Parsons, James (1747) *Human Physiognomy explained: in the Crounian Lectures on Muscular Motion for the year MDCCXLVI read before the Royal Society*, London: C. Davis.

Patrides, C.A. (1969; repr. 1980) *The Cambridge Platonists*, London: Edward Arnold (repr. Cambridge University Press).

Peacham, Henry (1622; 3rd edn 1661) *The Compleat Gentleman*, London: F. Constable (3rd edn London: Richard Thrale).

Pennington, Donald and Thomas, Keith (eds) (1978) *Puritans and Revolutionaries: Essays in Seventeenth Century History presented to Christopher Hill*, Oxford: Clarendon Press.

Pernetti, J. (1746) *Lettres philosophiques sur les phisionomies*, La Haie: J. Néaulme.

Pernety, A.J. (1769) *Discours sur la physionomie et les avantages des connaissances physionomiques*, Berlin: G.J. Decker.

Peschel, Oscar (1876) *The Races of Man and their Geographical Distribution*, London: Henry S. King.

Phayre, T. (1545) *The Regiment of Life whereunto is added a treatise of the pestilence with the boke of children newly corrected and enlarged*, London: n.p.

Pickering, C. (1854) *The Races of Man; and their Geographical Distribution*, London: H.G. Bohn.

Pinel, Philippe (transl. D. Davis) (1806) *A Treatise on Insanity in which are contained the principles of a new . . . nosology of maniacal disorders*, London: Cadell & Davies.

Pitcher, George (1977) *Berkeley*, London: Routledge & Kegan Paul.

Pliny the Elder (1601) *The Historie of the World Commonly called the Naturall Historie of C. Plinius Secundus*, transl. Philemon Holland, London: Andrew Islip.

Pollard, A.W. and Redgrave, G.R. (rev. W.A. Jackson, F.S. Ferguson and K.F. Pantzer (1986, 1976) *A Short-Title Catalogue of Books Printed in England, Scotland & Ireland and of English Books printed abroad, 1475–1640* (2 vols), London: Bibliographic Society.

Porta, Giovanni Battista della (1586) *De Humana Physiognomia Libri IIII*, Apud J. Cacchium: Vici Aequensis.

Porta, Giovanni Battista della (1658) *Natural Magick . . . in twenty bookes*, London: T. Young & S. Speed.

Porter, Roy (1983), 'The Rage of Party', *Medical History*, vol. 27, pp. 35–50.

Porter, Roy (1984), 'Sex and the Singular Man: The Sexual Ideas of James Graham', *Studies on Voltaire and the Eighteenth Century*, vol. 228, pp. 3–24.

Porter, Roy (1985a) 'Making Faces: Physiognomy and Fashion in Eighteenth-Century England', *Études Anglaises*, XXXVIIIe Année (4), pp. 385–96.

Porter, Roy (1985b) '"Under the Influence", Mesmerism in England', *History Today*, vol. 35, pp. 22–29.

Porter, Roy (1982) 'Mixed Feelings: The Enlightenment and Sexuality in Eighteenth Century Britain', in P.G. Boucé (ed.) *Sexuality in Eighteenth Century Britain*, Manchester: Manchester University Press, pp. 1–27.

Porter, Roy (1986) 'Love, Sex, and Madness in Eighteenth-Century England', *Social Research*, vol. 53 (2), pp. 211–42.

Porter, Roy (1988) *Mind-Forg'd Manacles, a History of Madness from the Restoration to the Regency*, Boston, MA: Harvard University Press.

Porterfield, William (1759) *A Treatise on the Eye, the Manner and Phaenomena of Vision* (2 vols), Edinburgh: for A. Millar at London and G. Hamilton & J. Balfour at Edinburgh.

Prichard, James Cowles (1835) *A Treatise on Insanity and other disorders affecting the Mind*, London: Sherwood, Gilbert & Piper.

Prichard, James Cowles (1836, 3rd edn; 1st edn 1813) *Researches into the Physical History of Mankind* (2 vols), London: Sherwood, Gilbert & Piper.

Prichard, James Cowles (1848, 3rd edn) *The Natural History of Man*, London: Hippolyte Baillière.

Priestley, Joseph (1762) *A Course of Lectures on the Theory of Language and Universal Grammar*, Warrington: W. Eyres.

Prochaska, George (1851; 1st Latin edn 1784) *De Functionibus Systematis Nervosa*, transl. and ed. Thomas Laycock as *A Dissertation on the Functions of the Nervous System*, London: Sydenham Society.

Quick, R.H. (1890) *Essays on Educational Reformers*, London: Longmans Green.

Rand, B. (1923) 'The Early Development of Hartley's Doctrine of Association', *Psychological Review*, vol. XXX, pp. 306–20.

Rauch, Frederick A. (1844, 3rd edn; 1st edn 1841) *Psychology; or a view of the Human Soul; including Anthropology, adapted for the use of Colleges*, New York: M.W. Dodd.

[Record, Robert] (1556) *The Castle of Knowledge*, London: Reginalde Wolfe.

Reeves, Joan Wynn (1958) *Body and Mind in Western Thought*, Harmondsworth: Penguin.

Reid, Thomas (1863, 6th edn) *The Complete Works of Thomas Reid D.D. Now fully collected, with selections from his unpublished letters. Preface, notes and supplementary dissertations, by Sir William Hamilton*, Edinburgh: Maclachlan & Stewart.

Reil, J.C. (1803) *Rhapsodien über die Anwendung der psychischen Curmethode auf Geisteszerrüttungen*, Halle: Cursche Buchhandlung.

Reiss, T.J. (1982) *The Discourse of Modernism*, Ithaca, NY and London: Cornell University Press.

Renaker, D. (1971) 'Robert Burton and the Ramist Method', *Renaissance Quarterly*, vol. xxiv, part 2, pp. 210–20.

Reynoldes, Edward (1640) *A Treatise of the Passions and Faculties of the Soule of Man with the Dignities and Corruptions thereunto belonging*, London: Robert Bostock.

Ribot, T.A. (1870) *La Psychologie anglaise contemporaine (école expérimentale)*, Paris: Ladrange.

Richards, Graham (1987a) 'Of What is the History of Psychology a History?', *British Journal for the History of Science*, vol. 20, pp. 201–11.

Richards, Graham (1987b) *Human Evolution: An Introduction for the Behavioural Sciences*, London: Routledge.

Richards, Graham (1989a) *On Psychological Language*, London: Routledge.

Richards, Graham (1989b) 'Human Behavioural Evolution: A Physiomorphic Model', *Current Anthropology*, vol. 30 (2), pp. 244–55.

Rigotti, F. (1986) 'Biology and Society in the Age of Enlightenment', *Journal of the History of Ideas*, vol. 47, pp. 215–33.

Roback, A.A. (1928) *The Psychology of Character with a survey of Temperament*, London: Kegan Paul, Trench & Trübner.

Robins, R.H. (1967) *A Short History of Linguistics*, London: Longmans.

Robinson, Daniel N. (1981, rev. edn) *An Intellectual History of Psychology*, New York: Macmillan.

Robinson, Daniel N. (1982) *Toward a Science of Human Nature: Essays on the Psychologies of Mill, Hegel, Wundt and James*, New York: Columbia University Press.

Robinson, Daniel N. (1986) 'The Scottish Enlightenment and its mixed bequest', *JHBS*, vol. 22, p. 171–7.

Rogers, G.A.J. (in press) 'Locke, Anthropology, and Models of the Mind', *History of the Human Sciences*.

Romanyshyn, R.D. (1982) *Psychological Life: From Science to Metaphor*, Milton Keynes: Open University Press.

Rose, Nikolas (1985) *The Psychological Complex: Psychology, Politics and Society in England 1869–1939*, London: Routledge & Kegan Paul.

Rose, Nikolas (1990a) 'Psychology as a 'Social' Science', in I. Parker and J. Shotter (eds), pp. 103–16.

Rose, Nikolas (1990b) *Governing the Soul: The Shaping of the Private Self*, London: Routledge.

Rosenow, Eliyahu (1980) 'Rousseau's *Emile*, an Anti-Utopia', *British Journal of Educational Studies*, vol. XXVIII (3), pp.

212–24.

Ross, George M. (1984) *Leibniz*, Oxford: Oxford University Press.

Ross, George M. (1988) 'Hobbes and Descartes on the Relation between Language and Consciousness', *Synthèse*, vol. 75, pp. 217–29.

Ross, Helen E. and George M. (1976) 'Did Ptolemy Understand the Moon Illusion?', *Perception*, vol. 5, pp. 377–85.

Rousseau, G.S. and Porter, Roy (eds) (1987) *Sexual Underworlds of the Enlightenment*, Manchester: Manchester University Press.

Rousseau, Jean-Jacques (1762) *Emile, ou de l'Education* (4 vols), Amsterdam: J. Néaulme; transl. (1966) Barbara Foxley, London/New York: Everyman's Library.

Rousseau, Jean-Jacques (1913; 1st French edn 1762) *The Social Contract, Discourses*, transl. and intro. G.D.H. Cole, London: Dent.

Rousseau, Jean-Jacques (1947) *The Social Contract*, ed. Charles Frankel, New York: Hafner.

Rousseau, Jean-Jacques (1782) *Les Confessions, suivies des Rêveries du Promeneur Solitaire* (2 vols), Geneva: n.p.

Rudwick, Martin J.S. (1972) *The Meaning of Fossils: Episodes in the History of Palaeontology*, London: Macdonald.

Ruskin, John (1909) *The Complete Works of John Ruskin* (39 vols), vol. 36, ed. E.T. Cook and Alexander Wedderburn, London: George Allen.

Russell, Bertrand (1946, repr. 1962) *History of Western Philosophy and its Connection with Political and Social Circumstances from the Earliest Times to the Present Day*, London: Allen & Unwin.

Ryle, Gilbert (1963; 1st edn 1949) *The Concept of Mind*, Harmondsworth: Penguin.

Salmon, Paul B. (1989) 'Also Ran: Some Rivals of Herder in the Berlin Acaedmy's 1770 Essay Competition on the Origin of Language', *Historiographica Linguistica*, vol. XVI (1/2), pp. 25–48.

Salmon, Vivian (1974) 'John Wilkins' *Essay* (1668): Critics and Continuators', *Historiographica Linguistica*, vol. I (2), pp. 47–63.

Sampson, Edward E. (1990) 'Social Psychology and Social Control', in I. Parker and J. Shotter (eds), pp. 117–26.

Saunders, J.W. (1983) *A Biographical Dictionary of Renaissance Poets and Dramatists, 1520–1650*, Sussex: Harvester Press.

Schaffer, Simon (1987) 'Godly Men and Mechanical Philosophers: Souls and Spirits in Restoration Natural Philosophy', *Science in Context*, vol. 1 (1), pp. 55–85.

Schappert, David G. (1987) 'Selected Bibliography of Primary Materials', in C. Fox (ed.), pp. 303–46.

Schultz, Duane (1975, 2nd edn) *A History of Modern Psychology*, New York: Academic Press.

Schwarz, Hans (1981) 'Darwinism between Kant and Haeckel', *Journal of the American Academy of Religion*, vol. xlviii (4), pp. 581–602.

Scull, Andrew T. (1979; repr. 1982) *Museums of Madness: The Social Organization of Insanity in Nineteenth-Century England*, London: Allen Lane; repr. Harmondsworth: Penguin.

Séguin, Edouard (1846) *Traitement moral, hygiène et éducation des idiots, et des autres enfants arrièrés ou retardés dans leur développement*, Paris.

Senault, Jean F. (1649) *The use of the passions*, London: J.L. & Humphrey Moseley.

Shand, A.F. (1910; 2nd edn 1926) *The Foundations of Character: Being a Study of the Tendencies of the Emotions and Sentiments*, London: Macmillan.

Shapin, Steven (1991) 'A Scholar and a Gentleman: The Problematic Identity of the Scientific Practitioner in Early Modern England', *History of Science*, vol 29 (3), pp. 279–327.

Shapiro, Barbara (1969) *John Wilkins 1614–1672: An Intellectual Biography*, Berkeley and Los Angeles: University of California Press.

Sheridan, Thomas (1769; 1st edn 1756) *British Education: or the Source of the Disorders of Great Britain*, London: E. & C. Dilly.

Sheridan, Thomas (1769) *A Plan of Education for the Young Nobility and Gentry of Great Britain*, London: E. & C. Dilly.

Sherrington, Charles (1906) *The Integrative Action of the Nervous System*, New Tork: Charles Scribner's Sons.

Shorter, Edward (1975) *The Making of the Modern Family*, New York: Basic Books.

Shortland, Michael (1987) 'Courting the Cerebellum: Early Organological and Phrenological Views of Sexuality', *British Journal for the History of Science*, vol. 20 (2), pp. 173–200.

Shotter, John (1990) 'Social Individuality versus Possessive Individualism: The Sounds of Silence', in I. Parker and J. Shotter (eds), pp. 155–69.

Sicard, R.A.C. (1800) *Cours d'Instruction d'un Sourd-muet de naissance, pour servir à l'éducation des sourds-muets*, Paris: Le Clere.

Singer, Bernard R. (1976) 'Robert Hooke on Memory, Association and Time Perception (1)', *Notes and Records of the Royal Society of London*, vol. 31(1), pp. 115–31.

Singer, Charles (1928) *A Short History of Medicine*, Oxford: Clarendon Press.

Singer, Charles (1931) *A Short History of Biology*, Oxford: Clarendon Press.

Skultans, Vieda (1975) *Madness and Morals: Ideas on Insanity in the Nineteenth Century*, London: Routledge & Kegan Paul.

Skultans, Vieda (1979) *English Madness: Ideas on Insanity 1580–1890*, London: Routledge & Kegan Paul.

Slaughter, M.M. (1982) *Universal Languages and Scientific Taxonomy in the Seventeenth Century*, Cambridge: Cambridge University Press.

Smith, Adam (1853; 1st edn 1759) *The Theory of Moral sentiments*, London: Henry G. Bohn.

Smith, Adam (ed. A. Skinner) (1974; 1st edn 1776) *The Wealth of Nations*, Harmondsworth: Penguin (1st edn London: W. Strahan & T. Cadell).

Smith, C. Hamilton (1852; 1st edn 1848) *The Natural History of the Human Species, its typical forms, primaeval distribution, filiations, and migrations*, London: Henry G. Bohm (1st edn Edinburgh: W.H. Lizars).

Smith, C.U.M. (187) 'David Hartley's Newtonian Neuropsychology', *JHBS*, vol. 23, pp. 123–36.

Smith, N. (ed.) (1983) *A Collection of Ranter Writings from the 17th Century*, London: Junction Books.

Smith, R. (1988) 'Does the History of Psychology Have a Subject?', *History of the Human Sciences*, vol. 1 (2), pp. 147–77.

Solly, S. (1836) *The Human Brain*, London.

Spencer, Herbert (1855) *The Principles of Psychology*, London: Williams & Norgate.

Spinoza, B.B. (1959) *Spinoza's Ethics and Treatise on the Correction of the Understanding*, London: Dent (*Ethics* 1st edn 1677).

Spoerl, Howard D. (1936) 'Faculties versus Traits: Gall's Solution', *Character and Personality*, vol. 4 (3), 216–31.

Spufford, Margaret (1981) *Small Books and Pleasant Histories: Popular*

Fiction and its Readership in Seventeenth-Century England, London: Methuen.

Stearns, Samuel (1791) *The Mystery of Animal Magnetism Revealed to the World, containing Philosophical Reflections on the publication of a pamphlet entitled, 'A True & Genuine Discovery of Animal Electricity and Magnetism'*, London: 'sold by Mr Parsons'.

Stewart, Dugald (1818, 3rd edn; 1st edn 1810) *Philosophical Essays*, Edinburgh: Archibald Constable *et al.*

Stewart, W.A.C. (1972) *Progressives and Radicals in English Education 1750–1970*, London: Macmillan.

Stich, Stephen P. (1983) *From Folk Psychology to Cognitive Science: The Case against Belief*, Cambridge, MA: MIT Press.

Stock, R.D. (1982) *The Holy and the Dæmonic from Sir Thomas Browne to William Blake*, Princeton, NJ: Princeton University Press.

Stocking, G.W. Jr (1968) 'The Persistence of Polygenist Thought in Post-Darwinian Anthropology' in G.W. Stocking Jr, *Race, Culture, and Evolution: Essays in the History of Anthropology*, New York: Free Press.

Stone, Lawrence (1977) *The Family, Sex and Marriage in England 1500–1800*, London: Weidenfeld & Nicolson.

Störring, Gustav (transl. T. Loveday) (1907) *Mental Pathology in its relation to Normal Psy-chology. A Course of Lectures delivered at the University of Leipzig*, London: Swan Sonnenschein.

Sutton, Geoffrey (1981) 'Electric Medicine and Mesmerism', *Isis*, vol. 72, pp. 375–92.

Swift, Jonathan (1751; 1st edn 1711) 'A Meditation upon a Broomstick', in *Miscellanies by Dr. Swift, Dr. Arbuthnot, Mr Pope and Mr Gay*, vol I, pp. 204-5, London: Charles Bathurst.

Swift, Jonathan (1712) *A Proposal for Correcting, Improving, and Ascertaining the English Tongue: in a Letter to the Most Honourable Robert Earl of Oxford and Mortimer, Lord High Treasurer of Great Britain*, London.

Taine, Hippolyte (transl. T.D. Haye) (1871) *On Intelligence*, London: L. Reeve.

Tarde, Gabriel (1890) *Les Lois de l'imitation. Etude sociologique*, Paris: Alcan.

Temkin, Otto (1947) 'Gall and the Phrenological Movement', *Bulletin of the History of Medicine*, vol. 1, pp. 275–321.

Temkin, Otto (1953) 'Remarks on the Neurology of Gall and Spurzheim', in E.A. Underwood (ed.) *Science, Medicine and History; Essays in Honor of Charles Singer* (2 vols), London: Oxford University Press, vol. 2, pp. 282–9.

Tetens, J.N. (1777) *Philosophische Versuche über die menschliche Natur und ihre Entwicklung*, Leipzig: Weidmanns Erben & Reich.

Thomas, Keith (1971) *Religion and the Decline of Magic*, London: Weidenfeld & Nicolson.

Toland, John (1696) *Christianity not Mysterious*, London: Sam. Buckley.

Tooke, Horne (1786; Part II & rev. Part I, 1798–1805) *Επεα Πτεροεντα, or the Diversions of Purley, Part I*, London: J. Johnson.

Topinard, P. (1890) *Anthropology*, London: Chapman & Hall.

Townshend, Rev. C.H. (1844; 1st edn 1839) *Facts in Mesmerism with Reasons for a Dispassionate Inquiry into it*, London: Baillière.

Trumbach, R. (1990) 'Sodomy Transformed: Aristocratic Libertinage, Public Reputation and the Gender Revolution of the 18th Century', *Journal of Homosexuality*, vol. 19 (2), pp. 105–24.

Truzzi, Marcello (1966) 'Adam Smith and Contemporary Issues in Social Psychology', *JHBS*, vol. 2, pp. 221–4.

Tuke, D. Hack (1884) *Influence of the Mind upon the Body*, London.

Tuke, Samuel (1813) *Description of the Retreat*, York: W. Alexander.

Turk, Christopher (1988) *Coleridge and Mill: A Study of Influence*, Hampshire: Avebury.

Tyacke, N. (1978) 'Science and Religion at Oxford before the Civil War', in *PR*, pp. 73–93.

Tylor, E.B. (1878) *Researches into the Early History of Mankind and the Development of Civilization*, London: John Murray.

Tyson, Edward (1699) *Orang-Outang, sive Homo Sylvestris: or the Anatomy of a Pygmie compared with that of a monkey, an ape, and a man*, London: T. Bennett & D. Brown.

Tytler, G. (1982) *Physiognomy in the European Novel: Faces and Fortunes*, Princeton, NJ: Princeton University Press.

Unzer, Johann Augustus (1851; 1st German edn 1771) *Grundrisse eines Lehrgebäudes von der Sinnlichkeit der thierschen Körper*, transl. and ed. Thomas Laycock as *The Principles of Physiology*, London: Sydenham Society.

Upham, T.C. (1831) *Elements of Mental Philosophy* (2 vols), Portland and Boston.

Verdon, Michel (1982) 'On the Laws of Physical and Human Nature: Hobbes' Physical and Social Cosmologies', *Journal of the History of Ideas*, vol. 43 (4), pp. 653–63.

Vickers, Brian (ed.) (1984) *Occult and Scientific Mentalities in the Renaissance*, Cambridge: Cambridge University Press.

Vickers, Brian (1985) 'Public and Private Life in Seventeenth-Century England: The Mackenzie–Evelyn Debate', in Brian Vickers (ed.) *Arbeit Musse Meditation: Betrachtungen zur Vis activa und Vita contemplativa*, Zurich: Verlag der Fachverein, pp. 257–78.

Villa, G. (1903) *Contemporary Psychology*, London: Swan Sonnenschein/New York: Macmillan.

Vincent, B. (1910, 25th edn) *Haydn's Dictionary of Dates and Universal Information relating to all ages and nations*, London: Ward Lock.

[Walker, Obadiah] (1683; 1st edn 1673) *Of Education. Especially of Young Gentlemen*, Oxford: Amos Curtyene.

Walsh, Anthony A. (1971) 'George Combe: A Portrait of a Heretofore Generally Unknown Behaviorist', *JHBS*, vol. 7, pp. 269–78.

Warner, Francis (1885) *Physical Expression: Its Modes and Principles*, London: Kegan Paul, Trench & Co.

Warnock, G.J. (1953) *Berkeley*, Harmondsworth: Penguin.

Warren, H.C. (1933) *Dictionary of Psychology*, London: Allen & Unwin.

Warwick, Eden (1848) *Nasology: or Hints towards a classification of noses*, London: Richard Bentley.

Watson, H.C. (1836) *Statistics of Phrenology; being a Sketch of the Progress of that Science in the British Isles*, London.

Watson, R.I. (1968, 2nd edn) *The Great Psychologists, Aristotle to Freud*, Philadelphia and New York: B. Lippincott.

Webb, M.E. (1988) 'A New History of Hartley's *Observations on Man*', *JHBS*, vol. 24, pp. 202–11.

Wecker, J. (1660) *18 Books of the Secrets of Art & Nature*, London: Simon Miller.

Wells, R.B.D. (n.d.; *c.*1890) *A New Illustrated Hand-Book of Phrenology, Physiology and Physiognomy*, London: H. Vickers.

Whytt, Robert (1751, 2nd edn 1763) *An Essay on the Vital and Other Involuntary Motions of Animals*, Edinburgh: G. Balfour.

Wilkins, John (1668) *An Essay Towards a Real Character and a Philosophical Language*, London: for S. Gellibrand and J. Martyn.

Willey, Basil (1934; repr. 1977) *The Seventeenth-Century Background*, London: Chatto & Windus (repr. New York: Columbia University Press).

Willis, Thomas (Latin, 1664; Eng. transl. 1681; repr. 1684; facs. repr. 1965) *The Anatomy of the Brain in The Remaining Medical Works of that Famous and Renowned Physician Dr Thomas Willis*, transl. Samuel Pordage, London: T. Dring, C. Harper, J. Leigh and S. Martyn; facs. edn ed. William Feindel, Montreal: McGill University Press.

Wilson, C. (1988) 'Visual Surface and Visual Symbol: The Microscope and the Occult in Early Modern Science', *Journal of the History of Ideas*, vol. XLIX (1), pp. 85–108.

Wilson Hayes, T. (1979) *Winstanley the Digger: A Literary Analysis of Radical Ideas in the English Revolution*, Cambridge, MA and London: Harvard University Press.

Wimsatt, W.K. (1948, repr. 1968) *Philosophic Words. A study of style and meaning in the Rambler and Dictionary of Samuel Johnson*, Newhaven, CT: Yale University Press.

Winstanley, Gerrard (1651; repr. 1973 ed. C. Hill) *The Law of Freedom and Other Works*, Harmondsworth: Penguin.

Wise, M. Norton (1990) 'England in Prussia: The Steam Powered Garden', unpublished conference paper, Achievement Project Conference, Windsor, UK, December.

Wittgenstein, Ludwig (1968) *Philosophical Investigations*, Oxford: Basil Blackwell.

Wittgenstein, Ludwig (1980) *Culture and Value*, Oxford: Basil Blackwell.

Wolff, Christian F. von (1732) *Psychologia empirica methodo scientifica pertracta*, Frankfurt & Leipzig.

Wolff, Christian F. von (1734) *Psychologie rationalis methodo scientifica pertracta*, Frankfurt & Leipzig.

Wood, P.B. (1990) 'The Natural History of Man in the Scottish

Enlightenment', *History of Science*, vol. XXVII, pp. 89–123.

Worsaae, J.J.A. (1849) *The Primeval Antiquities of Denmark*, London: John Henry Parker.

Wright, Thomas (1601) *The passions of the minde*, London: V. Sims.

Wundt, Wilhelm (1862) *Beiträge zur Theorie der Sinneswahrnehmung*, Leipzig and Heidelberg: C.F. Winter.

Wundt, Wilhelm (1863) *Vorlesungen über die Menschen- und Thierseele* (2 vols), Leipzig: L. Vosz.

Wundt, Wilhelm (1874) *Grundzüge der physiologischen Psychologie*, Leipzig: W. Engelmann.

Yates, Frances A. (1964) *Giordano Bruno and the Hermetic Tradition*, London: Routledge & Kegan Paul.

Yates, Frances A. (1966) *The Art of Memory*, London: Routledge & Kegan Paul.

Yates, Frances A. (1972) *The Rosicrucian Enlightenment*, London: Routledge & Kegan Paul.

Yolton, John W. (1956) *John Locke and the Way of Ideas*, Oxford: Oxford University Press.

Yolton, John W. (1984) *Perceptual Acquaintance from Descartes to Reid*, Oxford: Basil Blackwell.

Young, Robert M. (1970) *Mind, Brain and Adaptation in the Nineteenth Century: Cerebral Localization and its Biological Context from Gall to Ferrier*, Oxford: Clarendon Press.

Young, Robert M. (1972) 'Franz Joseph Gall', entry in C.C. Gillespie (ed.), *Dictionary of Scientific Biography*, New York: Scribner's.

Zilboorg, Gregory (1941) *A History of Medical Psychology*, New York: W.W. Norton.

The Zoist (1846–1848*) Nos 13–23, London: Baillière.

* Author's copy of a bound set including nos 13–15, 17, 19, 21, 23 only, April 1846–October 1848.

Proper Name Index

Aarsleff, H., 59, 60, 110, 114–5, 119, 121–2
Abercrombie, J., 326, 331
Adam, 113, 363
Agrippa, C., 275
Alexander, F.G., 309, 311, 313
Alison A., 100, 412 n.4
Allport, G.A., 169
Apel, K.O. 7, 8, 174
Aristotle, 27, 41
Arnauld, A., 49
Arnold, T., 201–6
Ascham, R., 20
Ash, M.G., 5
Aubrey, J., 63
Avernarius, R., 323
Averroës, 22
Avicenna, 22

Baader, F.X., 302
Babbage, C., 86
Bacon, F., 15, 16–18, 20, 62, 69, 89, 91–3, 102, 164, 394, 399, 401
Bain, A., 169, 171, 237, 249, 251, 258, 261–4, 285, 331, 332, 340, 347, 356, 361, 372–3
Bakan, D., 85, 265, 270
Barbu, Z., 48, 242
Barfield, O., 128
Battie, W., 196, 200, 204, 311
Baugh, A.C., 21
Baumgarten, A.G., 133, 294, 303
Bayle, P., 49
Beattie, J., 119, 142
Beck, C., 58
Bell, C., 198, 240, 256–7, 260, 304, 326, 328, 357–361, 382
Bell, J., 273–4
Beneke, F.E., 298–9, 302, 323
Bennington, G., 62
Bentham, J., 115, 130, 144, 175, 188–93, 349
Bentham, S., 188
Bergson, H., 381
Berkeley, G., 79, 98, 100, 134, 138, 139, 141, 144–150, 159, 164, 165–6, 236–7, 240, 338
Bernard, C., 377
Bernheim, H., 284
Bichat, M.F.X., 195, 257, 375, 378
Binet, A., 284, 387–8
Binswanger, L., 310
Biran, M. de, 375, 378–9, 388
Blake, W., 99, 124, 131, 208, 210, 229, 250, 254, 256
Bloom, L., 246
Blumenbach, Baron J.F. von, 256, 260, 321, 363, 365–7
Boas, F.S., 22
Boehme, J., 59
Boerhaave, H., 151, 153, 403
Bonnet, C., 100, 176, 253–4, 272, 356
Boole, G., 86
Bopp, F., 124, 321
Borelli, G.A., 39
Boring, E.G., 23, 79, 81, 146, 302, 305, 380, 390
Bossuet, J.B., 177
Boswell, J., 209, 219
Boyle, R., 31, 38, 48, 64, 75, 395

Braid, J., 273, 278–83, 357
Braubach, 302
Brentano, F., 323
Brett, G.S., 293, 339, 381
Broca, P.P., 261, 382
Brodie, B., 361
Bronowski, J., 254
Brontes, the, 370
Brookes, H., 279
Brooks, G.P., 169
Brooks-Davies, D., 208
Broughton, J., 135, 136, 141, 237
Broussais, F.J.V., 378
Brown, T., 115, 153, 164, 171–2, 325, 329, 332–41, 344, 346–7, 383, 403
Browne, P., 62, 112, 137–9, 141, 149, 237
Browne, T., 51, 52, 54, 371
Brücke, E.W. von, 318, 328
Bryson, G., 168, 236
Buckingham, Duke of, 60
Buckland, W., 328
Buffon, G.L.C., 175, 232, 382
Buikerood, J.G., 27
Bulwer, J., 18, 70–73, 90, 168
Burchell, Mr, 367
Burgess, T., 356
Burke, E., 100, 101, 247
Burton, R., 15, 23, 26, 51–2
Busby, T.L., 371
Bynum, W.F., 200
Byrom, J., 113
Byron, G.G., 124

Cabanis, P.J.G., 100, 198–9, 257, 270, 272, 375, 378
Calvin, J., 30
Camper, P., 260, 363
Cardano, G., 252
Carpenter, W.B., 326, 340, 361, 372
Cassirer, E., 84, 99, 294
Cavendish, H., 101
Cavendish, M. (Duchess of Newcastle), 52, 69
Chadwick, O., 192
Chambers, R., 326–7, 363
Chambre, M.C. de la, 79–80, 253
Charcot, J.M., 284, 290, 377
Chaucer, G., 398
Chesterfield, Earl of, 125, 272
Cheyne, G., 195
Chiarugi, V., 376
Chiaverini, L., 269
Chomsky, N., 105
Christie, J.R.R., 119–20
Clarke, E., 213
Clarke, S., 49
Cleland, J., 208
Clifford, W.K., 159
Cobbett, W., 245
Cole, G.D.H., 181
Coleridge, S.T., 101, 105, 124, 128–31, 132, 150, 153, 171, 191, 236, 246, 291, 325, 327, 346, 373
Combe, G., 171, 240, 241, 251, 262, 264–5, 326–8, 349–50, 363–4
Comte, A., 269, 373, 380–1, 387
Comenius, J.A., 58, 212, 214, 224
Condillac, E.B. de, 34, 100, 105, 108–10, 113, 117, 123, 193, 378, 396
Connolly, J., 352
Cooper, Ashley (Lord Shaftesbury), 139–40, 142, 184, 193
Cooter, R., 249, 258, 265–8, 270, 347–8, 372
Copernicus, 64
Coste, P., 49
Cournot, A., 381, 387
Cousin, V., 375, 379–80, 391
Coward, W., 135, 136, 154
Cowling, M., 251, 257
Crichton, A., 202, 205
Crombie, A.C., 79

Cromwell, O., 53
Cubi i Solar, M., 269
Cudworth, R., 30, 215
Cue, Mr, 275
Curie, M., 399
Cuvier, G.C.L.D., 382–3, 388

D'Alembert, J.R., 96
Dalgarno, G., 58, 59
Dalton, J., 114
Danziger, K., 102, 152, 173–4, 197, 199, 241, 290, 304, 329, 388
Darlington, C.D., 364
Darwin, C., 32, 72, 177, 241, 255, 257, 331, 358–9, 370, 372, 395, 399
Darwin, E., 247, 272, 383
Davidson, J., 302
Davies, T., 59
Da Vinci, L., 84
Dawkins, R., 177
Day, T., 217
Debus, A., 74
Decker, H.S., 318
Defert, D., 91
Defoe, D., 247
Degerando, Jh. M., 131
Democritus, 51
Dennis, W., 336
Derham, W., 98
Derrida, J., 134, 388
Descartes, R., 4, 6, 8, 15, 18, 20, 23, 24, 25, 27–31, 33, 36–43, 45, 49, 56, 57, 64–7, 73–5, 77–8, 80, 82, 93, 136, 155, 165, 168, 196, 198, 241, 394, 396
Desmoulins, A., 383
Dessoir, M., 295
Dewey, J., 306, 361, 405
Diamond, S., 79–80
Dickens, C., 370
Diconson, T., 71
Diderot, D., 234, 268, 394, 396
Digby, K., 69
Dilthey, W., 299, 323
Doerner, K., 200, 305, 309–12, 315–6, 319, 323
Doherty, H., 387
Dollond, J., 396
Donne, J., 22, 51, 54, 209
Dostoievsky, F., 251
Drever, J., 167, 172
Drobisch, M.W., 302
Dru, N.-P. le, 271
Dubois, E.F., 355–6
Du Bois-Reymond, E.H., 318, 328
Dumont, E., 192
Dunkel, H.B., 301–2
Dunn, R., 361
Dupotet, J., 273
Durkheim, E., 383

Earle, J., 21
Eden, R., 90
Edgeworth, H., 101, 210, 219, 225, 227
Edgeworth, M., 210, 213, 219, 224–7
Edgeworth, R.L., 213, 219, 224–7
Edwards, J., 9
Einstein, A., 84, 399
Elias, N., 242, 373
Eliot, G., 251, 370
Elliotson, J., 262, 273, 278
Elyot, T., 20, 21, 22
Emerson, R.W., 9
Ennemoser, J.E., 284
Epicurus, 166
Epstein, W., 79
Esdaile, J., 273, 278, 282
d'Eslon, Dr, 275
Esquirol, J.E.D., 264, 353, 375–7, 382
Eve, 363
Evelyn J., 52, 53
Everett, C.W., 190
Exner, S., 302

Falconer, W., 275
Falret, J.P., 269, 377
Faria, Abbé, 281
Faust, 399
Fechner, G., 173, 299, 303, 319
Féré, C., 284
Ferguson, A., 142, 174, 181–4, 187, 193, 236, 401
Ferrier, D., 262
Fichte, E.H., 298, 346, 373
Fitzroy, R., 255
Flourens, M.J.P., 198, 241, 261, 304, 359, 375, 383
Fludd, R., 275
Flugel, J.C., 251, 261
Fontana, F., 197
Forster, T.I.M., 260
Foucault, M., 101, 132, 188, 196, 200, 206, 242, 309, 352, 375, 377, 388
Fourier, C., 375, 383–7, 395
Foville, A., 264
Fowler, O.S., 270
Fox, C., 5, 65, 73, 97, 101
Frankel, C., 181
Frankenstein, Dr., 399
Franklin, B., 272
Freud, S., 88, 245, 246, 310, 313, 315, 318, 319
Fries, J.F., 298–9
Fritsch, G., 261
Froebel, F., 306–9, 313–4, 322, 370, 378
Fuseli, H., 253

Galileo, G., 18, 29, 57
Gall, F.J., 97, 103, 169–70, 195, 232, 241, 250, 253, 255, 257–70
Galton, F., 329, 345, 372, 388
Garrick, D., 220
Gassendi, P., 23, 49, 77, 99
Gay, Rev., 150
Gibson, J.J., 169
Gilpin, W., 212
Glanville, J., 54, 69, 99
Godwin, W., 247, 273
Goethe, J.W. von, 250, 255, 291, 319
Goffman, E., 242
Graham, H.G., 141, 172
Graham, J., 243, 272
Grainger, R.D., 360
Graunt, J., 329
Grave, S.A., 117, 167–8
Gregory, J., 18, 229, 233, 236–7, 240, 364
Gregory, T.S., 82
Griesinger, W., 311, 316–8, 320
Grimaldi, Father, 77
Grimm, J.L. & W.K., 124, 321
Guggenbühl, J.J., 370

Hacking, I., 85
Hailmann, W.N., 308
Haldane, E.S., 40
Hall, G.S., 308–9
Hall, M., 198, 326, 357, 359–361, 364
Hall, T.S., 273, 281
Haller, A. von, 42, 198–9, 201, 259
Hamilton, E., 210, 213, 219, 226–8
Hamilton, W., 116, 165, 168, 171, 263–4, 270, 295, 325, 332, 338, 340, 346, 348, 371, 383
Harris, J., 105, 117–8, 120, 130
Harte, R., 279
Hartley, D., 6, 100, 105, 110–13, 115, 128, 134, 141, 149–153, 154, 163, 189, 195, 201, 232–3, 236–7, 272, 333–4, 394
Hartlib, S., 58, 212, 214
Harvey, E.R., 22
Harvey, W., 64
Harvier, Father, 274
Haslam, J., 104, 274, 277
Hatfield, G.C., 79

Hearnshaw, L., 80, 83, 130, 171, 241, 380
Hebb, D.O., 151, 152
Hegel, G.W.F., 269, 298–9, 321, 346, 373, 379
Heinroth, J.C., 309, 311, 313–5, 319, 380, 391
Helmholtz, H., 88, 290, 298, 303–5, 318
Helmont, J.B. van, 275
Helvétius, C.-A., 189
Henry, C.S., 379
Henry, J., 37–8
Henshall, S., 115
Hensler, P.G., 284
Herbart, J.F., 85, 298–303, 305–6, 308, 321–3, 370
Herder, J.G., 105, 123–4, 131, 193, 250, 298, 321
Hill, C., 47
Hill, R., 252
Hitzig, E., 261
Hobbes, T., 4, 6, 15, 16, 20, 23, 26, 28–31, 37, 43–45, 47, 49, 54–8, 62, 65–7, 73, 75, 77, 93, 98, 106, 113, 152, 174, 177, 179, 221, 241, 255, 394
Hodgen, M.T., 90
Hoffmann, C.L., 271
Holland, H., 361
Holland, P., 89, 401
Hollingworth, H.L., 295
Holloway, Mr, 275
Home, H. (Lord Kames), 142, 164, 166, 171–2, 175, 184, 193, 236–7, 240, 401
Hooke, R., 31, 37, 38, 66–9, 92, 98, 394
Horney, K., 79
Howell, F., 254
Huarte, J., 23, 63, 80
Humboldt, W. von, 124
Hume, D., 6, 18, 97, 98, 100, 134, 141–2, 149, 153, 155–163, 165–7, 169, 171, 189, 229, 236–7, 240, 242, 332, 340, 401
Hundert, E.J., 177
Hunt, J., 330
Hunter, I., 265
Hunter, R., 200
Husserl, E., 323, 329
Hutcheson, F., 100, 140–44, 149, 164–5, 184, 189, 193, 233, 236, 240, 394, 401
Huxley, A., 218

Isidore of Seville, 90
Itard, J.M.G., 228

Jackson, H., 262
Jackson, S., 200
Jacob, M., 35, 48
Jaensch, E.R., 319
James I, 125
James II, 31–2
James, W., 152, 263, 297, 298, 329, 332
Janet, P., 284, 315
Jaspers, K., 310, 319
Jaynes, J., 101, 196
Jevons, W.S., 86
Jones, E., 315
Jones, W., 115
Johnson, S., 97, 125–8, 131, 164, 219, 397
Jouffroy, T.S., 381
Jung, C.G., 87, 88, 310, 315, 319

Kant, I., 85, 100, 101, 103, 128, 133, 135, 148, 167, 175, 269, 293–303, 310, 321, 325, 345, 378
Kantor, J.R., 4
Karpf, F.B., 321
Kassler, J., 86, 234
Keats, J., 124
Kelly, G., 406
Kepler, J., 93

Keynes, J.M., 189
Kidd, J., 370
Kierkegaard, S., 256
King, I., 306
Kinner, C., 58
Kirby, W., 370
Klein, D.B., 82, 83, 88, 291, 294–5, 332, 336, 379–80
Kluge, K.A.F., 284
Koffka, K., 152
Kovach, J.K., 83, 294, 304, 380
Kraepelin, E., 310, 318, 319
Krafft-Ebing, R. von, 246
Kretschmer, E., 310, 319

Lacan, J., 388
Lafontaine, M., 279
Lamarck, J.B.P.A. de M., 383
La Mettrie, O. De, 100, 149, 154–5, 195, 196, 268, 394, 396, 403
Lambert, C.F., 294
Land, S.K., 105, 117, 119
Lange, K., 85
Lanteri-Laura, G., 269
Laromiguière, M., 378
Latham, R.G., 363
Lavater, H., 253
Lavater, J.C., 97, 103, 242, 250–8
Lavoisier, A.-L., 114
Lawrence, W., 177, 326–7, 363–9, 372, 383
Layard, A.H., 326
Laycock, T., 198, 346, 353–6, 361, 371–2
Lazarus, M., 85, 320
Lazarus, M.E., 387
Leahey, T.H., 4, 23, 80, 83, 148, 162–3
Leary, D.E., 296–300, 302, 345
Le Bon, G., 284, 287
Leibniz, G.W., 4, 8, 15, 23, 37, 50, 63, 81, 84–9, 100, 117, 291–2, 295, 394, 404
Leigh, D., 200, 205, 281
Lélut, M., 269
Lessing, G.E., 294
Lévi-Strauss, C., 383, 388
Lévy-Bruhl, L., 383
Lichtenberg, G.C., 253
Liddell, E.G.T., 197
Liébeault, A.A., 282, 284
Linneaus, C. von, 60, 76
Locke, J., 4, 8, 15, 23, 26, 27, 31–6, 44–45, 48–50, 60, 62–64, 67, 69, 79, 86, 91–3, 99, 104–9, 114, 116, 134, 135–7, 139–41, 144, 145, 153, 155, 163, 169, 189, 190, 195, 201, 207, 213–6, 222–4, 226, 234–6, 240, 292, 346, 379, 405
Lodowyck, F., 63
Lombroso, C., 256, 269–70
Lotze, H., 85, 298, 303, 305
Loutherbourg, Mr de, 275
Lovejoy, A.O., 192
Lower, R., 73
Lowthorp, J., 78
Ludwig, C., 328
Luther, M., 30
Lyell, C., 326

Macalpine, I., 200
M'Cosh, J., 340
MacDonald, M., 47–8
McDougall, W., 82, 306, 345
Mach, E., 159, 323, 380
Mack, M.P., 189–91
Mackay, C., 371
Mackenzie, G., 53
Mackenzie, H., 256
Mackintosh, J., 172
McKusick, J.C., 128–9
M'Nish, R., 356
Macpherson, C.B., 242
Magendie, F., 198, 260, 357–8, 375, 382
Mainauduc, Dr de, 274
Magritte, R., 406

Malebranche, N. de, 15, 23, 49, 99, 136, 152, 165
Malinowski, B., 345
Mandeville, B. de, 125, 131, 174, 176–8, 182, 183, 193
Manson, D., 212
Mantegazza, P., 256
Martin, J., 274–5
Martineau, J., 346
Marvell, A., 209
Matthews, J.T., 274, 277
Mauduyt de la Verenne, P.J.C., 271–2
Mayhew, H., 371
Mayne, Z., 139, 141
Mayow, J., 38, 73
Mazarin, G. (Cardinal), 79
Mead, R., 272
Mendelssohn, M., 294
Mersenne, M., 58
Mesmer, A., 271–2, 275, 277, 395
Micale, M.S., 200
Michotte, A., 388
Midgley, M., 161
Mill, J., 6, 105, 115, 134, 150, 153, 163, 164, 169, 171–2, 191, 325, 336, 340–1, 346, 349, 383
Mill, J.S., 6, 130, 150, 153, 163, 172, 191, 261, 325, 327–8, 332, 336, 339–47, 349–50, 371–3, 381
Millar, J., 175
Miller, J., 273
Milton, J., 47, 126, 214, 223
Molière, J.B.P., 37
Molyneux, W., 27, 76–79, 145
Monboddo, Lord (James Burnet), 105, 110, 119, 123, 124, 142, 175, 229, 236
Montaigne, M.E., 16, 50, 53
Montesquieu, C.L. de S., 175, 193, 220, 232
More, Hannah, 210, 213, 219, 225, 227–8, 245
More, Henry, 30, 67, 69
More, T., 20, 21, 22, 50
Morel, B.A., 269, 352, 377
Morell, J.D., 302. 346–7, 373
Morgagni, G.B., 195
Morgan, C.L., 306
Morgan, J., 6, 26, 46
Moriarty, M., 234
Morison, A., 256
Morse, D., 26, 50–3
Mudie, R., 326, 331
Mulcaster, R., 20, 22
Müller, F.M., 110
Müller, G.E., 323
Müller, J., 145, 261, 290, 303–4, 359–60
Munro, A., 196, 200
Murphy, G., 23, 83, 294, 304, 380
Murray, A., 115
Murray, D.J., 85, 171
Murray, E.R., 306–9

Napier, R., 48
Nashe, T., 22
Neuberger, M., 272
Newton, I., 8, 35, 37, 38, 48, 60, 84, 151, 166, 337, 338, 394, 395, 396
Nicholl, C., 22
Nichols, T.L., 246
Nicolai, F.C., 253
Nietszche, F., 189
Noah, 129, 363
Noble, D., 372
Nollet, J.-A., 272
Norton, D.F., 49, 99
Nye, R.A., 389

Oken, L., 299, 330, 373
Ørsted, H.C., 271
Orwell, G., 218
Owen, R., 212, 330, 348–50, 351

Paine, T., 181, 247

Paracelsus, P.A.T., 275
Parker, I., 132
Parsons, J., 253
Pascal, B., 15, 49, 53
Paschal, A., 63
Pasteur, L., 399
Pearson, J., 274, 275
Pearson, K., 329, 388
Peirce, C.S., 169
Pepys, S., 52, 60
Perkins, E., 272
Pernetti, J., 253
Pernety, A.J., 253
Pestalozzi, J.H., 227, 301, 306, 370, 378
Petty, W., 58, 329
Phayre, T., 20
Piaget, J., 306, 379, 388
Piéron, H., 388
Pigott, T., 63
Pinel, P., 206, 311, 352–3, 375–6
Pliny, 89, 401
Pope, A., 98
Pordage, S., 64
Porta, G.B. della, 252
Porter, R., 195, 196, 200, 207–8, 273
Porterfield, W., 145–6
Preyer, W., 323
Prichard, J.C., 201, 264, 273, 280–1, 313, 326, 328, 352–4, 363, 367–9
Priestley, J., 114, 115, 150, 153, 213, 247, 272
Prochaska, G., 198–9, 260, 270, 272, 281, 354, 360
Ptolemy, 76
Purkinje, J.E., 197–8
Puységur, Marquis de, 274, 395

Quetelet, A., 329, 388

Rabelais, F., 59
Radcliffe-Brown, A., 345
Ramus, P., 51
Rand, B., 150
Rauch, F., 9
Ray, J., 60, 63
Reeves, J.W., 390
Reichenbach, Baron von, 282
Reid, T., 9, 100, 105, 110, 116–7, 121–2, 131, 137, 139, 142, 144, 163–72, 184, 203, 229, 235–7, 240, 241, 247, 263, 294, 332, 338, 346, 378, 381, 401
Reil, J.C., 309, 311–313, 315, 319, 320
Renaker, D., 51
Ribot, T., 284, 375, 380, 387
Riccioli, 77
Richards, G.D., 2, 3, 5, 6, 64, 271
Richelieu, A.J. du P. (Cardinal), 79
Roback, A.A., 375, 384, 387
Robins, R.H., 124
Roinson, D.N., 23, 28, 167, 172, 340, 346, 372
Rochester, J.W., 208
Rolando, L., 195
Romanyshyn, R.D., 64
Rose, N., 5, 6, 7, 93, 101, 231, 242–3
Rosenow, E., 178, 217–9, 225
Ross, B.C., 65
Ross, G.M., 24, 28, 57, 76, 84, 86
Ross, G.R.T., 40
Ross, H.E., 76
Rousseau, J.-J., 99, 105, 174–5, 176, 178–81, 184, 192, 213, 216–9, 224–5, 227–8, 232, 301, 306, 370, 378, 395
Royer-Collard, P.P., 378
Rush, B., 9
Russell, B., 81–3, 85
Ryle, G., 380

Sade, Marquis de, 363
St. Augustine, 30, 181
St. Hilaire, G., 383

St. Thomas Aquinas, 4, 22
Sampson, E.E., 243–4
Sartre, J.-P., 388
Schaffer, S., 38, 67
Schelling, F.W.J. von, 128, 298–9, 313, 373
Schiller, J.C.F. von, 319
Schubert, G.H., 302
Schultz, D., 23, 101
Scull, A., 196, 200, 350–1
Séguin, E., 370, 378, 388
Selesnick, S.T., 309, 311, 313
Shakespeare, W., 22, 54
Shand, A., 345
Shapin, S., 398
Shapiro, B., 59
Shelley, P.B., 124, 208, 210, 373
Sheridan, R.B., 219
Sheridan, T., 104, 105, 125, 213, 219–24, 228
Sherrington, C., 262, 361
Shotter, J., 101, 132, 242–3
Sidney, P., 126
Siemers, C.S., 284
Singer, B.R., 68, 69
Singer, C., 39
Skinner, B.F., 83, 148, 218
Skultans, V., 200, 350, 353, 356
Smith, A., 110, 119–20, 142, 161, 175–8, 185–8, 193, 236–7, 240, 242, 401
Smith, R., 3, 6, 10
Solly, S., 356
Spearman, C., 388
Spencer, H., 249, 251, 258, 261–2, 285, 328, 330–1, 372–3, 381
Spenser, E., 21
Spinoza, B.B., 8, 15, 23, 50, 81–3
Spoerl, H.D., 168–70
Sprat, T., 58
Spurzheim, G., 250, 258, 263, 266–7, 270
Stahl, G.E., 39, 42, 43, 154, 198, 303
Stearns, S., 274–7
Steffans, H, 302
Steiglitz, J., 281
Steinthal, H., 85, 320
Sterne, L., 247
Stewart, D., 100, 105, 110, 117, 121–2, 142, 164, 169–70, 233, 235, 237, 241, 247, 294, 325, 332, 336, 370, 378, 381, 383, 401
Stewart, W.A.C., 217, 219
Stillingfleet, E., 31, 35
Stone, L., 53, 207–9
Störring, G., 318
Stout, G.F., 306–7, 345
Strangelove, Dr, 399
Stumpf, C., 323
Sutton, G., 272
Swammerdam, J., 39
Swedenborg, E., 254
Swift, J., 105, 125, 131, 223

Taine, H., 375, 380, 387
Tarde, G., 284, 375, 387
Temkin, O., 257
Tetens, J.N., 100, 133, 228, 293–4, 297
Theophrastus, 254
Thoreau, H., 9
Tillotson, J., 31
Titchener, E.B., 148
Toland, J., 35, 135, 137
Tooke, H., 105, 106, 113–115, 122, 128–9, 131, 164, 190, 232, 370
Topinard, P., 383
Tracy, D. de, 378
Traherne, T., 52
Trimmer, S., 210, 227
Tuke, D.H., 72
Tuke, S., 350
Tuke, W., 206, 350, 353, 376
Tyson, E., 75–6, 90
Tytler, G., 249, 251, 255–6, 258

Unzer, J.A., 198–9, 271, 303, 354
Upham, T.C., 331
Ure, A., 267
Urquhart, T., 59
Ussher, J., 58

Verdon, M., 29, 57
Vickers, B., 53
Victor (Wild Boy of Aveyron), 228
Victoria (Queen), 251, 349, 364
Villa, G., 293
Virey, J.J.V., 383
Virgil, 222
Volkmann, W.F., 323
Voltaire, F.M.A. de, 365

Waite, A.E., 281
Waitz, T., 302
Walker, O., 213
Wall, Dr, 77
Wallis, J., 58, 60, 70, 75
Walsh, A.A., 264–5
Ward, S., 75
Warnock, M., 145–6
Watson, J.B., 2
Watson, R.I., 5, 83, 251
Watson, W., 272
Watt, J., 197
Webb, M.E., 150
Weber, E.H., 198, 290, 303–5, 323, 359
Weber, M., 242
Wecker, J., 38
Weiss, C., 302
Wesley, J., 219
West, D.J., 251
Whewell, W., 191, 326, 328, 330
Whichcote, B., 140
Whiter, W., 115
Whytt, R., 85, 97, 152, 173–4, 194, 198–9, 201, 232, 236, 241, 259
Wilberforce, S., 32
Wilberforce, W., 348, 350
Wilkins, J., 26, 38, 54, 58–63, 65, 70, 75, 84, 92, 98, 106, 112, 113, 118, 125–6, 221, 255
William of Orange, 31
Williams, D., 212
Willis, F., 312
Willis, T., 23, 39, 42, 43, 64, 73–5, 89, 154, 195, 401
Willoughby, F., 60
Wittgenstein, L.W., 1
Wolff, C., 86, 100, 133, 135, 292–5
Wollstonecraft, M., 213, 227–8, 247
Wood, P.B., 18, 130, 175
Woodward, W.R., 5
Wordsworth, W., 124
Worsaae, J.J.A., 326
Wren, C., 63
Wundt, W., 85, 148, 290, 299, 303–5, 319–20, 322–4, 381

Yeldal, Dr, 275
Yolton, J., 33
Young, R.M., 249, 257–63
Young, T., 272, 397

Zilboorg, G., 309, 311, 376

Subject Index

Entries in italic refer to discussion of the word or concept (except when referring to book and journal titles or foreign terms).

Abstract Ideas: Berkeley's attack on, 146–7
adaptationism, 162–3, 240, 262–3, 270
aesthetics, 97–8, 100, 236, 358, 412 n.4
affection, 185–6; Brown, T.'s adoption of, 334–5, 337; principle of unity of mankind, 182, 187
affections, 140, 142, 144, 173
affordances, 308
alchemy, 22, 74
animal magnetism (*See* Mesmerism)
animal spirits, 40, 64, 73–4, 151, 198
animals: Lavater on, 252
anthropology/*Anthropologie*/ ethnology, 11, 72, 75–6, 80, 90, 97, 102, 175, 236, 250, 260, 269, 293, 297, 321, 326, 329, 345, 370; British, 362–9; French, 382–3; Lawrence, W.'s views, 364–7; Prichard's views, 367–9
Antichrist, 47
apperception, 85–6, 295, 300–1
archaeology, 326, 372
Argument from Design, 98, 156, 327–8
Association: Laws of, 158–9, 161, 163, 333-6, 340–1, 344
Associationism/-ists, 23, 36, 100, 105, 110–11, 113, 115, 121, 134–5, 137, 145, 150–3, 155, 164, 169, 171–2, 191, 193, 204, 226, 231, 233, 236–9, 240–1, 246, 250, 260, 261–3, 294, 325, 328–9, 332–3, 336, 339–41, 345, 371
attention, 67–8, 85, 379

Bath, 207
Behaviorism/behaviourism, 2, 23, 37, 40, 44, 66, 148, 162, 264, 361, 380
Bethlem, 350–1
Bicêtre, 206, 376
blemmys, 72, 90
blushing, 356
brain (*See also* phrenology, physiology), 73–4, 78, 89–90, 151, 153, 194–5, 198, 200, 241, 257, 259–61, 263–4, 304, 333–4, 355, 357–8, 360–2, 367, 382, 401; speech area of b., 261, 382
Bridgewater Treatises, 327
Bushmen & Hottentots, 365, 367–8

canonical texts, 6, 9–10; construing, 92–3; French, 387
cause, 155, 159–60
chemistry: influence on linguistics, 114–5
child development (*See also* education), 5, 16, 100–1, 169, 206,

225, 228–30, 237, 299, 308–9, 322, 378, 379, 388–9, 395, 401; Froebel on, 306–9; Gregory, J. on, 229; Locke on, 214–6; wickedness of children, 219
childhood, 229–30
chimpanzee: similarity to *Homo*, 75–6
Chinese, 109
Civil War (English), 28, 47, 89, 125
classification, 59–60
Cognition: Kant's use of, 297
cognitive Psychology, 85–6
'Common Sense' School, 100, 113, 116–7, 139, 164–172, 325, 332; evaluation of role, 169, 171–2, 371
comparative Psychology, 233, 264, 299, 370
conatus, 29, 57
consciousness, 137–9
consciousness, 88, 108, 154, 197, 260, 300, 307, 321–3, 355, 371, 405; Cousin's view of, 379– 80; Heinroth's view of, 313–4; Marxist view of, 266, 268; 'scientific', 66, 404–6; 'synthesis' of c. lost in madness, 311
The Constitution of Man, 264, 363–4
craniology (*See also* phrenology), 257, 260

deconstructionism, 132
deductive method in Mill, J.S., 342–3
degeneration, 352, 377, 395
Delphigamy, 386
delusions: Arnold's examples of, 203–4
desire, 142–4, 297
developmental Psychology (*See* child development)
deviance: Psychology originating in need to control, 102, 242, 372, 402

Eclectics, 380, 381
Economics, 176, 178
education (*See also* child development), 5, 36, 80–1, 97–8, 103, 207, 212–230, 237, 241, 242, 250, 269, 322, 370, 387, 395, 401, 402; Edgeworths on, 224–6; eighteenth century British, 212–3; female, 212, 227–8, 419 n.26; Froebel on, 306–9, 322; Hamilton, E. on, 226–8; Herbart on, 301–2, 308–9, 322; Locke on, 213–6, 227; Rousseau on, 213, 216–9, 224–5, 227, 301; Sheridan, T. on, 125, 219–224, 232
electricity, 151, 198, 271–2
electrifying, 272, 397
emotions, 24–5, 39–40, 82, 102, 143–4, 155, 158, 259, 308, 316, 333, 336, 358–9; James–Lange theory anticipated, 82, 358
empiricism, 23, 29, 63, 108, 134–6, 141, 144, 166, 171–2, 293, 299, 305, 329
Empiricists, 99, 298, 346
English, 19–22; Elyot, T.'s neologisms, 21; an imperial language, 90; More, T.'s neologisms, 21; potential superiority to all other languages, 221–2
'epistemization', 25, 55, 66; in Europe, 49
epistemology, 16, 27, 29, 32–6, 63, 93, 99, 120, 139, 145, 156, 158, 173, 193, 203, 258, 293, 345, 403; emergence as central, 29, 32
ESP, 69
ethical relativism, 161
ethics, 83, 140, 153

Ethology: Mill, J.S.'s concept of, 343–5, 347, 426, n.15
etymology (*See also* philology), 110, 114, 122, 125, 128–9
eugenics, 229
evolutionary theory, 85, 193, 241, 247, 262–3, 326–8, 359, 369–70, 372, 387; Spencerian view of, 262–3, 328–30
experiment, 173; in Hume, 156–8; in Reid, 165–6
experimental Psychology, 290, 299, 302; absence of in eighteenth century, 100–101; German, 321–4
expression, 71–2, 108, 307, 358–9

faculties, 17, 173, 226, 259, 337; German views, 294, 296–7, 340–7; phrenological, 258–9, 266–7; traditional quartet, 169
feeling, 116, 307, 333; in Kant, 296–7
female sexuality and roles in eighteenth century, 209–11, 245
feminism, 206, 213
Finnegan's Wake, 52
free will, 84, 152, 172, 297–8, 344
frogs, 199
functionalism, 257–9, 263, 270, 294

Geisteswissenschaften, 299, 319, 320, 324, 383
'general will', 179–181, 217
gesture, 70–71, 108; deaf and dumb, 70
God, 26–32, 35, 59, 91, 113, 129, 260, 314, 399
Grace, 26, 45–6
grammar, 117–20, 123, 129; universal g., 117–8, 130
Great Chain of Being, 176, 192–3, 254, 260, 362, 395

habit, 162
hedonism, 161, 189–90, 210
homosexuality and lesbianism in eighteenth century, 211
Hottentots (*See* Bushmen)
Humanism, 20, 22
Humanistic Psychology, 7–8, 163, 299
humanitarianism, 132, 188, 193, 206, 219, 232, 244, 256, 352
humanity, 132
humours, 64–5
hypnotism, 282
hypnotism (*See also* Mesmerism), 273, 278–83, 357, 377, 387; Braid's medical uses of, 282; neurological basis of, 280–1
hypochondria, 65, 317–8, 350, 354–5
hysteria, 200, 203, 354–5

idea, 24, 33, 94, 116, 153, 173, 237
Idealism, 129, 138, 141, 146–9, 164, 250, 284, 298–9, 301, 313, 339, 375, 378–80
Idealrealismus, 302–3, 305, 346
'ideas', 92; Arnold on, 201; Berkeley's concept of, 145–7, 400; Browne's attack on Locke's concept, 112, 137–8; Hartley's concept of, 110; Hooke's concept of, 68; Hume's concept of, 158–9; innate, 29, 32–3, 258, 260; Locke's concept of, 23, 33–4, 44, 108, 134–5, 137; Mill, J. & J.S. on, 340–1; Reid's rejection of concept, 167; source of psychological (*See also* language: psychological (PL)), 22, 390–1, 393–401
'Ideas of Reflection', 34, 108; absurd concept, 137–8; in Hume,

158
Idéologie/idéologues, 258, 305, 328, 375, 378, 429 n.6
Idols of the Mind, 16
imagination, 17, 28, 43–4, 109, 129, 167, 262, 276
imitation, 169; Tarde's laws of, 387
impressions, 110–1, 134, 153, 158, 173, 237, 308
Industrial Revolution, 8, 188, 242, 266, 329, 351
information processing, 26
instinct, 229, 262, 264, 326, 381
intelligence testing, 378
introspection, 148, 173, 293, 297, 380–1
irritability, 85, 197, 199, 259-60

j.n.d.'s, 305
Journal of the History of the Behavioral Sciences, 5, 264

kindergarten, 306, 308

language (*See also* linguistics), 16, 26; Bentham on, 190–1; Coleridge's neologisms, 128–9; Condillac on, 108–110; figurative (inc. metaphor), 56–8, 61–2, 90, 112–3, 122, 138–9, 235, 393; Hartley on, 110–12; Hobbes on, 55–8, 106, 112–113, 223; Johnson, Dr. on, 125–8; Locke on, 106–8, 234; Mandeville on 178; nature of, 2; origin of, 59, 104, 108–10, 113–4, 117–8, 119–20, 123; psychological (PL), 2–3, 22, 24–25, 40, 54–5, 57, 60–66, 92, 102, 104–7, 111–12, 114–6, 120–2, 124, 128–30, 132–3, 173, 191, 193, 199, 223, 231, 233–6, 246–7, 391, 393, 396–8, 403, 407 n.2; private l. argument, 2; Reid, T. on, 116–7, 168–9; Sheridan, T. on, 221–3; Smith, A. on, 110; universal (*See also* Wilkins on), 70–2, 84, 110; Whorfian view of, 124; Wilkins on, 57–62, 106, 112–113, 118, 131, 223, 393
Latin, 20–1, 129, 221, 392
laws (*See also* Natural Law): empirical and causal in J.S. Mill, 341–4; moral, 193
learning, 5
Lebenskraft, 311
legislation: central to Bentham's view, 189, 192
liberation, forms of, 316–7
limen, 301, 305
linguistics (*See also* language), 103–124, 370; Coleridge, S.T. view of, 124, 128–30; eighteenth century schools of, 105, 130–1; literary school, 125–8, 223; materialist sensationalist view of, 106–116, 235; Romantic view of, 118, 123–4, 235; structuralist view of, 116–122, Whorfian theories, 124
literacy, 21
Logical Positivism, 380
lypemania, 376

madness/insanity (*See also* psychiatry), 47–8, 98, 194–6, 199–206, 242, 250, 327, 331, 401, 402; Arnold, T.'s classification of, 201–4; Battie's view of, 200; Crichton's classification of, 202, 205; cultural meanings of, 48, 356–7; Esquirol's view of, 375–6; Griesinger on, 316–8; Heinroth on, 313–5, 353; Laycock on, 354–6; modern classification terms, 203; Prichard on, 353–4; psychosomatic model

anticipated, 354– 6; Reil's therapy 311–2
magic, 38
'Man': treated zoologically, 364–7
manic depression, 317, 320
marriage/family, 53, 179–80; in eighteenth century, 175, 205–6, 208–211, 245, 256
Marxism, 7, 266, 268
masturbation, 209, 211, 245, 353
matter: active or passive?, 29, 37; Berkeley on, 147–8; nature of, 38–9, 151, 154, 173
meaning: picture theory of, 62
mechanism/ mechanization of the mind, 23–5, 29, 31–2, 35, 36–45, 49, 64–5, 73, 84, 91, 93–4, 100, 114, 144, 149, 196–7, 234, 241, 268, 393–4, 396–7, 405; La Mettrie's, 154–5, 234; physiological m., 196–9, 271; varieties of, 37–39
melancholy, 51–2, 54, 195, 201, 203, 317–8, 350
memory, 17, 23, 43, 66–69, 92, 102, 109, 167, 260, 262, 295, 335, 394
Mesmerism (*See also* hypnotism), 102, 232, 243, 249, 271–285, 355, 395; anaesthetic use, 273, 278; arrival in Britain, 273–278; dangerous to women, 275; French, 283–4, 377, 388; German, 283–4; hypnotism, difference from M., 279; a panacea, 276; 'passes', 274; second phase in Britain, 278–283
methodologies: empiricism vs intuitionism, 329; Mill, J.S.'s view of, 343–4; national differences, 290; physiological, 303–5, 359
metaphor (*See also* language), 138, 334
mind–body problem, 2, 28, 34, 82, 152, 173–4, 196, 259, 295, 304, 320
monogeny vs polygeny controversy, 330, 362–3, 365–9, 382–3, 401, 427 n.37; Lawrence, W.'s monogenism, 365–6; Prichard's monogenism, 367–9
monomania, 376
Moon Illusion, 76–8, 145, 415 n.8
moral, 353–4
moral evaluation: Smith, A.'s account, 185
moral imbecility, 314
'Moral Insanity', 201, 313, 352–4
moral philosophy, 29, 140, 142–4, 157–8, 163, 172, 240; phrenology as, 264, 266
moral scepticism, 177–8
Moral Sense/perception, 143, 153, 176
'Moral treatment/ therapy', 196, 206, 243, 312, 329, 350–2, 376; and the doctors, 352
morality, 161, 193, 402–3; Ferguson's refutation of Mandeville, 182–3; Mandeville's scepticism, 177–8
motivation, 5
multiple personality, 320
musical instrument metaphor, 234–5, 396

Natural History, 130, 175, 232, 233, 383
Natural Law, 98, 141, 173, 176, 193, 267, 327–8
Natural Religion, 98, 136, 327
Natural Theology, 330, 359
Naturphilosophie, 9, 99, 128, 210, 251, 285, 299, 307, 313–4, 322, 327, 330
Naturwissenschaften, 299, 319, 324, 383
Neo-Platonism, 30–31, 69, 140,

215
nerves, 197–8
neurology (*See* physiology)
neuroses, 312, 318
New Lanark, 348
noses, 421 n.11
the novel, 251, 257, 370–1

Occasionalism, 152
'Operations of the Mind', 121, 165; listed, 167
oratory, 125, 220–222

'pain', 168, 190; not an idea, 138
Panopticon, 188, 192
passions, 16, 19, 23–5, 39–42, 79–80, 94, 111, 140, 144, 158, 161, 173, 184, 205; Descartes' classification of, 41–2; Fourier, C. on, 384–6
perception, 5, 23–4, 44, 69, 77–9, 86–7, 102, 144–8, 159–60, 167, 169, 193, 206, 303–4, 308, 331, 337–8, 396–7; Divine p., 147–8
Perkinism, 272
personality/ individual differences (*See also* phrenology, physiognomy), 237, 250–1, 254, 257, 299, 370; Fourier, C.'s view of, 384–7
Phanerophily, 386
phenomenology, 329
philology (*See also* etymology), 76, 110, 115, 120, 122, 321–2
philosophy (*See also* Associationism, Empiricism, Rationalism *etc*): British in early nineteenth century, 331–348; evaluation of Psychological character of p. in eighteenth century 172–4; French in early nineteenth century 375, 378–81; German tradition, 292–303
Phrenological Journal, 262
phrenology, 9, 97, 102, 174, 195, 232, 241, 243, 247, 249–50, 253, 257–270, 285, 304, 326–7, 329–30, 347, 349, 351, 359, 361–2, 371–2, 380, 381, 383, 397, 401; attacks on, 263–4; coinage of term, 260; a *faux pas*, 251; in France, 269; functionalist character, 270; Gall's materialism, 258; in Germany, 269; influence of neurology, 262; influence on Psychology, 249, 261–3, 285; in Italy, 269–70; legacy of p., 270; organic character, 267–8; *Phrenological Society*, 250; social impact and appeal, 264–8, 285; in U.S.A., 270, 285
phrenomagnetism, 273, 281
physiognomy, 16, 73, 82, 97, 102, 235, 241, 243, 249–257, 259, 270, 359, 371; and art, 257; and the literature, 251, 255, 257; and madness, 256; popularity of, 254–5; pre-Lavater, 252–3, 421 n.8; post-Lavater, 256–7
physiological language, 195
physiology/ neurology (*See also* phrenology), 22–3, 37, 39–41, 42– 44, 63–5, 71–5, 77–8, 92, 97, 98, 101, 102, 173–4, 194–9, 232, 235, 236, 241, 257–61, 289, 316–7, 326–7, 341, 397; in Britain, 340, 356–62, 372; Brown, T.'s attack on Hartley's p., 333–4; electricity in, 271–2; of emotion, 358–9; in France, 382–3; in Germany, 303–5, 322–3; Hartley's p., 149–53; of hypnotism, 280–1, 284; La Mettrie's p., 154–5; Müller, J.H.'s influence, 303–4; and psychiatry, 316, 318, 354–6, 377; Hall, M. on reflex action, 357– 61; sensory & motor nerves

distinguished, 198, 357–8, 382; specific nerve energies, 314, 357–8
physiomorphism, 3, 11, 54–5, 57, 68, 92, 122, 129, 266, 268, 271, 391, 395, 397
pleasure, 43, 143, 161, 177, 237, 299; Bentham's analysis, 190; Hartley's account of, 153
Pneumatology, 19, 31, 67, 97, 393
political and social philosophy, 29, 98, 102,130,174–192, 231, 242
positivism, 148, 159, 190–1, 240, 303, 316, 318, 328, 380; Mill, J.S.'s attack on Comte's, 381
'Powers of the Mind' (*See also* 'Operations of the Mind'), 121, 168–70, 193, 204, 237, 263, 394
Pragmatism, 169
presentism, 10
privacy, 26, 50–54, 92; and Protestantism, 53
Protestantism, 26, 29–30, 45, 49, 53, 88
Psychiaterie, 311
psychiatry (*See also* madness/insanity) 196, 200, 207, 241, 327–8; British, 350–7; French, 375–8, 387; German, 309–20, 402; History of, 357
psychoanalysis, 7, 313–5
psychodrama, 313
psychology: defining, 1–2, 19; difference from Psychology, 10, 25, 194, 407 n.1, 408 n.4
psychology/ Psychologie, 73–4, 128, 141, 246, 321, 402
Psychology: absence of in seventeenth century, 15–18, 246–7; empirical vs rational, 292–3; German: limitations of, 322; goals of, 7, 174; history of problematic, 4–7, 23–25, 99–103, 232–3, 390–3; Kant's view of, 101, 295; national traditions, 289; North American, 9; reflexivity of (*See also* reflexive discourse), 2; its subject matter, 1; tensions in British situation, 327–31
psychometry, 169, 233, 292, 295
psychoneuroses, 312
psychophysics, 233, 241, 299, 301, 305, 320, 322–3, 382–3
psychoses, 376
psychotherapy (*See also* madness), 42, 313, 315, 320
Puritanism, 26, 45–6, 52, 208

radicalism, 330
Rational Religion, 31, 35, 47–8, 92, 94
Rationalism, 84, 94, 134–6, 253
Rationalists, 99
Reason (*See also* faculties), 28, 34, 46, 63, 108, 155, 160–2, 173, 216, 259–60, 262, 296–7, 310, 371, 380–1, 399, 404; in the child, 214–5; supremacy of, 29–30, 99, 391; tension with Faith, 46, 48
redintegration, 292, 295, 334, 339–40
reflex, 23, 37, 39–40, 44, 262, 264, 357–61, 394; r. arc, 359–60, 405, 427 n.34; r. function, 360
reflexive discourse, 3, 6, 19, 24, 97, 240, 246, 371, 402–4; French, 389; in seventeenth century, 16, 19–22, 92
relation: Brown, T.'s use of, 335–6
religion, 26–8, 45–50, 93, 173, 226–7, 256
The Retreat (asylum at York), 206, 350
rhetoric, 62, 80, 97, 178, 221–2; r. of middle-class self righteousness, 244–5

Romanticism, 99, 105, 113, 118, 123–4, 131, 133, 140, 188, 193, 206, 208, 210, 236, 250, 253, 255–6, 284–5, 298, 305, 309, 315, 319, 327, 330, 373, 395; R. view of madness, 311–3, 315
Rousseauism/Rousseaumania, 213, 217
Royal Society, 58–60, 63, 67, 76, 399

Saint-Simonians, 386
Salpetrière, 376
Satan, 48
scepticism: Hume's, 159–162
'Science of Man', 97, 101–2, 226, 233, 255–6, 265, 293, 383, 394, 403–4, 419 n.27; Bacon's view of, 16–18; Hume's view of, 158, 163
'Science of Mind', 98, 101–2, 115, 135, 233, 331, 347, 361, 371, 394, 404; Brown, T.'s concept of, 335–9; contradiction in Brown, T.'s concept of, 337–9, 403; Mill, J.S.'s concept of, 341–5
'scientific psychology', 404–6
Scottish Enlightenment, 9, 18, 120, 130, 135, 142, 168, 171, 175, 229, 231–2, 235–238, 240–41, 243, 401, 403; concept of Natural Philosophy, 168; coverage in history texts, 239
'secularization' in late Renaissance Britain, 434
self, 139, 160, 231, 243
self-contained/ autonomous individuality, 101, 132–3, 231–2, 242–5, 310, 373, 391, 400
selfishness/self-interest, 177, 182–3, 187–8, 294
sense/sensation, 33–4, 44, 56, 74, 92, 94, 108, 110, 112, 116, 134, 137, 150, 153, 158, 160, 167, 173, 237, 327
sensibility: physiological sense, 85, 197, 199, 259; psychological sense, 256
sentiment, 173
sex, 102, 173, 194, 246, 314; contraception, 208; eighteenth century attitudes towards, 206–12; s. therapy, 243, 272, 313
Shaking Quakers, 276–7, 284
'Signal mode', 146, 148
The Social Contract, 178–81
social distance, 185
social Psychology, 187, 237, 298–9, 320, 370–1, 403
social roles, 398–400; of scientist, 399–400, 404–6
socialism, 330, 348, 372
sociobiology, 178
sociology, 182, 236, 380
soul, 16–9, 25–6, 28–9, 34–5, 40–2, 67–9, 72, 74, 78, 87, 91, 94, 109, 129, 135–6, 138, 154, 173, 195–7, 199, 252, 260, 271, 293–4, 296, 298, 360, 393
statistics, 329, 376, 388
stimulus, 197, 199, 205
'Stream of Thought', 332
Structuralism (nineteenth-century), 148
subnormality, 5, 242, 327, 370, 378
substance and accidents, 136
suggestibility, 283–4, 377
suggestion: Brown, T.'s concept of, 332–6, 339, 348
surgical instruments, 186
sympathy, 153, 161, 184–7, 243

Theology, 26, 28, 30–32, 35, 97–8, 155, 371; t. motives of Berkeley, 146–8
Third Reich, 322

Tollheit, 314
Tunbridge Wells: promiscuity in, 207

Ultra-ethereal eye, 386
unconscious, 82, 204, 361, 389, 397; Herbart's concept of, 300–1; Leibniz's concept of, 85–8; Wolff's concept of, 295
universities, 212–3, 291, 318–9, 403
Utilitarianism, 143, 175, 186, 188–92, 340, 345, 347, 349, 401

Verdrängung, 300
vibration, 151–2, 154, 333–4
vibratiuncles, 110, 151, 233, 394
virtue, 140, 143
vis nervosa, 198
Völkerpsychologie, 298–9, 320–1, 323, 383
Vorstellungen, 300–1

war, 183
will (*See also* faculties), 28, 143, 191, 259–61, 297–8, 307, 379–80

Zeitgeist, 390
The Zoist, 262, 278